THE AUTHORITATIVE GUIDE

NEW DEVELOPMENTS IN THE
BIOLOGY OF
MENTAL
DISORDERS

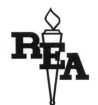

Research & Education Association

NEW DEVELOPMENTS IN THE BIOLOGY OF MENTAL DISORDERS

1997 PRINTING

Printed in the United States of America

Library of Congress Catalog Card Number 94-67652

International Standard Book Number 0-87891-960-0

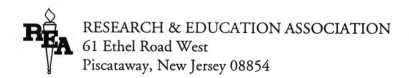 RESEARCH & EDUCATION ASSOCIATION
61 Ethel Road West
Piscataway, New Jersey 08854

PREFACE

Almost one in three American adults will experience a mental disorder during his or her lifetime.

It is estimated that 50 million Americans are affected each year by disorders and disabilities that involve the brain, including major mental illnesses; inherited and degenerative diseases; stroke; epilepsy; addictive disorders; injuries resulting from prenatal events, environmental conditions and trauma; speech, language, and hearing; and other cognitive disorders.

Among this group of 50 million Americans are about 2.4 million Americans who currently suffer from disabling mental disorders.

It is estimated that costs associated in dealing with mental disorders produce an economic burden of $305 billion annually.

At least 20 Federal agencies support research devoted to brain and behavioral research with expenditures exceeding well over 1 billion annually.

These statistics have given rise to the rapidly growing field of neuroscience. The neuroscience field is an area of interdisciplinary research focused on how the nervous system works and how disease affects it. Neuroscience has in recent times drawn in a large number of new workers as evidenced by the rapid growth in the membership of the Society for Neuroscience, and the increased number of papers that have been published in neuroscience and behavioral research.

Exciting research advances have been carried out on the brain, and they have produced effective treatments of disorders and disabilities that affect the brain.

Scientific information on the brain is amassing at an enormous rate, made possible by the level of sophistication reached in the computer field. Advances in mathematics and physics have also contributed significantly to facilitate the study of the brain.

With current technological advances, moreover, it is possible to study the workings of the living brain non-invasively and in very substantial detail.

This book defines mental disorders and describes what they are. The genetics of mental disorders is also discussed. Government policies and issues are summarized. Research efforts and issues are reported. From these considerations, it is possible to assess the potential and opportunities offered by the growing neuroscience field.

The material presented in this book is thoroughly supported by references. A glossary, acronyms, and an index are included.

Acknowledgements

The material in this book has been produced by the staff of the U.S. Office of Technology Assessment under the directions of Roger C. Herdman, Michael Gough, David R. Liskowski, and Laura Lee Hall.

Contents

A more detailed Table of Contents is given at the beginning of each chapter.

Chapter 1

Summary, Policy Issues, and Options for Congressional Action

CONTENTS OF CHAPTER 1

Boxes

Figures

Tables

Summary, Policy Issues, and Options for Congressional Action

Mental disorders can strike with savage cruelty, producing nightmarish hallucinations, crippling paranoia, unrelenting depression, a choking sense of panic, or inescapable obsessions. The sheer number of Americans with mental disorders transforms this personal tragedy into a widespread public health problem. Nearly one in three American adults will experience a mental disorder during his or her lifetime, whether one of the disorders considered in this report [schizophrenia, bipolar disorder (commonly known as manic depression), major depression, obsessive-compulsive disorder, and panic disorder; table 1-1], or one of a variety of other conditions, including cognitive impairment (as in Alzheimer's disease), substance abuse or dependence, phobias, and antisocial personality disorder. Moreover, approximately 1.7 to 2.4 million Americans currently suffer from a persistent and severely disabling mental disorder, such as schizophrenia or bipolar disorder.

What are the costs of this public health problem? The most recent and comprehensive estimate of the total costs of mental disorders—for fiscal year 1985—added up to $103.7 billion (figure 1-1) (box 1-A). When adjusted for inflation, this figure reaches $136.1 billion in 1991. However, dollar figures alone, no matter how large, do not convey the toll mental disorders take. These disorders can be extremely disabling, significantly compromising productivity and the ability to work. It has been estimated that individuals with mental disorders fill 25 percent of all hospital beds and, further, that one-third of these persons suffer from schizophrenia. Mental disorders account for an even larger percent-

age of hospital beds in Department of Veterans Affairs (VA) hospitals: Fully 40 percent of all VA inpatient care is for persons with mental disorders. Perhaps most tragically, approximately one-third of homeless single adults and 10 to 15 percent of individuals who are incarcerated in jails and prisons have a severe mental disorder such as schizophrenia or bipolar disorder.

One of the most powerful factors affecting people with mental disorders and their families is the stigma often attached to these conditions. While the public's attitudes and knowledge about mental disorders have improved during the last 30 years, negative attitudes toward and ignorance of these disorders still abound. A sizable number of people continue to be frightened by the notion of mental illness. The public fears that people with mental disorders are violent and dangerous and perceives them to be dirty and unattractive, therefore often treating them with disrespect, if not rejecting them outright. Furthermore, despite gains in knowledge about specific

Table 1-1—Prevalence of Severe Mental Disorders

Disorder	Adults diagnosed with disorder during their lifetimes (%)
Schizophrenia	1.0
Bipolar disorder	0.8
Major depression	4.9
Obsessive-compulsive disorder	2.6
Panic disorder	1.6

SOURCE: L.N. Robins and D.A. Regier, *Psychiatric Disorders in America, The Epidemiologic Catchment Area Study* (New York, NY: Free Press, 1991).

Figure 1-1—The Cost of Mental Disorders, 1985
(in billions of dollars)

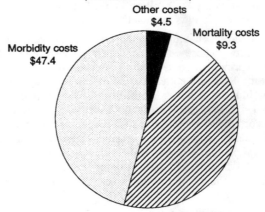

In 1985, mental disorders cost the United States more than $103 billion. Approximately 41 percent of that cost—$42.5 billion—stemmed from hospital care, medication costs, and other treatment costs. Nearly half of the costs of mental disorders—$47.4 billion—derives from lost productivity.

SOURCE: D.P. Rice, S. Kelman, L.S. Miller, et al., *The Economic Costs of Alcohol and Drug Abuse and Mental Illness*, report submitted to the Office of Financing and Coverage Policy, Alcohol, Drug Abuse, and Mental Health Administration, U.S. Department of Health and Human Services (San Francisco, CA: Institute for Health and Aging, University of California, 1990).

Box 1-A—The Cost of Mental Disorders

How big a problem do mental disorders present to our Nation? What priority should these disorders receive in the outlay of government funds for research and services? The answers to these questions are often sought in terms of a dollar figure. However, estimating the toll of mental disorders, or any illness, in economic terms is no easy or straightforward task. Everything from the cost of hospitalization, which is relatively easy to estimate, to the cost of reduced productivity, which is more difficult to assess, may be evaluated. And while rarely included in studies, the psychological and social tolls on an individual's life are substantial, though not easily quantified.

During the last 40 years, studies have reported that mental disorders cost the Nation from $3.6 billion to more than $100 billion each year. The variation in estimates reflects changes over time as well as the use of different methods of calculation and sources of data. Dorothy Rice and colleagues have derived the most comprehensive estimate, based on the most recently available survey data. They estimate the total costs of mental disorders—including schizophrenia, major depression, bipolar disorder (manic-depressive illness), anxiety disorders, somatization disorder, antisocial personality disorder, and cognitive impairment—to be $103.7 billion for the year 1985. When adjusted for inflation, this figure reaches $136.1 billion in 1991.

These costs include health-related, or core, costs—that is, the expenditures made and resources lost as a consequence of having a mental disorder. Such costs make up 96 percent of the total estimated costs for 1985, or $99.2 billion. Health-related costs can be broken down further into direct and indirect costs.

Direct health-related costs—$42.5 billion in 1985 and more than $58 billion in 1991—include all expenditures related to the treatment and support of persons with mental disorders. The vast majority of these direct costs—92 percent—are related to treatment and involve expenditures on hospital and nursing home care, physician and other professional services, and drugs (figure 1-1). More than 50 percent of the treatment costs—almost $22 billion in 1985—were spent on care in institutional or hospital settings, such as Department of Veterans Affairs (VA) hospitals, State and county psychiatric hospitals, private psychiatric hospitals, residential treatment centers for emotionally disturbed children, and short-stay (general) hospitals. The costs of care provided by office-based physicians, psychologists, and social workers amounted to approximately $5.7 billion in 1985. Approximately $1.5 billion was spent on prescription drugs, including minor tranquilizers, antidepressants, and antipsychotics. The estimate reached more than $2.2 billion in 1991, when adjusted for inflation. Support costs, which equaled approximately $3.2 billion in 1985, include expenditures for research, physician and nurse training, and program administration (as for health insurance).

Indirect health-related costs estimate the burden of increased morbidity and mortality that accompanies mental disorders. These estimates, which are based on the National Institute of Mental Health's Epidemiologic Catchment Area prevalence data, include the value of lost output caused by decreased productivity, lost work days, or premature death. Rice and colleagues do not include measures of the psychological and social effects of mental disorders on the individual's life. Morbidity and mortality costs were estimated at $47.4 billion and $9.3 billion, respectively, in 1985. For 1991, estimates were $60.0 billion for morbidity costs and $11.7 billion for mortality costs. Thus, according to these data, lost or diminished productivity is the most costly outcome of mental disorders, with morbidity accounting for nearly 50 percent of the total costs of mental disorders. Furthermore, the cost of morbidity is not primarily due to institutionalization. Additional analysis, which considers such factors as the prevalence of mental disorders in various demographic groups, the type of disorder, and income levels, shows that a very large share of the morbidity costs—$44.1 billion in 1985 and $55.8 billion in 1991—derives from noninstitutionalized individuals.

Mental disorders have other, nonhealth-related effects that impose a cost on society. Nonhealth effects lead to public and private expenditures on crime control and social welfare administration, the sum of which was estimated at $1.7 billion by Rice and colleagues. Furthermore, the value of reductions or losses in productivity due to either incarceration for a criminal offense or time spent to care for a family member with a mental disorder exacts a price, estimated at approximately $2.8 billion.

SOURCES: D.P. Rice, S. Kelman, L.S. Miller, et al., *The Economic Costs of Alcohol and Drug Abuse and Mental Illness: 1985*, report submitted to the Office of Financing and Coverage Policy, Alcohol, Drug Abuse, and Mental Health Administration, U.S. Department of Health and Human Services (San Francisco, CA: Institute for Health and Aging, University of California, 1990); The National Foundation for Brain Research, *The Costs of Disorders of the Brain* (Washington, DC: 1992).

disorders and their treatment, considerable public ignorance about mental disorders persists. Although the stigma attached to mental disorders is complex in its makeup and effects, negative attitudes and ignorance have contributed to discrimination in research support, treatment availability, funding of mental health care, housing, and employment.

The reality of mental disorders—their symptoms, prevalence, costs, and associated stigma—commands the Federal Government's attention. Despite the fact that Federal, State, and local governments spend more than $20 billion each year on mental health services, with approximately 40 percent of these public funds derived from Federal sources, the consensus is that mental health policy is fragmented and mental health services often deficient. Fundamental to improving the Nation's efforts on behalf of people with mental disorders is increasing public understanding of these conditions. More than a decade ago the President's Commission on Mental Health wrote, "Expanding our understanding of the functioning of the mind, the causes of mental and emotional illness, and the efficacy of various treatments is crucial to future progress in mental health." This report from the Office of Technology Assessment (OTA) offers an appraisal of current knowledge about biological factors in severe mental disorders—schizophrenia, bipolar disorder, major depression, obsessive-compulsive disorder, and panic disorder.[1] It also reviews support for that research and considers some of the social implications of data from biological research into mental disorders.

DECADE OF THE BRAIN

An atmosphere of enthusiasm surrounds neuroscience—an area of interdisciplinary research focused on how the nervous system works and how it is affected by disease. Neuroscience is a rapidly growing field, as reflected in the membership of the Society for Neuroscience: This professional organization grew from 1,100 members at its inception in 1970 to more than 17,000 in 1990 (figure 1-2). The 1980s saw a nearly 70 percent increase in the number of papers published in neuroscience and behavioral research. At least 20 Federal organizations support research devoted to brain and behavioral research (figure 1-3), with total Federal expenditures just exceeding $1 billion in 1990.

Figure 1-2—Membership in the Society for Neuroscience

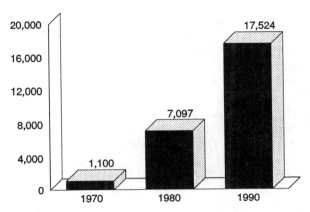

Membership in the Society for Neuroscience has grown dramatically since its inception in 1970.
SOURCE: Society for Neuroscience, 1991.

Figure 1-3—Distribution of Federal Support of Neuroscience Research, Fiscal Year 1990

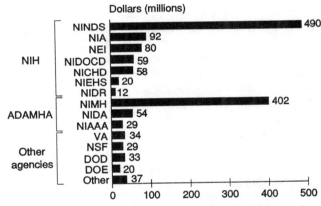

Funding of neuroscience research by various Federal agencies.

KEY: NIH = National Institutes of Health; ADAMHA = Alcohol, Drug Abuse, and Mental Health Administration; NINDS = National Institute of Neurological Disorders and Stroke; NIA = National Institute on Aging; NEI = National Eye Institute; NIDOCD = National Institute on Deafness and Other Communication Disorders; NICHD = National Institute on Child Health and Human Development; NIEHS = National Institute on Environmental Health Sciences; NIDR = National Institute of Dental Research; NIMH = National Institute of Mental Health; NIDA = National Institute on Drug Abuse; NIAAA = National Institute on Alcohol Abuse and Alcoholism; VA = U.S. Department of Veterans Affairs; NSF = National Science Foundation; DOD = U.S. Department of Defense; DOE = U.S. Department of Energy; Other = National Institute on Disability and Rehabilitation Research, National Aeronautics and Space Administration, Environmental Protection Agency, U.S. Department of Agriculture, Centers for Disease Control, and U.S. Food and Drug Administration.
[a]Fiscal year 1991.
SOURCE: Office of Technology Assessment, adapted from E. Pennisi and D. Morgan, "Brain Decade Scientists Court Support," *The Scientist* 4:8, 1990.

---

[1] Addictive disorders, Alzheimer's disease, and developmental disorders such as autism have been or are being discussed in other OTA reports, and therefore are not considered in this report.

Advances in scientific methods and techniques have fueled the dramatic increase in neuroscience research during the last 15 years. Improved methods for staining nerve cells have made it possible to pinpoint their precise location in the brain. The electrical activity of a single channel in a nerve cell's membrane—less than one-trillionth of an inch in diameter—can be measured. Advances in computing, microscopy, and especially imaging technology underlie the spectacular ability to observe living brain tissue—from single nerve cells to the intact human brain. The development of psychological tests has enabled researchers to correlate observed brain activity with specific behaviors and thought processes. And molecular biology has revolutionized the study of the brain, producing monoclonal antibodies that allow labeling of specific nerve cells, the cloning of proteins involved in brain function, and the search for specific genes.

The rapid growth and productivity of neuroscience spearheads, in large measure, the general interest in the biology of mental disorders and Congress' request for this study. Modern neuroscience research is an important part of the contemporary effort to expose the causes of mental disorders. The National Institute of Mental Health (NIMH), the primary source of Federal funding for research into mental disorders, has focused a major portion of its research plan on the basis of developments in neuroscience. By strongly supporting neuroscience research, NIMH aims to "understand the workings of the human brain in sufficient detail to effectively treat or prevent the broad variety of behavioral disorders and mental illnesses." The spectacular growth of neuroscience also distinguishes the current focus on the biology of mental disorders from that of previous eras. While biological models of mental disorders have been emphasized time and again in the past, today's research into the brain's functions in mental disorders is supported in a qualitatively and quantitatively new way by an expanding base of knowledge about the brain and behavior.

SCHIZOPHRENIA

Schizophrenia "is arguably the worst disease affecting mankind."[2] It is not, as commonly misconstrued, split personality. Although important questions remain about its classification, its characteris-

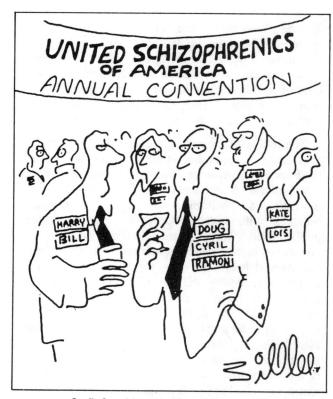

Credit: Copyright © 1992 Bill Lee. Reprinted with permission.

This cartoon, provided by O. Wahl, illustrates the commonly held misperception that schizophrenia is multiple personalities.

tic symptoms are well defined. Positive symptoms, which typify psychosis, include hallucinations and delusions, as well as bizarre behaviors and dissociated or fragmented thoughts. Negative symptoms include impaired emotional responsiveness, loss of motivation, general loss of interest, and social withdrawal.

Schizophrenia is a common disorder, with approximately one in every 100 persons developing it during the course of his or her lifetime; approximately 1.2 million people have schizophrenia in the United States at the present time. While schizophrenia does not invariably follow a deteriorating course, there are substantial and enduring consequences for many people with this condition. Its onset typically occurs during the late teens and early 20s, with a generally younger age of onset and worse prognosis in men. The expressed symptoms of schizophrenia may combine in various ways, their severity and duration fluctuating over time. Schizophrenia is associated with an increased risk of suicide; approx-

---

[2] *Nature*, editorial, 336:95, 1988.

Box 1-B—The Final Symptom: Mental Disorder and Suicide

In 1987, 11.7 people in every 100,000—more than 30,000 people—killed themselves in the United States, making it the eighth leading cause of death in the nation. While many factors are associated with suicide, including medical illness, availability of firearms, or stressful events such as a divorce or loss of a job, data indicate that mental disorders are a significant antecedent to many suicides in the United States. About 50 percent of all suicide victims may have suffered a mood disorder, and an estimated 5 to 10 percent of suicide victims suffered from schizophrenia.

Among people with schizophrenia, suicide is the number one cause of premature death, with the estimated age-adjusted suicide rate averaging 90 per 100,000 women with schizophrenia and 210 per 100,000 men with the disorder; 10 to 15 percent of individuals with schizophrenia commit suicide. The higher rate of suicide among men versus women with schizophrenia not only mirrors the suicide statistics in the general population, but also reflects the more severe symptoms that men usually suffer. Some people with schizophrenia may commit suicide as a result of a psychotic episode—in response to a hallucinatory command. More commonly, however, people with this condition take their lives early in the course of the illness during a relatively stable period following a recent hospitalization.

Approximately 15 percent of people with mood disorders will commit suicide, with the suicide rates for men and women with major mood disorders averaging 400 and 180 per 100,000, respectively, 30 times higher than the rate in the general population. The link between mood disorders and suicide is well recognized, with recurrent thoughts of suicide or a suicide attempt being one diagnostic criterion for these conditions. Other mental disorders, such as panic disorder, also appear to be correlated with suicide. Although there is little information available concerning the number of people with panic disorder who actually commit suicide, survey data show that approximately 20 percent of people with this condition will attempt suicide during their lifetime.

High rates of suicide among individuals with major mental disorders like schizophrenia or major depression provide chilling evidence of the distressing nature of mental disorders. Furthermore, the strong correlation between mental disorders and suicide indicates that general suicide prevention efforts must include strategies to improve the treatment of mental disorders.

SOURCES: C.B. Caldwell and I.I. Gottesman, ''Schizophrenics Kill Themselves Too: A Review of Risk Factors for Suicide,'' *Schizophrenia Bulletin* 16(4):571-589, 1990; F.K. Goodwin and K.R. Jamison, *Manic-Depressive Illness* (New York, NY: The Oxford University Press, 1990); J. Johnson, M.M. Weissman, and G.L. Klerman, ''Panic Disorder, Comorbidity, and Suicide Attempts,'' *Archives of General Psychiatry* 47:805-808, 1990; E.K. Moscicki, chief, Prevention Research Branch, National Institute of Mental Health, U.S. Department of Health and Human Services, personal communication, Apr. 30, 1991; U.S. Department of Health and Human Services, Public Health Services, National Center for Health Statistics, *Monthly Vital Statistics Report* 40(8 suppl. 2), 1992.

imately 10 to 15 percent of individuals with this disorder take their own lives (box 1-B).

Currently, there is no way to prevent or cure schizophrenia; however, treatments that control some of its symptoms are available. The optimal treatment generally integrates antipsychotic drugs and supportive psychosocial treatment. Individuals acutely ill with schizophrenia may require hospitalization. Furthermore, rehabilitation is generally necessary to enhance social and occupational outcomes.

The complexity of expressed symptoms and the likelihood that the disorder encompasses various subtypes, which are not yet reliably distinguishable, have slowed progress in understanding schizophrenia. Nonetheless, converging research data point to the alteration of specific brain chemicals and regions as the biological substrate of the schizophrenia*s*.

Investigators have examined the possible role of several brain chemicals in schizophrenia, including serotonin, norepinephrine, various neuropeptides, and, most recently, glutamate. The most venerable theory concerning the chemistry of schizophrenia implicates the brain chemical dopamine. Dopamine-releasing drugs, such as amphetamines, can induce a psychotic state, and drugs reducing dopamine function have antipsychotic effects. However, studies looking for simple changes in dopamine levels in the brain have provided inconsistent results. Thus, even though there is a consensus that dopamine plays a role in schizophrenia, the specifics of this brain chemical's action remain unknown.

Various studies of the function and structure of the brain in schizophrenia point to the involvement of two specific areas, namely, the frontal cortex and the limbic system (figure 1-4). The limbic system seems to be involved in the positive symptoms and the frontal cortex in the negative symptoms of schizophrenia. The precise interaction between these specific brain regions, as well as the possible involvement of other areas of the brain, still need to be clarified.

In addition to pinpointing the regions and chemicals in the brain that underlie the symptoms of schizophrenia, researchers have put forward several hypotheses concerning the cause or causes of this disorder. Information about the course of schizophrenia, its epidemiology, and specific biological measures suggests that a virus or immune system problem is a possible culprit. Another hypothesis asserts that injury to the brain early in life is the critical factor. Support for this viewpoint stems from various observations, including the higher rate of birth complications among individuals with schizophrenia and subtle deviations in neurological and psychological functions that sometimes precede the full expression of schizophrenia. Evaluation of the prevalence and pattern of schizophrenia among related individuals shows that genetic factors contribute to this disorder; however, the inheritance of schizophrenia is quite complicated, and nongenetic factors also play a role. The location of specific genes involved in schizophrenia remains unknown.

MOOD DISORDERS: MAJOR DEPRESSION AND BIPOLAR DISORDER

Mood disorders, which are also referred to as affective disorders, are characterized by extreme or prolonged disturbances of mood, such as sadness, apathy, or elation. These disorders can be divided into two major groups: bipolar and depressive disorders. The occurrence of manic symptoms distinguishes bipolar disorders from depressive, or unipolar, disorders.

The most severe depressive disorder is major depression. While it has proven difficult to discern whether depression is a single disorder or a collection of disorders, its expression is well characterized. Box 1-C is a personal account of the symptoms of depression. Various psychological and somatic symptoms accompany episodes of depression, including profoundly depressed mood, the complete loss of interest or pleasure in activities, weight gain or loss, insomnia or excessive sleepiness, slowed or

Figure 1-4—PET Scan of an Individual With Schizophrenia

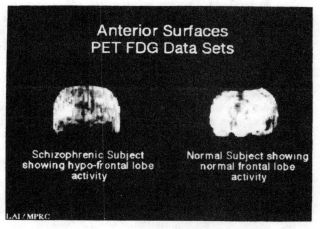

Brain activity in an individual who does not have schizophrenia (right) and a person who does (left). The frontal cortex shows more activity in schizophrenia (white areas).
SOURCE: W. Carpenter, Maryland Psychiatric Research Center and H. Loats, Loats Associates, Inc.

agitated movement, diminished energy, intense feelings of guilt or worthlessness, a diminished ability to concentrate, and recurrent thoughts of death or suicide (see box 1-B).

Major depression is a prevalent disorder: Nearly 5 percent of the population will develop it and the risk is twice as great for women as for men. Furthermore, its occurrence seems to be increasing among young people. Major depression typically has its onset in the late 20s, although it can emerge at any age. More than 50 percent of patients will have more than one bout of depression, the average being five or six episodes during a lifetime. Approximately 15 percent of persons suffering from the symptoms of depression will die by suicide.

Major advances have taken place in the pharmacological treatment of depression during the last decade. Various forms of psychotherapy—either alone or as an adjunct to medication—are also important to treatment. Severe cases may require hospitalization; electroconvulsive therapy may be used in severe cases. In depression that recurs each fall and winter, known as seasonal affective disorder, or SAD, light therapy can be useful.

Bipolar disorder is a severe mood disorder characterized by manic and depressive episodes. Although its symptoms are quite well known, questions remain about how it relates to other disorders, such

Box 1-C—*Darkness Visible—A Personal Account of Depression*

Depression is a disorder of mood, so mysteriously painful and elusive in the way it becomes known to the self—to the mediating intellect—as to verge close to being beyond description. It thus remains nearly incomprehensible to those who have not experienced it in its extreme mode, although the gloom, 'the blues' which people go through occasionally and associate with the general hassle of everyday existence are of such prevalence that they do give many individuals a hint of the illness in its catastrophic form. But at the time of which I write I had descended far past those familiar, manageable doldrums. . . .

It was not really alarming at first, since the change was subtle, but I did notice that my surroundings took on a different tone at certain times: the shadows of nightfall seemed more somber, my mornings were less buoyant, walks in the woods became less zestful, and there was a moment during my working hours in the late afternoon when a kind of panic and anxiety overtook me, just for a few minutes, accompanied by a visceral queasiness—such a seizure was at least slightly alarming, after all. . . .

I felt a kind of numbness, an enervation, but more particularly an odd fragility—as if my body had actually become frail, hypersensitive and somehow disjointed and clumsy, lacking normal coordination. And soon I was in the throes of a pervasive hypochondria. Nothing felt quite right with my corporeal self; there were twitches and pains, sometimes intermittent, often seemingly constant, that seemed to presage all sorts of dire infirmities. . . .

It was October, and one of the unforgettable features of this stage of my disorder was the way in which my own farmhouse, my beloved home for 30 years, took on for me at that point when my spirits regularly sank to their nadir an almost palpable quality of ominousness. The fading evening light—akin to that famous 'slant of light' of Emily Dickinson's, which spoke to her of death, of chill extinction—had none of its familiar autumnal loveliness, but ensnared me in a suffocating gloom. . . . That fall, as the disorder gradually took full possession of my system, I began to conceive that my mind itself was like one of those outmoded small-town telephone exchanges, being gradually inundated by flood waters: one by one, the normal circuits began to drown, causing some of the functions of the body and nearly all of those of instinct and intellect to slowly disconnect. . . .

What I had begun to discover is that, mysteriously and in ways that are totally remote from normal experience, the gray drizzle of horror induced by depression takes on the quality of physical pain. But it is not an immediately identifiable pain, like that of a broken limb. It may be more accurate to say that despair, owing to some evil trick played upon the sick brain by the inhabiting psyche, comes to resemble the diabolical discomfort of being imprisoned in a fiercely overheated room. And because no breeze stirs this cauldron, because there is no escape from this smothering confinement, it is entirely natural that the victim begins to think ceaselessly of oblivion.

SOURCE: Quoted from W. Styron, *Darkness Visible* (New York, NY: Random House, 1990). Copyright © 1990 by William Styron. Reprinted by permission of Random House, Inc.

as major depression and schizophrenia. The depressive episodes in bipolar disorder are similar to those seen in major depression. During a manic episode, an individual's mood is extremely elevated, expansive, or even irritable, and his or her self-esteem is elevated. There is diminished need for sleep, energy abounds, and thoughts race. Individuals are extremely talkative and distractible and stereotypically indulge in unrestrained buying sprees or sexual activity. Psychotic features (i.e., delusions and hallucinations) are not uncommon during a manic episode.

Bipolar disorder afflicts approximately 0.8 percent of the population, with men and women being affected equally. It emerges relatively early in life, usually during the mid-20s. Episodes of mania or depression occur every several months to every year

or more, with periods of recovery typically separating the mood swings. This disorder continues throughout an individual's lifetime.

Treatment for bipolar disorder is aimed at ending a manic or depressive episode and preventing its recurrence. Medication is typically required, and hospitalization may be required for acute episodes. The specific symptoms are treated: depressive episodes with antidepressant drugs; psychosis with antipsychotic medication; and manic symptoms and relapses with lithium, or, less frequently, carbamazepine. Supportive psychotherapy is generally required to help patients understand and deal with the symptoms of bipolar disorder.

The typical symptoms and course of major mood disorders have led to their being conceptualized as biologically based conditions. Since the discovery of clinically useful mood-altering medications 30 to 40 years ago, research has focused intensely on the biology of these conditions. Although the causes of these disorders remain obscure, studies of brain chemistry and function, other physical correlates, and genetic research provide clues about the biology of major mood disorders. The most consistent of these observations are discussed below.

A number of different brain chemicals appear to be involved in mood disorders. The most prominent hypotheses have focused on a group of brain chemicals called monoamines, especially norepinephrine and serotonin, because clinically effective antidepressant medications influence the levels of these chemicals. While neither depression nor mania seems to result from a simple decrease or increase of these chemicals, there is sufficient evidence to implicate monoamines in mood disorders.

Hormonal abnormalities are common in depression. Many of the symptoms associated with mood disorders—changes in appetite, sleep patterns, and sex drive—may be related to these hormonal changes. One of the most consistent findings in this regard is an elevation of cortisol in severely depressed individuals. Also, altered mood sometimes accompanies reproductive events in women—menstruation, pregnancy, childbirth, menopause—suggesting an association between reproductive hormonal alterations and mood disorders.

Individuals with mood disorders typically have sleep disturbances. Insomnia or excessive sleeping often occurs in depression, with REM sleep, during which dreaming occurs, frequently disrupted. The sleep of individuals with bipolar disorder is often affected; during depressive episodes, people may sleep excessively, and when manic, little or not at all.

Other functions that cycle over time may be disrupted in mood disorders. For example, many people with depression exhibit daily and seasonal fluctuations in mood. Some data suggest that circadian rhythms—biological and behavioral functions that repeat roughly every 24 hours—are disrupted in mood disorders. Furthermore, animal studies indicate that some antidepressant medications have an effect on the organization of circadian rhythms.

Episodes of mania and depression increase in frequency over time. And while environmental factors appear to be important in triggering periods of altered mood in the early stages of bipolar disorder, mood swings become automatic later on. The increasingly frequent and spontaneous nature of mood cycling has led to the development of a hypothesis about the recurrent nature of bipolar disorder: the kindling and sensitization hypothesis. Kindling refers to an experimental model for epilepsy, in which spontaneous seizures occur after repeated stimulation of a particular region of the brain. Behavioral sensitization refers to an increasing behavioral response to the same dosage of a drug following repeated administration. It is possible that similar brain mechanisms underlie mood swings. While additional information is needed to confirm this hypothesis, it is interesting to note that the medications used to treat bipolar disorder—carbamazepine and lithium—can block kindling and behavioral sensitization.

The most clearly established biological observation about mood disorders, and especially bipolar disorder, is that genetic factors play a role. Identical twins more frequently share mood disorders than do fraternal twins (figure 1-5). Also, parents, siblings, and children of individuals with bipolar disorder or major depression more commonly develop these conditions. Family and twin studies support a genetic link between depression and bipolar disorder, although the genetic overlap is not complete.

Clearly, genetic factors are important in both bipolar disorder and major depression. However, studies do not reveal a simple pattern of inheritance, nor do they necessarily implicate the action of a single gene. Data also indicate that nongenetic factors must play a role. While many studies have attempted to locate specific genes that lead to mood disorders, some with positive results, no strong evidence fixes a gene for mood disorders to a specific location.

ANXIETY DISORDERS: OBSESSIVE-COMPULSIVE DISORDER AND PANIC DISORDER

Anxiety is a normal human emotion, familiar to us all. However, anxiety can become extreme, leading to a disabling feeling of panic, a constant sense of apprehensiveness, or unrelenting worry about a possible mishap or accident. The current diagnostic system for mental disorders distinguishes several specific anxiety disorders, including panic disorder,

Figure 1-5—Mood Disorders Among Twins

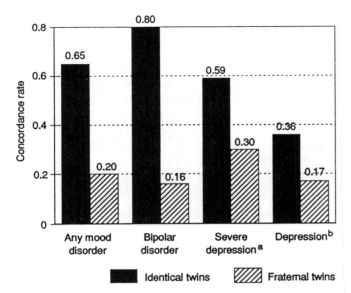

Graphically depicted data were derived from evaluation of 110 pairs of twins. Identical twins shared mood disorders, and especially bipolar disorder, more frequently than fraternal twins.

[a]Three or more episodes of depression.
[b]Less than three episodes of depression.

SOURCE: Adapted from A. Bertelsen, B. Harvald, and M. Hauge, "A Danish Twin Study of Manic-Depressive Disorders," *British Journal of Psychiatry* 130:330-351, 1977.

phobias, obsessive-compulsive disorder, posttraumatic stress disorder, and generalized anxiety disorder. This report considers two of these conditions—obsessive-compulsive disorder and panic disorder—in which the role of biological factors has been more fully explored.

Obsessive-compulsive disorder (OCD) is characterized by the presence of recurrent and persistent thoughts, images, or ideas that are experienced by the afflicted individual as intrusive and senseless (obsessions) and stereotypical, repetitive, and purposeful actions perceived as unnecessary (compulsions) (table 1-2). A common manifestation of this disorder is the obsessional feeling of being dirty or contaminated, which leads to the compulsion of repeated hand washing. Many individuals with OCD have another diagnosis, most often depression. Other problems that may be associated with OCD include other anxiety disorders, eating disorders, alcohol abuse, and Tourette's syndrome.

Once thought to be quite rare, OCD has been found by more recent epidemiological studies to affect approximately 2 to 3 percent of the U.S.

population. Males and females appear to be afflicted equally. The symptoms of OCD begin in childhood or adolescence in one-third to one-half of all individuals who develop the disorder; the average age of onset is 20. Although the symptoms of OCD sometimes recede completely with time, most patients suffer chronically from OCD, with a waxing and waning course.

Currently there are two primary treatment approaches for OCD: behavioral therapy and medication. Behavioral therapy entails repeated exposure of the patient to the stimulus that sets off ritualistic acts. For example, if an individual has a compulsion that causes him to wash his hands 20 or 30 times a day, his hands may be deliberately dirtied, after which he is prevented from washing them. Medications affecting the brain chemical serotonin have proven effective, with clomipramine (Anafranil) being commonly used to treat OCD.

As with the other mental disorders considered in this report, biological factors appear to have a role in OCD. The fact that drugs which act on the brain chemical serotonin are sometimes effective in treating OCD implicates biological factors. Studies have not, however, uncovered a specific abnormality in serotonin metabolism or activity. Other studies implicate a genetic component in OCD.

Several lines of evidence indicate that a specific region of the brain—the basal ganglia—mediates the symptoms of OCD. Damage to the basal ganglia can lead to compulsive behavior. And OCD is sometimes associated with Tourette's syndrome, which also involves this region of the brain. These observations, coupled with data from studies that show increased activity in the basal ganglia and in another region of the brain, the orbital system in the frontal cortex, have led to the hypothesis that OCD results from the abnormal interaction of these two regions of the brain (figure 1-6). According to this hypothesis, the basal ganglia and frontal cortex, which normally modulate actions based on thoughts or impulses, do not work properly in OCD.

While controversy remains as to whether panic disorder is a distinct entity, clinicians have long recognized panic attacks and the extensive morbidity associated with them. The hallmark symptoms of a panic attack include a sudden and inexplicable bout of intense fear associated with strong bodily symptoms. A panic attack typically unfolds quite

Table 1-2—Obsessions and Compulsions

Obsessions	Reported symptom at initial interview[a]	
	(no.)	(%)
Concern with dirt, germs, or environmental toxins	28	(40)
Something terrible happening (fire, death, or illness of self or loved one)	17	(24)
Symmetry, order, or exactness	12	(17)
Scrupulosity (religious obsessions)	9	(13)
Concern or disgust with bodily wastes or secretions (urine, stool, saliva)	6	(8)
Lucky or unlucky numbers	6	(8)
Forbidden, aggressive or perverse sexual thoughts, images, or impulses	3	(4)
Fear might harm others or oneself	3	(4)
Concern with household items	2	(3)
Intrusive nonsense sounds, words, or music	1	(1)

Compulsions	Reported symptom at initial interview	
	(no.)	(%)
Excessive or ritualized hand washing, showering bathing, tooth brushing, or grooming	60	(85)
Repeating rituals (going in or out of a door, up or down from a chair)	36	(51)
Checking (doors, locks, stove, appliances, emergency brake on car, paper route, homework)	32	(46)
Rituals to remove contact with contaminants	16	(23)
Touching	14	(20)
Measures to prevent harm to self or others	11	(16)
Ordering or arranging	12	(17)
Counting	13	(18)
Hoarding or collecting rituals	8	(11)
Rituals of cleaning household or inanimate objects	4	(6)
Miscellaneous rituals (such as writing, moving, speaking) ...	18	(26)

[a]The most frequent obsessions and compulsions among 70 children and adolescents who were diagnosed as having OCD by the author and her colleagues at the National Institute of Mental Health. The proportions total more than 100 percent because many sufferers have more than one symptom.

SOURCE: J.L. Rapoport, "The Biology of Obsessions and Compulsions," *Scientific American* 260(3):83-89, 1990.

rapidly; in just a few minutes an extreme sense of fear overtakes an individual, his or her heart begins racing, the individual begins to perspire, sometimes profusely, and he or she has trouble breathing. A single attack is short-lived, lasting 20 minutes to an hour, on average. These symptoms often leave a person believing that he or she is suffering from a heart attack or is losing his or her mind. In fact, many individuals with panic disorder seek general medical care at an increased rate. Panic attacks occur, on average, about two times a week, although the frequency varies considerably among individuals. People with panic disorder often exhibit other disorders as well. They may fear being in a public place from which escape is difficult—agoraphobia. Depression and substance abuse are also common among individuals with panic disorder.

Data show that approximately one to two persons in every hundred will develop panic disorder during their lifetimes, with women being twice as likely as men to develop the disorder. The disorder usually first appears during young adulthood, with an average age of onset of 24 years. Data suggest that many patients suffer chronically from this condition.

Panic disorder is treated with medication and/or psychotherapy. Antidepressant drugs and antianxiety agents, such as the benzodiazepine alprazolam, are used with some effectiveness in panic disorder; behavioral or cognitive therapy may prove useful in diminishing the severity or frequency, or both, of panic attacks.

There are several psychological and biological theories about the origin of panic disorder. For example, one cognitive theory posits that individuals may misinterpret normal physiological changes, such as an increase in heart rate, as dangerous, thus inducing anxiety and precipitating a panic attack. Several observations are consistent with a role for biological factors in panic disorder. Data from

Figure 1-6—PET Scan of an Individual With Obsessive-Compulsive Disorder

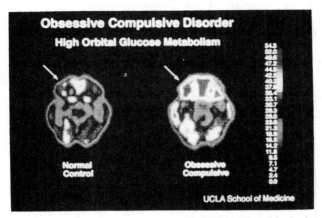

Brain activity in the brain of a person with OCD (right) and the brain of a person without OCD (left). In OCD, there is increased activity in a region of the brain called the frontal cortex.

SOURCE: L. Baxter, UCLA Center for Health Sciences, Los Angeles, CA.

genetic studies indicate that panic disorder may, in part, be inherited. The action of antianxiety medications has led to hypotheses that naturally occurring anxiety-provoking chemicals underlie panic disorder or, conversely, that a deficit of natural anxiety-blockers is at the root of the disorder. To date, however, no such substances have been identified. Research data have also implicated a particular region of the brain, the limbic system, in anxiety and possibly panic disorder.

Whatever the cause, several lines of evidence point to the role of a particular brain region (the locus ceruleus) and a specific chemical (norepinephrine) in mediating panic attacks. Antidepressant drugs, which act on norepinephrine, are an effective treatment for panic disorder. Various drugs and other substances that stimulate the locus ceruleus and increase norepinephrine production can also trigger panic attacks. Continuing research is aimed at clarifying what role the locus ceruleus plays in panic disorder, how it might relate to the limbic system (which is involved in anxiety), and what other chemicals and regions of the brain may be involved.

A SYNTHESIS: UNDERSTANDING THE ROLE OF BIOLOGY

What can we conclude about the role of biology in mental disorders? In its review of research, OTA found the following evidence that biological factors

are involved in schizophrenia, bipolar disorder, major depression, OCD, and panic disorder:

- Medications can suppress symptoms associated with these disorders.
- Specific mental disorders can often be typified by distinguishable clinical features, such as age of onset, symptoms, and course.
- These disorders may have associated ''physical'' symptoms, such as altered sleep patterns in depression.
- Known physical agents and drugs can produce some symptoms of mental disorders, demonstrating that biological factors can in fact be causative.
- Genetic studies show that the disorders are influenced by inheritance.
- Other areas of research provide evidence about correlated biological factors and suggest testable hypotheses as to causation.

Some researchers and advocates conclude from this evidence that biological factors are the predominant cause of severe mental disorders and that the medical model is the best way to conceive of them. In contrast, others deplore the talk of ''brain disease,'' citing the incomplete state of our knowledge about what causes these conditions and even how best to categorize them. The majority of experts and interested parties—and OTA—recognize that research data increasingly show that biological factors play an important role in these disorders. Furthermore, OTA concludes that advances in biological research will serve as the linchpin in improving our understanding of these conditions.

Biological research has not ruled out a role for psychosocial factors in the mental disorders considered in this report. In fact, it is clear that mental disorders cannot be understood or treated in biological terms only. Nor does biological research necessarily implicate biological treatments. Environment, education, and culture exert powerful influences, and psychological interventions are important for treatment. Experts increasingly recognize the essential error of discussions that pit biology against psychosocial factors: The two are obviously and inextricably interrelated. Sorting out their relative roles and how they interact in different conditions will be critical for the development of research and treatment strategies.

Many questions remain about the biology of mental disorders. In fact, research has yet to identify specific biological causes for any of these disorders. Why do we not know more about the biological causes and correlates of these conditions? One reason stems from the complexity of these disorders and the difficulty of categorizing them. Individuals often exhibit symptoms that reach across categories of disorders. And a single diagnostic category may encompass multiple conditions. Furthermore, we do not completely understand the relationship among different disorders.

Another reason is our incomplete understanding of the brain. The brain and behavior are immensely complicated, and our knowledge of them is still scant in comparison to what we have yet to learn. With advancing knowledge about the brain, more sophisticated hypotheses about mental disorders—involving how the many chemicals in the brain work, and how nerve cells and discrete regions of the brain interact—will be propounded. Given our nascent understanding of the brain, it will be necessary to stay the course in what is likely to be a slow unveiling of the biology of mental disorders.

The search for specific genes involved in mental disorders has also proven a difficult task. Attempts to locate specific genes have alternately produced acclaimed reports of success and contradictory data followed by the withdrawal of results. While these events impugn the theory of a simple relationship between one gene and a particular mental disorder, they do not rule out the need for further genetic studies: Evidence from many sources clearly indicates that mental disorders have a genetic component. Nor do past problems necessarily rule out the action of a major gene in the development of a mental disorder, at least in some cases. Like the investigations of other common diseases with complex genetics (e.g., Alzheimer's disease, diabetes mellitus), future studies must take into account the complicated pattern of inheritance, the likely role of more than one gene operating within different families and individuals, questions as to what is inherited, and the undeniable role of nongenetic factors.

THE RESEARCH ENTERPRISE

The pursuit of knowledge about the biological aspects of mental disorders rests upon an adequate research capacity, which in turn is subserved by a complex enterprise that makes funds available, sets research priorities, attends to relevant ethical and policy issues, outfits researchers with equipment and other resource needs, and provides for education and training. The answers to three questions shed light on factors that influence this research enterprise: What level of public concern motivates research into mental disorders? What is the level of research support? What factors form barriers to research?

What Level of Public Concern Motivates Research Into Mental Disorders?

Several studies and mental health advocates have claimed that research into mental disorders is underfunded, attributing the deficiency to the low priority assigned to these conditions by the public and policymakers. This assertion stems from three observations: 1) the Federal investment, as reflected in the NIMH budgets, declined significantly between the late 1960s and early 1980s; 2) Federal support for research on mental disorders is comparatively less than its support of other areas of health research; and 3) there are limited nonFederal sources of funding, especially from private foundations.

A seminal report from the Institute of Medicine concluded in 1984 that the:

> . . . real buying power of research funding for mental disorders has dropped sharply during the past 15 years, even as available personnel and basic knowledge about brain function have expanded dramatically.[3]

OTA evaluated the NIMH research budget since 1980, to gauge recent Federal support (figure 1-7). Between 1980 and 1992,[4] NIMH funding of research, including funding of extramural basic and clinical research, intramural research, and research training, increased by 6.7 percent annually.[5] The rate of growth from 1986 to 1992 was substantially higher, at 11.5 percent.[6]

---

[3] Institute of Medicine, *Research on Mental Illness and Addictive Disorders: Progress and Prospects* (Washington, DC: National Academy Press, 1984).

[4] Fiscal years are indicated.

[5] This is the average annual real rate of increase, determined by converting the NIMH budget in current dollars into constant 1987 dollars, using the gross domestic product deflator as the price index.

[6] Based on estimates, the increase in NIMH's research budget slowed to 7.7 percent between 1991 and 1992.

Figure 1-7—NIMH Budget, Fiscal Years 1980-92

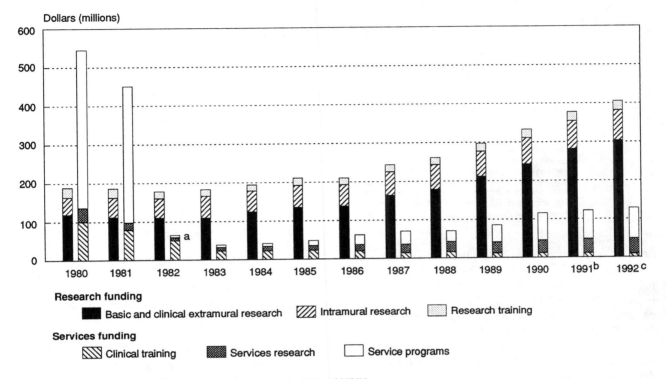

Funding of the components of the research and services budgets of NIMH.

NOTE: Figures converted to constant 1987 dollars using the 1992 gross domestic product deflator.
aDecrease reflects initiation of State block grants.
b1991 and 1992 figures are estimates.
c1992 figures based on assumption of constant price index.
SOURCE: Office of Technology Assessment from figures supplied by National Institute of Mental Health, 1992.

Despite the increases, various measures indicate that during the 1980s the relative investment in research on mental disorders was considerably less than that for other diseases. OTA compared the relative support for research to the total costs of mental disorders, cancer, and heart disease (table 1-3).[7] For every $100 of costs imposed by mental disorders, $0.30 was spent on research. In comparison, for every $100 of costs of heart disease and cancer, $0.73 and $1.63, respectively, were spent on research. It is of interest to note, however, that the Federal Government's purchasing power for mental disorders research increased faster in the 1980s than did its purchasing power for cancer research.

Previous studies have also called attention to the historic neglect of research into mental disorders by private foundations and voluntary health agencies,

which currently form a relatively small, but important source of support for biomedical research. The 1980s did witness new sources of private support for research into the biology of severe mental disorders, with the formation of the National Alliance for Research on Schizophrenia and Depression (NARSAD) in 1986 and the establishment of the National Alliance for the Mentally Ill's (NAMI's) Stanley Awards Program. Still, support from such organizations for mental disorder-related research stands at a much lower level than private foundation support for other diseases. For example, in fiscal year 1991, the American Cancer Society spent nearly $91 million dollars on research, compared to NARSAD's $3.3 million.

What can we conclude about the level of public concern that surrounds mental disorders, as meas-

---

[7] The analysis used the most comparable and recent data, which stemmed from 1985.

Table 1-3—Comparison of Costs and Research Funding, Fiscal Year 1985

Illness	Costs[a] ($ millions)	Total budget of principal Federal institution[b] ($ millions)	Dollars spent on research per $100 of cost to society
Mental disorders	103,691[c]	310[d]	0.30
Cancer (malignant neoplasms only)	72,494	1,184	1.63
Heart disease	69,000	501	0.73

[a]D.P. Rice, S. Kelman, L.S. Miller, et al., *The Economic Costs of Alcohol and Drug Abuse and Mental Illness: 1985*, report submitted to the Office of Financing and Coverage Policy, Alcohol, Drug Abuse, and Mental Health Administration, U.S. Department of Health and Human Services (San Francisco, CA: Institute for Health and Aging, University of California, 1990); D.P. Rice, T.A. Hodgson, and F. Capell, "The Economic Burden of Cancer, 1985: United States and California," *Cancer Care and Cost: DRGs and Beyond*, R.M. Scheffler and N.C. Andrews (eds.) (Ann Arbor, MI: Health Administration Press Perspectives, 1989); T. Thom, Health Statistician, Division of Epidemiology and Clinical Application, National Heart, Lung, and Blood Institute, National Institutes of Health, personal communication, 1991.
[b]National Institute of Mental Health, National Cancer Institute, and National Heart, Lung, and Blood Institute budgets.
[c]Costs of mental disorders include costs of dementia.
[d]Figure includes $29 million for funding of dementia research by the National Institute on Aging.
SOURCE: Office of Technology Assessment, 1992.

ured by research support? As others have noted, the historical lack of support for this research was reversed somewhat in the 1980s: Federal funding for research into mental disorders increased significantly, and new private sources of funding developed. Even with the increased funding of the 1980s, however, support for research into mental disorders falls short of that for other conditions in relation to their cost to society.

What Is the Level of Research Support?

How much of NIMH's increasing funding goes to support the areas of research considered in this report? OTA examined extramural research funding in two major divisions of NIMH: the Division of Basic Brain and Behavioral Sciences (DBBBS) and the Division of Clinical Research (DCR). In 1991, these divisions accounted for 74 percent of the extramural research budget—some $287.2 million.

As indicated by its name, DBBBS supports basic research aimed at furthering the understanding of basic brain mechanisms and behavior related to mental disorders. Over the last few years, DBBBS has received increasing support, with its research budget reaching $117.6 million in 1991 (figure 1-8). Specific areas of neuroscience, including molecular and cellular biology, cognitive neuroscience, neuroimaging, and psychopharmacology research, have been particularly favored. The annual rate of increase in its budget was 14.5 percent between 1988 and 1992.

DCR consists of six research-oriented branches; its total research budget in 1991 was $169.6 million.

Two branches—the Schizophrenia Research Branch and the Mood, Anxiety, and Personality Disorders Research Branch—target the disorders considered in this report and receive 50.3 percent of DCR's research budget. Between 1986 and 1992, both of these branches experienced above average funding increases (figure 1-9). The DCR's emphasis on schizophrenia and mood disorders is further reflected in the fact that 16 of its 23 research centers focus on these disorders.

What Factors Create Barriers to Research?

Funding is not the sole determinant of research capacity. Various other factors, ranging from the availability of animals to the number of trained researchers, influence the success of the research enterprise. OTA has identified several areas that, if neglected, can create barriers to research.

Several issues common to all biomedical research come to bear on research into mental disorders. For instance, support for facilities and equipment affects mental disorders research. Efforts to contain health-care costs also affect clinical research, since third-party payers typically cover the costs of clinical care in research. Another general issue for mental disorders research centers around the representation of all members of society in research, regardless of age, sex, race, or ethnic group; concerns about fairness and the ultimate implications for health and the advancement of knowledge have driven congressional and executive branch action. Finally, because the use of animals, especially nonhuman primates, is critical for neuroscience and research into mental

Figure 1-8—Funding of the Division of Basic Brain and Behavioral Sciences, Fiscal Years 1988-92

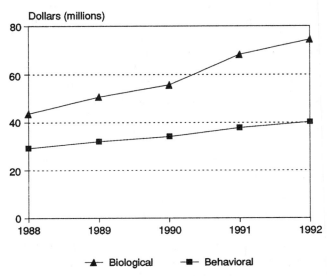

The funding of the Division of Basic Brain and Behavioral Sciences broken down into biological and behavioral research (see text).

NOTE: Figures converted to constant 1987 dollars using the 1992 gross domestic product deflator.

SOURCE: Office of Technology Assessment from figures supplied by National Institute of Mental Health, 1992.

disorders, developments concerning the use of animals in research, including tightening regulations and increased cost, raise concern.

The fact that mental disorders disrupt human cognitive, emotional, and social capabilities presents special challenges for researchers. For example, how can these complicated effects be studied or modeled in animals? Also, the unique nature of mental disorders raises ethical concerns in clinical research, requiring a careful balancing of individuals' needs and interests and the need for continued research. While these issues cannot be eliminated, investigators can devise ways of dealing with them effectively. Finally, the stigma attached to and the ignorance surrounding mental disorders influence research in a variety of ways, from hindering recruitment of subjects to amplifying privacy concerns.

OTA considered, in some detail, three issues identified as significant obstacles to research on mental disorders: the difficulty of obtaining postmortem brain tissue, the cost of hospitalization, and the number of clinician-researchers.

Figure 1-9—Funding of the Division of Clinical Research, Fiscal Years 1980-92

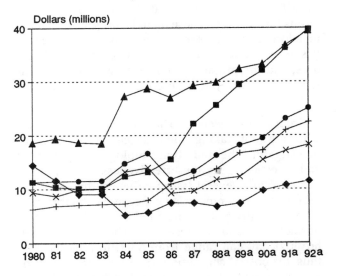

Funding of the six research branches of the Division of Clinical Research.

NOTE: Figures converted to constant 1987 dollars using the 1992 gross domestic product deflator.
aFigures include research training.

SOURCE: Office of Technology Assessment from figures supplied by National Institute of Mental Health, 1992.

The expansion of biological research into mental disorders makes the availability of postmortem brain tissue increasingly important. While there are two federally sponsored brain bank centers in the United States, as well as an informal supply, the amount of tissue available for research is simply inadequate. Improving the banking of brains requires consideration of several factors: funding, standardization of tissue retrieval and handling methods, attracting tissue donors, the need for complete medical histories, and safeguarding confidentiality. In an effort to improve the acquisition process and to better disseminate information about the availability of sources of brain tissue from various centers, NIMH has created a task force to make recommendations on how to coordinate these efforts. A number of suggestions are under consideration, including the use of a private institution under contract to NIMH as a clearinghouse for the collection and distribution of brain tissue. The NIMH task force is also identifying other needs related to the collection of brains for research. These include designing systems to address the problem of the limited samples of tissue available from persons with specific disorders, and the pressing need for tissue from normal individuals that can be used as experimental controls.

Studies of subjects who have mental disorders and who are not taking medications are critical in investigating the underlying biology of a disorder and in establishing the effectiveness of new treatments. While several issues influence this research, the cost of care for medication-free research subjects—who generally require hospitalization—is a major obstacle to clinical research. The cost of each hospital day can range from $300 to over $1,000; thus, the cost of supporting a single research bed for a year can range from $109,500 to $365,000. NIMH funding can be used to support bed costs, but generally this is not a realistic option, since it would divert an enormous proportion of funds from other research activities.

Many experts and organizations have drawn attention to the apparent shortage of clinician-researchers—namely, psychiatrists and psychologists—in the United States. Recently, NIMH convened a task force to make specific recommendations about the recruitment of investigators into clinical research careers. While the need for clinician-researchers is not peculiar to mental health research, some factors make the situation particularly acute in this field. Few students in mental health professional training programs receive formal exposure to research. And financial issues, including expected salary levels and the need to pay off medical and/or graduate school debts, tend to forestall the choice of a research career.

IMPLICATIONS OF BIOLOGY

Support for neuroscience research, in general and as it is applied to the study of mental disorders, stems from a palpable enthusiasm for advances in understanding the human brain. Support for research into the biology of severe mental disorders is also intimately linked to the hope for improved treatments for these disorders. While treatments exist, they are not effective in all cases, and side effects, some of which are serious, are common. Although a detailed analysis of the development of new treatments lies outside the purview of this report, OTA finds that the development of new drugs to treat mental disorders is one of the greatest promises that biological research holds. History bears out this potential, as does the number of drugs being developed and tested (table 1-4). The increasing and more precise understanding of the action of chemicals in the brain has facilitated and will continue to facilitate the development of new medications for mental disorders. At the same time, important issues that cannot be overlooked—cost, side effects, forced treatment—accompany the development and use of psychoactive medication.

The zeal associated with the current focus on the biology of mental disorders may benefit from some tempering. Scientific advances can lead to better treatment, diagnostic tests, cures, and preventive measures. However, most new treatments will reflect incremental advances: Significant improvements in the understanding and treatment of mental disorders are likely to require years, even decades, to unfold. Some observers have noted that fostering expectations of rapid progress in discerning the biological underpinnings of mental disorders or developing new treatments may provoke impatience, disappointment, or even a backlash against this research. Perhaps most important, exclusive emphasis on biological factors could divert resources from other important areas of research and the provision of care for people currently suffering from these conditions.

Biological research into mental disorders has influenced the mental health care finance debate, as exemplified by recent court cases and State laws. Coverage for mental health care in both the public and private sectors is generally lower than coverage for ''physical'' illnesses. In order to gain parity in insurance coverage and to help defray the costs of these chronic and often severe disorders, some advocates have emphasized the biological basis of certain mental disorders, thus invoking the traditional medical model of illness as the most appropriate one for treatment. Also, emphasizing the biological basis of a disorder underlines the fact that the disorder is outside the control of the individual and invokes society's perceived responsibility for providing care. Biological research may also help insurers in objectively determining an insurable event, by identifying biological markers for certain mental disorders, along with effective treatments.

Table 1-4—Drugs in Development for
Mental Disorders

Disorder	United States	Other countries
Schizophrenia	76	42
Mood disorders	83	61
Anxiety disorders	91	46

SOURCE: PJB Publications, *Pharmaprojects* (Surrey, England: PJP Publications, 1992).

Data from research point increasingly to the importance of biological factors in certain mental disorders. This has given rise to other concerns, however, including coverage of ''nonbiological'' disorders or interventions. Furthermore, there is heightened concern about the cost of health care. Given the public health problem that severe mental disorders present and the complex issues involved in health care finance, the way in which care for persons with these disorders is financed warrants full evaluation.

OTA has identified ways in which information from research into the biology of mental disorders is used to counter the ignorance and negative attitudes that have long been attached to these conditions. Mental disorders have often been and continue to be perceived as a sign of moral or personal weakness. Biological explanations for mental disorders are used to counter the view that these conditions are based in moral turpitude, thus exculpating individuals whose disorders may lead to unusual, erratic, or frightening behavior. Also, the assertion that biological factors contribute to the development of mental disorders refutes the once-reigning and stigmatizing notion that bad parenting is the essential, causative factor. Despite the fact that little or no scientific evidence supports theories of bad parenting as a sufficient or necessary cause of severe mental disorders considered in this report, these theories continue to shape the attitudes of the public and even some experts.

The increased emphasis on biological aspects of mental disorders, while helpful in dismantling some negative attitudes, is not without limitations. Perceptions of what causes mental disorders are not the sole source of stigma; other factors, such as personal experiences and media portrayals (box 1-D), influence public attitudes as well. Also, with the increased publicity given biological research data, questions and worries may arise among individuals with mental disorders and their families. For example, many family members who have heard about genetic studies of mental disorders may overesti-

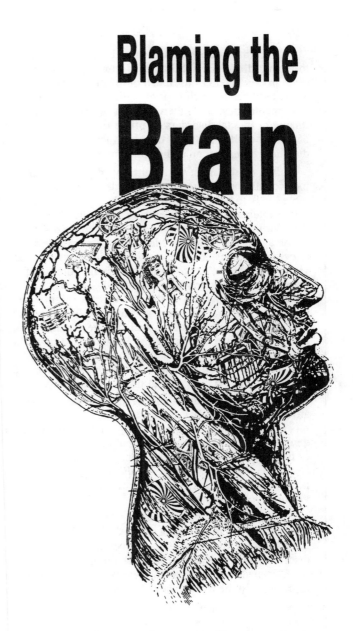

Blaming the Brain

Credit: Illustration by Robin Applestein, reprinted by permission of R. Applestein and The Washington Times.

Findings that biological factors underpin certain mental disorders help relieve individuals and their families from feelings of guilt.

mate their risk for these conditions. Furthermore, the perception that mental disorders are inherited could instill guilt among parents, who fear they might transmit ''flaws'' to their progeny. While our current understanding of the genetics of mental disorders makes unlikely the development of a single, highly

Box 1-D—Media Portrayals of Mental Disorders

Since the late 1950s and early 1960s, studies have consistently revealed a high incidence of media attention to mental disorders. While media attention contributed significantly to the end of mass warehousing of patients, often in cruel conditions, much of the information it provided about mental disorders was negative and inaccurate. Recent studies have shown that although there has been an increase in the frequency of portrayals of individuals with mental disorders, there has not necessarily been an increase in the accuracy of such portrayals. Surveys of images of mental disorders on prime-time television conducted in the 1980s found that between 17 and 29 percent of the shows had some portrayal of mental disorders. Unfortunately, much of that information concerning mental disorders is inaccurate and stigmatizing.

One of the most persistent and damaging inaccuracies conveyed by the media is the characterization of individuals with severe mental disorders as violent despite the fact that individuals with severe mental disorders are more likely to be withdrawn and frightened than violent and are more frequently victims than perpetrators of violent acts. Violence occurs on television at the rate of approximately six incidents per hour in prime time and 25 incidents per hour in children's daytime programming; a disproportionate number of these occurrences are either perpetuated by or against individuals identified as mentally disordered. In fact, characters labeled mentally disordered in television dramas are almost twice as likely as other characters to kill or be killed, to be violent or fall victim to violence. Efforts to combat this image are confounded by the fact that some individuals with mental disorders—particularly when untreated—are at risk of committing violent acts against themselves or others, or both. Perhaps more troubling is the fact that the stigmatizing equation of severe mental disorder with violence is not limited to fictional entertainment media. News stories and headlines identifying violent criminals on the basis of their mental health history, such as the recent Associated Press headline "Woman Who Shot at Restaurant Previously Committed to Mental Hospital," saturate the news media, while stories of successful recovery are rare. Such news stories are damaging to individuals with mental disorders because they suggest both an inescapable connection between mental disorders and violence and the incurability of mental disorder (that is, even *former*, treated mental patients remain prone to violence).

Do these inaccurate and negative depictions of individuals with mental disorders adversely affect public attitudes? Research has shown that television is able to influence viewers' attitudes in subtle ways, through the repetition of images not necessarily labeled as factual. Knowledge specifically concerning the impact of media depictions of mental disorders on public opinions is limited. Some studies have revealed that programming intended to increase knowledge of and improve attitudes toward individuals with mental disorders has a positive impact. However, data indicate that the damaging effects of negative portrayals overwhelm the benefits of the media's positive efforts. Negative mass media portrayals of persons with mental disorders generate negative attitudes among viewers, and corrective information, or disclaimers, has been shown to be largely ineffectual.

Advocacy groups are working to reduce inaccurate and stigmatizing depictions of individuals with mental disorders in the mass media. For example, the Alliance for the Mentally Ill of New York State operates a Stigma Clearinghouse that records and responds to inaccurate or stigmatizing media depictions of individuals with mental disorders, and the National Alliance for the Mentally Ill may soon launch a similar program nationwide. In addition, the Carter Center in Atlanta, Georgia, has held two conferences addressing the problems of stigma and mental disorders and the role of the mass media and has subsequently launched a media initiative to address these issues.

SOURCES: *Stigma and the Mentally Ill: Proceedings of the First International Rosalynn Carter Symposium on Mental Health Policy*, Nov. 15, 1985 (Atlanta, GA: Carter Center, 1985); L.R. Marcos, "Media Power and Public Mental Health Policy," *American Journal of Psychiatry* 146:1185-1189, 1989; A. Mayer and D. Barry, "Working With the Media To Destigmatize Mental Illness," *Hospital and Community Psychiatry* 43:77-78, 1992; Robert Wood Johnson Foundation, Program on Chronic Mental Illness, "Public Attitudes Toward People With Chronic Mental Illness," April 1990; O. Wahl, "Mental Illness in the Media: An Unhealthy Condition," *The Community Imperative*, R.C. Baron, I.D. Rutman, and B. Klaczynska (eds.) (Philadelphia, PA: Horizon House Institute, 1980); O. Wahl, Professor, George Mason University, personal communication, February 1992; O. Wahl and J.Y. Lefkowitz, "Impact of a Television Film on Attitudes Toward Mental Illness," *American Journal of Community Psychology* 17(4):521-528, 1989; O. Wahl and R. Roth, "Television Images of Mental Illness: Results of a Metropolitan Washington Media Watch," *Journal of Broadcasting* 28:599-605, 1982.

predictive genetic test that would be useful across the general population, the future possibility of genetic testing—even the perception that mental disorders are inherited—raises additional concerns about possible discrimination.

Biological data also may be simplified or misinterpreted. Attributing behavior to biological, especially genetic, factors may lead to the perception that human actions are predetermined. Thus, biological explanations of behavior encroach uncomfortably on our sense of free will and moral agency. Furthermore, some observers fear that biological theories of mental functions reduce human behavior to the output of the gray mass in our craniums, thus robbing human thought and emotion of meaning and import. Individuals with mental disorders may be especially vulnerable in a society seduced by notions of biological determinism and reductionism; in this case, not only are mental functions just the reflection of brain function, but the brain function is diseased. The meaning attached to a person's thoughts and actions, and the extent to which he or she is responsible for them, are complex issues requiring the consideration of biological as well as social, philosophical, legal, and moral issues, which are beyond the scope of this report. Nevertheless, it is important to debunk some of the myths that surround these issues. Biological theories of causation are not necessarily more damaging to the person afflicted with a mental disorder than other theories; one need only be reminded of the cruel and stigmatizing concepts of family causation. Nor is it true that a biological underpinning is immutable and an environmental one malleable. Recent advances in neuroscience do not suggest that our brains are biologically fixed; rather, results increasingly show the dynamic nature of nervous tissue and its responsiveness to environmental cues throughout life.

POLICY ISSUES AND OPTIONS FOR CONGRESSIONAL ACTION

The findings of this study attest to the recent growth of the neurosciences and to a corresponding surge of interest in the biology of mental disorders. Researchers have partially uncovered the biological substrates of some mental disorders and have propounded testable hypotheses about causes. The upshot of the scientific advances is expanded research opportunities, potential treatments, and new questions regarding how this knowledge is used. The potential consequences of biological research into mental disorders raise several policy issues of congressional interest:

- Federal support for research,
- implications of scientific advances, and
- dissemination of new information.

The following section covers each of these policy issues and sets forth several options for congressional action. Some options require direct congressional action, while others involve indirect efforts, such as oversight or direction of the executive branch. OTA has fashioned a list of reasonable responses to the policy issues that emerged during the course of this study. No priority is set nor course recommended; rather, an analysis of each option and its likely result is presented.

ISSUE 1: Federal Support for Research

Congress is faced with the question, *How should we support research on mental disorders?* The most important congressional response to this question is given annually, in the allocation to NIMH; several observations and results from this study may assist Congress with its funding decision.

Option 1: Support research at NIMH.

It is no exaggeration to state that advances in neuroscience have revolutionized the study of mental disorders. While the causes of mental disorders remain unknown, data from various and diverse studies illuminate the role of biological factors in schizophrenia, bipolar disorder, major depression, OCD, and panic disorder. Furthermore, the intense efforts and rapid progress in neuroscience portend increased knowledge about these disorders in the years to come. New technologies enable scientists to probe more thoroughly everything from the tiniest molecules to the interaction of large collections of nerve cells, giving us insights into the more than 100 billion nerve cells that together make up the brain. This confluence of technological advances, rapidly accruing knowledge in the neurosciences, and considerable excitement among researchers calls for, at the very least, a sustained level of funding for biological research into mental disorders; undoubtedly, this research enterprise could effectively use even higher levels of funding. To reduce funding would be to ignore the opportunities that exist at this time, thus failing to capitalize on the investment and gains to date.

While this report does not detail the research and development of specific treatments for mental disorders, OTA finds that one of the greatest promises of research into the biology of mental disorders is the development of more effective medications. The need for and promise of better medications also argue for continued or enhanced funding. New drugs resulting from the investment in research could more than pay for their development costs by offsetting some of the tremendous burden now borne by society. For example, it is estimated that the 1969 introduction of lithium to treat bipolar disorder resulted in average yearly savings in treatment costs of $290 million in the United States. It was also estimated that $92 million in lost wages was regained in the first year following the introduction of lithium. It is important to note, however, that the translation of new scientific findings into new treatments will probably take place over a period of years, if not decades. Therefore, this must be viewed as a long-term investment.

Although the social burden of mental disorders is difficult to compare with that of other types of illness, it is generally of the same magnitude as cancer and heart disease. Mental disorders lead to considerable suffering, disability, and death. These conditions take a large toll on society, afflicting millions of Americans and costing the nation more than $100 billion each year. Yet based on the costs of the disorders, research spending for mental disorders is lower than that for cancer or heart disease. Increased allocation of funds for mental disorders research would redress this inequity in funding and demonstrate the priority given to mental disorders by the Federal Government. The relative cost of a health problem cannot be the sole determinant of research funding; however, together with the fact that significant research opportunities exist in this field, it serves as a strong argument for increased funds.

It is apparent that several factors argue for continued, if not increased, funding of mental disorders research, but Congress must weigh the relative importance and need for this investment of Federal dollars against a host of competing programs. It is also important to note that additional funding would certainly enable researchers to pursue more scientific opportunities and would yield fruitful gains, but it would also enlarge the system and increase the number of deserving competitors for Federal support. Scientific research budgets, including that of the NIMH, have fared well during the past years of fiscal constraints; however, the growing Federal debt and mechanisms enacted to address it have sharpened the competition among federally financed programs. While a main conclusion of this report is that continued support for research into the biology of mental disorders is necessary in order to reap the potential benefits, this study did not assess the state of knowledge, relative promise, or warranted priority of other programs or fields of inquiry.

Whatever the level of support for mental disorders research, it is critical that funding go to the highest quality research. Given the state of knowledge and existing research opportunities, how are Federal monies best invested, with the highest likelihood of return? OTA finds that maintaining a broad portfolio of research is the key. Continued investment in basic research is central to this effort, given the rudimentary, if rapidly growing, state of our knowledge concerning the brain and its functioning. Basic neuroscience research will produce more sophisticated hypotheses and methods of analysis, which are essential to understanding the complex manifestations of mental disorders.

Disorder-targeted funding is also necessary. This report notes many areas that are prime for research and that are likely to improve public health. Various viable hypotheses have been put forth concerning the causes of mental disorders, but further information is needed concerning the specific manifestations of these conditions and their pattern of inheritance. Advances in molecular biology and imaging technologies make possible more detailed examination of brain function and structure in these disorders.

Support for disorder-targeted research encompasses clinical studies. Congressional support for clinical research can be shown in various ways, among them additional funding for NIMH. The options that follow are also means of supporting clinical research.

Option 2: Support clinical research by the VA.

Since the costs of medical care in clinical investigations at VA hospitals are charged to health care delivery funds rather than research dollars, a modest increase in research appropriations could significantly increase clinical research. Thus, Congress could enhance clinical research by increasing the VA's research budget. Furthermore, to foster mental disorders research, Congress could direct the VA to move forward on a recommendation from the VA Advisory Committee for Health Research Policy, which recommended the creation of a Health Research Advisory Council to identify and prioritize those areas with the greatest promise of enhancing VA health care. The council could be a useful mechanism for redressing the disparity between VA medical research expenditures for mental disorders and their clinical costs.

Option 3: Convene a task force to delineate mechanisms for underwriting bed costs.

Rapidly rising bed costs threaten clinical studies, which often require hospitalization of subjects during trials, as well as other persons who are free of medication. Bed costs can be included in the NIMH funding made available to the Clinical Research Centers. Yet few center directors choose to use funds in this fashion, since it would divert an enormous proportion of their total funding away from other priorities. The pharmaceutical industry has recently recognized the obstacle created by increasing bed costs; and while some companies have begun providing support, it is difficult to document the extent of such support. NIMH has not taken any direct action in regard to bed costs. In the absence of congressional action, it is unclear whether NIMH will address this issue. Thus, this acute need may go unmet.

Some virtually untapped resources exist to help defray the expense of bed costs in clinical research. In an effort to deal with the issue of bed costs, Congress could direct that a task force be established. The task force could include representatives of all parties who have a stake in this research and who can contribute to the solution: clinical investigators, NIMH, health insurance companies, private foundations, advocacy groups, pharmaceutical companies, State mental hospitals, the VA hospital system, and general and private hospitals. While it might be difficult for the many different parties involved to form a consensus, together they could devise a workable plan that would take advantage of existing and unutilized resources (e.g., VA hospitals, State hospitals). In addition to considering cost issues, the task force could explore research approaches that might be less expensive (e.g., day hospitals and partial-care centers). NIMH can be directed to follow the findings and recommendations of the task force.

Option 4: Fund the training of clinician-researchers.

The limited availability of researchers trained as clinicians has a continuing impact on the quality and quantity of clinical research. Professionals and policymakers acknowledge this problem, and NIMH is poised to address it by enhancing exposure to research for psychiatrists and psychologists during training. Support for research centers, which bring together clinicians and researchers with various skills to work together on research projects, also addresses the need for the clinician's expertise in studies.

Congress could, however, further respond to the need for clinician-researchers. Congress established the National Research Service Awards (NRSA) to provide for the training of clinician-researchers, but its appropriations for NRSA have not increased in the last 12 years. When adjusted for inflation, the 1991 training budget of $26.9 million is $2 million less than the 1980 budget. Increasing total funding and increases in the maximum salary for individual investigators could make this program more effective. Earmarked funds could also be directed to Research Career Awards and Scientist Development Award for Clinicians programs, which are generally considered successful, although underfunded. Simply providing additional training funds is not the whole solution, or even the most efficient mechanism for dealing with the problem. For example, forgiveness of medical school debt would be a powerful incentive. Congress may, therefore, want to link increased funds to such programmatic issues.

ISSUE 2: Implications of Scientific Advances

Advances in biomedical research during the latter part of the 20th century have raised new and difficult ethical, legal, and social questions; research into the biology of mental disorders is no different. In this study, OTA considered issues raised both by the conduct of research and by new findings.

Issues of informed consent and confidentiality inevitably emerge during the conduct of mental disorders research. While these issues are neither new nor entirely unique to the study of mental disorders, there are special concerns deriving from the nature of mental illness, its impact on the mind, and the associated stigma. Furthermore, scientific advances may add a new twist to these issues. For example, the process of gathering clinical information for genetic studies poses questions about what to tell relatives of individuals with mental disorders who are contacted for this research. Existing guidelines specify that an Institutional Review Board (IRB) review the medical, legal, and ethical aspects of proposed research projects that will involve human subjects.

The results of research into the biology of mental disorders also have ethical, legal, and social implications. For example, findings concerning the biology of mental disorders have become an issue in the mental health care financing debate. The development of new medication interfaces with ongoing concerns about the right to refuse treatment. Increased understanding of the genetics of mental disorders raises the specter of a new age of discrimination against individuals with mental disorders (box 1-E). Advances in brain research challenge our very conceptualization of the human mind, affecting such issues as personal responsibility and free will. Researchers, clinicians, advocates, policymakers, ethicists, and lawyers have addressed some of the implications of research findings. However, NIMH pays little formal attention to the ethical, legal, and social implications of the results of the research they sponsor.

Option 1: Direct NIMH to formalize consideration of ethical, legal, and social issues.

Congress could stipulate that NIMH devise a systematic plan to deal with the ethical, legal, and social implications of both the conduct and the results of mental disorders research. By mandating such a program and providing funds for it, Congress would draw attention to these issues and create a process of anticipating the social impact of research results. The structure of a program devoted to such issues could take various forms. It could be modeled after the National Institutes of Health-Department of Energy program that considers such implications of the Human Genome Project: the Ethical, Legal, and Social Implications, or ELSI, program. Like the ELSI program, it might fund research into the likely implications and conduct of biological research into mental disorders. The NIMH program would foster the development of knowledge upon which consideration of these issues can be based and would increase the number of professionals with expertise in this area.

Such a program is not without potential problems. Forecasting the impact of scientific advances is difficult. Also, without a specific focus and a specific charge, the program might be ineffectual. The ethical, legal, and social issues raised by research are complex and sometimes emotionally charged; they lie at the interface of scientific knowledge and social values and beliefs. Forming a consensus about these complex and sensitive issues is often hard, if not impossible. The resolution of these issues may be more properly dealt with, in a democratic society, by a political process such as in the U.S. Congress rather than an academic or bureaucratic one.

Option 2: Request topic-specific studies as issues arise.

Rather than erecting a bureaucratic structure to handle the ethical, legal, and social implications of research, Congress could request individual studies from various governmental or nongovernmental organizations. This strategy would permit timely identification of topics for consideration, and the issues and charges of the study could be clearly elucidated and circumscribed. While this mechanism would give Congress more direct control over individual studies and would serve to focus the studies, it could lead to a piecemeal approach that does not provide the continuity and comprehensiveness of a permanent program.

Option 3: Establish an advisory commission on the ethical, legal, and social implications of mental disorders research.

Individuals with various backgrounds and expertise who are not normally a formal part of the policymaking process have important insights into the ethical, legal, and social issues raised by mental disorders research. Furthermore, such persons have a stake in how the issues are addressed. In order to tap into the expertise and interests of these groups, Congress could establish an advisory commission to study and make recommendations on aspects of policy related to the implications of mental disorders research sponsored by the Federal Government. Such bodies, including the ongoing Advisory Panel on Alzheimer's Disease, have proven useful.

A successful panel would be composed of distinguished and expert representatives from biomedical research, the social sciences, the legal profession, care-providing professions, law enforcement, consumers, families, and relevant organizations and businesses. It is important that membership on the

Box 1-E—Eugenics and Mental Disorders

In Nazi Germany and the United States during the earlier part of this century, people with mental disorders were among the initial targets of eugenic policies. People with mental disorders were subjected to immigration restrictions, involuntary sterilization, and extermination. While moderns deny that such practices could be repeated, the record of eugenics and its historical link to mental disorders raise uncomfortable questions: Is the new age of genetics a harbinger of a new age of eugenics? Are people with mental disorders especially vulnerable?

Eugenics enjoys a long, well-bred intellectual pedigree, with the cousin of Charles Darwin, Sir Francis Galton, as its modern forefather. Galton coined the term "eugenics" in 1883, christening the scientific pursuit of improved inborn human qualities through judicious matings: positive eugenics. Prior to Galton, eugenic notions can be traced back as far as Plato's *Republic*, wherein the philosopher also proposes positive eugenic practices. Of course, the human genetic pool can be distilled by other means. Negative eugenics refers to the systematic attempt to minimize the passing of deleterious genes by reducing or preventing the reproduction of individuals carrying such genes.

A number of scientific discoveries planted the seeds of eugenic policies in the 19th and 20th centuries. Galton himself observed that many accomplished men of his day were linked by blood lines, which led to his belief that proper matings could produce a race with enhanced intellectual, behavioral, and physical characteristics. In addition, Galton, as well as others, developed statistical techniques that permitted the quantitative analysis of inherited traits.

While these and other scientific advances were the seeds of eugenics, they were not solely responsible for such policies in the United States. Social, political, and economic factors of the late 19th and early 20th centuries fertilized the growth of the eugenics movement. National attention was increasingly focused on social issues of unemployment, criminality, prostitution, and chronic alcoholism. Also, concerns arose that increased immigration from southern and eastern Europe was drawing the United States away from its "Anglo-Saxon superiority."

At the Federal level, eugenic policies took the form of increasingly restrictive immigration laws. Eugenicists, asserting the simple inheritance of such traits as lunacy, epilepsy, alcoholism, pauperism, criminality, and feeblemindedness, proffered scientific rationales for excluding individuals from entry to the United States. It is important to note that while authentic advances in genetics seeded the eugenics movement, they provided no evidence for the simple inheritance of the traits mentioned above.

Eugenic considerations also prompted States to enact laws regarding compulsory sterilization. In 1907, Indiana passed the first law legalizing the compulsory sterilization of inmates at the State reformatory; by 1931, 30 States had passed compulsory sterilization laws applying to individuals categorized as feebleminded, alcoholic, epileptic, sexually deviant, or mentally ill. Individuals with mental disorders made up half of the 64,000 persons in this country sterilized for eugenic reasons between 1907 and 1964. When eugenic sterilization laws were challenged in 1927, the Supreme Court ruled the practice was constitutional.

What is the current status of eugenic policies in the United States? While immigration laws still restrict the entry of people with mental disorders, denial of entry is not based on eugenic principles, but rather on concerns about whether behavior associated with a disorder poses a threat. State sterilization laws still stand, as does the 1927 Supreme Court ruling upholding them. As of 1987, compulsory sterilization laws remained on the books in 22 States; however, these laws are rarely invoked.

The current application of immigration and compulsory sterilization laws suggests that eugenics is not a major concern at this time. Furthermore, the understanding that mental disorders do not have a simple genetic basis and that nongenetic factors play an important role would seem to limit the potential of eugenic policies. Perhaps most important, Americans repulsion by the Nazi legacy and the emphasis in this country on individual reproductive rights also make State-determined eugenic policies unlikely. But indirect pressure not to have children may well come to bear on individuals seen to have a greater genetic risk of mental disorders; society may brand them irresponsible or immoral for transmitting disorders to their children. Given the financial strain posed by mental disorders today and the stigma attached to them, in conjunction with scientific advances, it is possible that these factors could unlock what some call a backdoor to eugenics.

SOURCES: T. Duster, *Backdoor to Eugenics* (New York, NY: Routledge, 1990); K.L. Garver and B. Garver, "Eugenics: Past, Present, and Future," *American Journal of Human Genetics* 49:1109-1118, 1991; I.I. Gottesman, *Schizophrenia Genesis: The Origins of Madness* (New York, NY: W.H. Freeman, 1991); D.J. Kevles, *In the Name of Eugenics* (New York, NY: Knopf, 1985); D. Suzuki and P. Knudtson, *Genethics: The Clash Between the New Genetics and Human Values* (Cambridge, MA: Harvard University Press, 1989); N.A. Holtzman, *Proceed with Caution: Predicting Genetic Risks in the Recombinant DNA Era* (Baltimore, MD: The Johns Hopkins University Press, 1989).

commission be balanced in terms of the points of view represented, something rarely achieved in mental health policy. This advisory commission could be established by the Secretary of Health and Human Services, or Congress itself, and could be assigned specific issues to address every year or two. The commission could then study the issue, identify the problems of concern, develop a consensus on how such problems can best be met, and present recommendations for legislation to the Congress and the States; the commission could also recommend executive branch regulations, activities, and other programs.

ISSUE 3: Dissemination of New Information

The Federal Government does not support research into the biology of mental disorders merely to gain new knowledge. Rather, Federal funds for this research reflect in large measure a desire for improved medications as well as for improved public perceptions of mental disorders and of individuals with these disorders.

The enthusiasm for and considerable gains in information about the brain and mental disorders that have accrued during the last several years speak to the potential gains in treatment and social handling of persons with mental disorders. However, to effect better treatment, care, and consideration of such individuals, the knowledge gained from biological research must be transferred to the public at large, including individuals with mental disorders and their families, as well as mental health professionals and policymakers.

There are many indications that the transfer of new knowledge to those who need and can act upon it is inadequate. Studies show that providers of mental health care are sometimes inadequately informed about the diagnosis and treatment of mental disorders or that they harbor some negative feelings about their patients. As noted earlier, the public at large commonly holds negative attitudes toward people with mental disorders or are ignorant about the prevalence, manifestation, or cause of these disorders. Such ignorance and attitudes have adverse consequences beyond stigmatizing people with mental disorders and their families. They also interfere with successful treatment: Individuals with

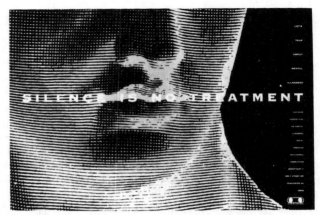

Photo credit: Courtesy of the American Psychiatric Association, 1992.

A recent public education campaign, sponsored by the American Psychiatric Association, highlighted the negative impact of stigma on treatment-seeking.

a mental disorder may avoid seeking treatment in order to avoid the associated stigma. Perhaps of most importance to Congress is the fact that uninformed and negative attitudes contribute to discriminatory public policies. A recent report by the Interagency Task Force on Homelessness and Severe Mental Illness highlights the malignant consequences of negative attitudes on public policy:

> Stigmatization, fear, and mistrust regarding people with severe mental illnesses. . .are commonplace in our Nation. Such reactions influence both the direct responses of community members to these individuals as well as the development of local, State, and Federal policies affecting them.

One conclusion that OTA draws from this analysis is that advances in knowledge about mental disorders do not in themselves ensure better diagnosis, care, or prevention; nor do they guarantee that public policy keeps abreast of research and development. Those improvements and informed policy also depend on the dissemination of accurate information about mental disorders.

The current excitement about brain research, already recognized by Congress' declaration of the 1990s as the Decade of the Brain, can provide both an impetus to and a focus for information dissemination efforts, which began in 1983. That year and every year since, Congress has passed legislation that designates one week as Mental Illness Awareness Week.[8] More recently, several members of the

---

[8] The first legislation, in 1983, authorized a National Mental Health Week. All subsequent resolutions fell under the designation of Mental Illness Awareness Week.

House of Representatives, who formed a working group on mental illness, see as one of their first tasks the education of the "Congress and the American people about the *causes* of mental illness and about *new breakthroughs* in research and treatment modalities, and to eliminate the *ignorance and stigma* surrounding mental illness" (emphasis added).

OTA identifies several options for congressional action to improve the publics', providers', and policymakers' understanding of mental disorders. These options are not mutually exclusive; in fact, a combination of them may best serve the ultimate goal of facilitating the transfer of accurate information to the various parties who affect mental health care and policy.

These options focus on Federal programs, but they can also influence other dissemination activities. OTA knows full well that there are many other sources of information about mental disorders. The media, which often provide a skewed or inaccurate view of mental disorders, are far and away the public's primary source of information about mental disorders (see box 1-D). Furthermore, virtually every major national mental health organization and organizations promoting research (e.g., the National Institute for Brain Research, the Society for Neuroscience) direct educational materials toward the public. All of these activities may benefit from improvements in Federal programs that pay attention to recent advances in research and the promise of more to come.

Option 1: Build upon existing and planned educational efforts on mental disorders supported by the Federal Government.

The primary Federal source of information on mental disorders is NIMH. While NIMH has supported an assortment of educational activities, the centerpiece of its educational effort is the DEPRESSION Awareness, Recognition and Treatment (D/ART) campaign, which was launched in 1986 (box 1-F). Only last year, NIMH announced a new and similar program on panic disorder.

Congress can build upon existing and planned Federal activities, namely the D/ART program, the panic disorder campaign, and the recommendations of the Interagency Task Force on Homelessness and Severe Mental Illness, to capitalize upon the strengths of programs already in place. For example, the use of multimedia presentations, the collabora-

tion with various private organizations, and the targeting of specific audiences (e.g., care providers) are all strong points of the D/ART program that could form a solid foundation for future educational efforts.

Expanding congressional support for ongoing Federal educational activities could take several forms. At the most basic level, Congress could augment the modest funding for these programs ($8.5 million for D/ART since 1986, or less than $2 million annually). Additional funds could ensure the expansion of existing programs and the full implementation of planned ones. Of particular importance to a successful public education campaign are evaluations of "outcomes." There has been less than adequate evaluation of the D/ART program's effectiveness, due at least in part to the expense of such research.

Money is not the only issue. To date, the entire D/ART program has been managed by only one and one-half full-time professional staff persons. Thus, Congress could urge NIMH to give a higher priority to educational activities in order to maximize the effectiveness of such programs.

Without establishing any new functions, Congress could direct NIMH to centralize all educational campaigns within a single office, thus improving the efficiency of the programs. At present, the panic disorder campaign, for example, will be administered separately from the D/ART program, even though both have similar goals and objectives: increased recognition and treatment of a disorder.

Option 2: Target educational activities at secondary schools.

Currently, students in junior high school and high school learn little, if anything, about mental disorders, despite the fact that adolescents are especially interested in the topics of health and human behavior. The Department of Education recognizes the importance of such instructional opportunities and includes some mental health information as part of the health curriculum. That information targets mental health in the context of family violence, rape, other emotional crises, the prevention of drug abuse, stress management, and assertiveness training rather than specific mental illnesses. Congress could direct the Department of Education, alone or in conjunction with NIMH, to initiate a grants program to develop model supplemental curricula on advances

Box 1-F—Educating the Public About Depression

Of the 15 million people who experience a major depressive disorder each year, four-fifths can be treated successfully; yet, only one-third of them seek treatment. Even when people seek treatment, symptoms of a depressive disorder are often unrecognized or inappropriately treated by health professionals. Given this level of ignorance, as well as the negative attitudes that surround mental disorders, the Federal Government sponsored its first major health education program about a specific mental disorder in 1986, with the initiation of the National Institute of Mental Health's (NIMH's) DEPRESSION Awareness, Recognition and Treatment (D/ART) program. The D/ART seeks to: 1) increase public knowledge of the symptoms of depressive disorders and the availability of effective treatment, 2) change public attitudes about depression so that there is greater acceptance of depression as a disorder rather than a weakness, 3) encourage changes in help-seeking behavior to reduce the number of untreated and inappropriately treated individuals, and 4) provide information to primary care physicians, mental health specialists, and medical students about advances in diagnosing and treating depressive disorders. The D/ART program will extend over a decade and consists of three components: a professional training program, a public education campaign, and a national worksite program.

For fiscal years 1986 to 1991, the D/ART program expended $4.5 million to train health professionals about recent advances in diagnosis and treatment of depressive disorders (table 1-5). Short-term training courses, developed for this purpose, have been used to train more than 11,000 primary care physicians, mental health professionals, and medical students about depressive disorders. In addition, the D/ART program sponsors continuing education programs in collaboration with professional associations.

In 1988, the D/ART program launched a two-part public education campaign consisting of a multimedia component to publicize messages about depressive disorders and a community partnership program to extend and reinforce the media messages at the local level. First, D/ART staff conducted 20 focus groups in nine geographically dispersed cities and contracted for a survey of 500 people in two cities (Indianapolis, IN and Sacramento, CA) to find out what people knew about depressive disorders. Furthermore, in the early stages of campaign development, the D/ART program organized a group of 45 campaign consultant organizations to advise about public education strategies. The group—comprised of representatives from the major mental health and medical professional associations as well as health and mental health organizations, businesses, labor, religious, and educational groups, mental health advocacy groups, foundations, and other Federal agencies—continues to provide advice on campaign policy matters and to disseminate information on depression.

The D/ART Public Education Campaign has expended $3.6 million in the past 5 years (table 1-5) to develop educational materials. For example, a total of 16 flyers, brochures, and booklets have been produced and distributed to more than 13 million people, with some of the publications geared toward the general audience and some to specific groups, such teenagers, college students, young African-Americans, and older people; some have been published in Spanish and five Asian languages. Also, close to 1,000 television and 9,000 radio stations have broadcast public service announcements (PSAs) about depression to as many as two-thirds of households nationwide. A number of the initial PSAs featured celebrity spokespersons to introduce the campaign.

A critical component of the D/ART program is its community partnership strategy. The Community Partnership Program consists of 32 mental health groups, mostly ''Mental Health Association'' and ''Alliance for the Mentally Ill'' organizations, located in 24 States and the District of Columbia. Community partners reproduce and distribute copies of print materials on depression; conduct public forums, worksite programs, and professional

Table 1-5—DEPRESSION Awareness, Recognition, and Treatment Program, Fiscal Years 1986-91

Area	($ thousands)						Total
	FY 86	FY 87	FY 88	FY 89	FY 90	FY 91	FY 86-91
Training	142	520	646	824	1,146	1,250	4,528 (53%)
Public education	292	924	447	745	616	631	3,655 (43%)
Worksite	N/A	N/A	50	50	100	100	300 (4%)
Total	434	1,444	1,143	1,619	1,862	1,981	8,483

SOURCE: I. Davidoff, Director, D/ART Campaign, National Institute of Mental Health, Rockville, MD, personal communication, Feb. 28, 1992.

seminars; develop videos; appear on television and radio talk shows; sponsor support groups and telephone hotlines, and carry out other varied educational activities, including brochure translations in five Asian languages. In 1990, the total dollar value of the programs that were offered and the partners' direct and in-kind contributions was estimated at nearly $1.3 million, about ten times the Federal investment in the Community Partnership Program. D/ART also recently initiated a Professional Partnership Program, through which depression-related community education activities similar to those offered by Community Partners will be developed by universities, foundations, and professional organizations.

In 1988, the D/ART program established a National Worksite Program as a collaborative effort between NIMH and the Washington Business Group on Health, a nonprofit health policy group composed of Fortune 500 employers. To date, $300,000 has been expended on this program component. The purpose of the worksite initiative is to assist employers in reducing the impact of depression on productivity, on health and disability costs, and on employees and their families. The program disseminates information about depressive disorders to employers and encourages corporate policies and programs that promote early recognition, quality cost-effective care, and on-the-job support for individuals experiencing depressive illnesses. The program has developed a "Management of Depression" model program and published a report based on the experience of seven large U.S. companies that contributed to development of the model. In 1992, the program will produce a training program for management personnel and occupational health professionals to improve early recognition and referral to appropriate care for depression.

Preliminary data suggest that the D/ART program has had some positive effects. For example, prior to the dissemination of any information, NIMH funded a 1987 telephone survey by the University of Michigan Institute of Social Research of 500 people (250 in Indianapolis, IN, and 250 in Sacramento, CA) to determine the extent of their knowledge about depression. The survey found that most people believed that depressed persons could get better on their own rather than by seeking treatment. In 1990, the American Medical Association conducted a followup survey of the same group of 500 people. A total of 210 of the original group responded; 40 percent of the respondees in Indianapolis and 25 percent of the respondees in Sacramento said they knew more about depression because of the D/ART campaign. AMA also surveyed a new group of 500 people (250 people from each of the two cities). Of this group, 34 percent of those in Indianapolis and 30 percent of those in Sacramento said they were aware of the D/ART campaign and its messages. Another survey in North Dakota found that the number of adults treated for depressive disorders increased 1.5 times and the number of children treated increased 3 times in Human Service Centers (akin to Community Mental Health Centers) for fiscal years 1986 to 1991. The increase was attributed in part to the D/ART public and professional education programs and to a State program to develop treatment teams specifically for children within the Human Service Centers.

Has the D/ART program been a success? While the limited data on the effectiveness of the D/ART program preclude a quantitatively based answer to this question, several aspects of the program clearly deserve commendation. With limited resources and personnel (the entire D/ART program is managed by one-and one-half full-time Federal professional staff persons), the D/ART program established an educational campaign that is solidly rooted in research advances; the D/ART program carefully devises the messages to be relayed, uses diverse media to disseminate the messages, and coordinates its efforts with people in the community. D/ART has also trained substantial numbers of health and mental health care providers through its own efforts and through collaborations with public and private organizations. Advancement of this pioneering educational effort on a mental disorder by the Federal Government—via further study of its effect on the level of awareness, prevalence and treatment changes, expansion of the program into other communities, and adapting its techniques for educating the public about other conditions—will require some combination of increased funds and personnel, as well as highlighting this activity as a priority at the NIMH.

SOURCES: J.E. Barham, Mental Health Consultant, personal communication, May 4, 1992; R. Brown, Senior Scientist, Department of Mental Health, American Medical Association, personal communication, June 23, 1992; I. Davidoff, Director, D/ART Campaign, National Institute of Mental Health, Rockville, MD, personal communication, June 1992; R. Kessler, Institute for Social Research, University of Michigan, personal communication, June 23, 1992; A. Koss, coordinator of State D/ART Program, Division of Mental Health, Department of Human Services, Bismarck, ND, personal communication, June 22, 1992; D.A. Regier, M.A. Hirschfeld, F.K. Goodwin, et al., "The NIMH Depression Awareness, Recognition, and Treatment Program: Structure, Aims, and Scientific Basis," *American Journal of Psychiatry* 145:1351-1357, 1988; D. Regier, Director, Division of Clinical Research, National Institute of Mental Health, personal communication, May 1992; U.S. Department of Health and Human Services, Public Health Service, Alcohol Drug Abuse and Mental Health Administration, National Institute of Mental Health, *Depression, Awareness, Recognition, and Treatment (D/ART) Fact Sheet*, DHHS Pub. No. (ADM) 90-1680 (Rockville, MD: U.S. DHHS, 1990).

in neuroscience and mental disorders. Outstanding materials, capturing the excitement and complexity of a scientific area, have been developed on other topics, including a recent supplement on the genome project and the ethical issues it poses.

It is important to note that model supplemental curricula do have some limitations. While they can be distributed to school districts nationwide, the law prohibits mandating the use of such materials. Also, supplemental materials may not be the most fruitful approach, given the need for comprehensive curriculum development in science education and the large number of competing supplements now available in the sciences and in health education.

Option 3: Direct the Federal Government to play a role in coordinating the training and level of knowledge of persons caring for individuals with mental disorders.

Optimal care for individuals with mental disorders relies on providers having accurate, up-to-date information. Yet, providers face a widening pool of knowledge from basic, clinical, and rehabilitative research. Furthermore, the extent to which this information is included in academic and training programs remains a matter of institutional choice. This report did not evaluate in detail the extent of provider knowledge about mental disorders; however, it did note research evidence that some providers have less than adequate knowledge about diagnosing and treating these conditions. As a first step toward ensuring that providers receive current and accurate information about mental disorders, Congress could commission a study on the level of knowledge of providers and the way in which these professionals are trained and licensed. Furthermore, Congress could request that such a study devise mechanisms for improving the transfer of knowledge to providers.

Option 4: Formalize a mechanism for improving information transfer and communication among Federal agencies concerned with mental disorders.

One goal of giving the public information about mental disorders is to make it easier to develop public policies that will help people with these conditions. While such efforts can be important in shaping the political will needed to bring about successful policy initiatives, public education is unlikely to solve many of the problems people with

mental disorders face, at least in the near term. Indeed, the mechanisms by which Federal policies on mental disorders are formed and implemented erect barriers to a rational problem-solving process. No single agency is primarily responsible for the issues that affect people with mental disorders; rather, it is scattered among various agencies, including several offices and institutes within the Departments of Health and Human Services (NIMH, Health Care Financing Administration, and others), Veterans Affairs, Justice, Labor, Education, Housing and Urban Development, and others. While NIMH has sometimes offered Federal leadership on policy issues related to mental disorders, there is clearly a need for better dissemination of new research findings, better communication about areas needing research, and better coordination of policy planning. This need is likely to become more acute with the reorganization of the Alcohol, Drug Abuse, and Mental Health Administration and separation of NIMH and the newly formed services agency, SAMHSA, Substance Abuse and Mental Health Services Administration.

NIMH, recognizing the need for information transfer, has set out to develop methods and a system by which knowledge exchange can proceed. Congress could build upon these plans and ensure the involvement of high-level officials in other Federal agencies and institutions, so as to create a mechanism for the exchange of information and development of policies and programs, by creating an Interagency Task Force or Council on Mental Disorders that would include representatives from all relevant agencies in the Federal Government. It could be directed to coordinate research and policy issues concerning mental disorders and to establish a mechanism for sharing information among all officers and employees of the departments carrying out programs that concern people with mental disorders.

Some mechanism for facilitating talk among Federal agencies is needed, given that no single agency has the jurisdiction or expertise to address thoroughly the issues associated with mental disorders. The composition of the task force is the single most important key to its success. Representatives from every relevant agency should be included. In addition, task force members should have adequate experience, expertise, and authority to devise and help implement policies and programs. The chair of the task force is also important; ideally, this person would bring personal dedication and sufficient authority to help drive the group's efforts. A clear charge is necessary to focus the work of the group. Congress could specify topics for study every year or two and request that a report be made at the end of that time. The report would elucidate the topic and provide for policy initiatives.

One topic could be consideration of the financing of mental health care. Research advances, whether the development of new treatments or changing conceptualizations of the causes of mental disorders, clearly have influenced and will continue to influence the issue of mental health care financing. A study involving NIMH and other agencies in the Federal Government with expertise in and jurisdiction over the financing of health care and the provision of services could review the relevant factors and issues and develop a cohesive Federal policy. A final point should be made: Even in the event of a successful effort on the part of the task force, certain policy and program suggestions may be forestalled until adequate funds are provided.

Chapter 2

Introduction

CONTENTS OF CHAPTER 2

Box

Figures

Table

Mental disorders can strike with savage cruelty, producing nightmarish hallucinations, crippling paranoia, unrelenting depression, a choking sense of panic, or inescapable obsessions. The sheer number of Americans with mental disorders transforms this personal tragedy into a widespread public health problem. Nearly one in three American adults will experience a mental disorder during his or her lifetime, including schizophrenia, mood disorders, anxiety disorders, antisocial personality disorder, substance abuse, or cognitive impairment (23,25) (table 2-1) (see ch. 3).[1] Altogether, approximately 1.7 to 2.4 million Americans currently suffer from a persistent and severely disabling mental disorder (15).

What are the costs of this public health problem? The most comprehensive estimate of the total costs of mental disorders—for the year 1985—is $103.7 billion (24) (figure 2-1) (box 2-A). A recent update of this figure estimated that the costs of mental disorders in 1991 reached $136.1 billion (20). Dollar figures alone, however, no matter how large, do not convey the toll that mental disorders take. It has been estimated that individuals with mental disorders fill 25 percent of all hospital beds and, further, that one-third of these persons suffer from schizophrenia (10,15). In 1986, more than 2 million episodes of inpatient care in the United States were provided for persons with mental disorders (16). Many such

Table 2-1—Prevalence of Severe Mental Disorders

Disorder	Adults diagnosed with disorder during their lifetime (%)
Schizophrenia	1.0
Bipolar disorder	0.8
Major depression	4.9
Obsessive-compulsive disorder	2.6
Panic disorder	1.6

SOURCE: L.N. Robins and D.A. Regier, *Psychiatric Disorders in America, The Epidemiologic Catchment Area Study* (New York, NY: Free Press, 1991).

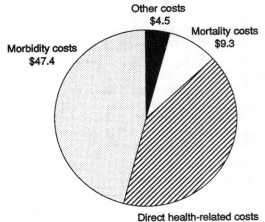

Figure 2-1—The Cost of Mental Disorders, 1985
(in billions of dollars)

Other costs $4.5
Mortality costs $9.3
Morbidity costs $47.4
Direct health-related costs $42.5

In 1985, mental disorders cost the United States more than $103 billion. Approximately 41 percent of that cost—$42.5 billion—stemmed from hospital care, medication costs, and other treatment costs. Nearly half of the cost of mental disorders—$47.4 billion—derives from lost productivity.

SOURCE: D.P. Rice, S. Kelman, L.S. Miller, et al., *The Economic Costs of Alcohol and Drug Abuse and Mental Illness*, report submitted to the Office of Financing and Coverage Policy, Alcohol, Drug Abuse, and Mental Health Administration, U.S. Department of Health and Human Services (San Francisco, CA: Institute for Health and Aging, University of California, 1990).

disorders, including depression, obsessive-compulsive disorder, and panic disorder, are associated with increased use of general health care services (25). Productivity and the ability to work are also significantly compromised by mental disorders (2, 19,44). For example, the results from one study indicate that major depression leads to a more than fourfold increase in disability days, defined as days "in which a person spent all or part of the day in bed due to illness or was kept from usual activities due to feeling ill" (4). Data show that approximately one-third of the homeless population and 10 to 15 percent of individuals incarcerated in jails and prisons have a severe mental disorder such as schizophrenia or bipolar disorder (i.e., manic-depressive illness).[2]

[1] Estimate derived from the National Institute of Mental Health's Epidemiologic Catchment Area (ECA) Program. Data resulted from interviews of more than 20,000 persons in five sites during the early 1980s. Some variation in prevalence estimates was reported between sites. See references 7 and 25 for discussion of the methods used in the ECA program.

[2] Research into the prevalence of mental disorders among the homeless population and among individuals in jails and prisons has resulted in divergent estimates, due to definitional problems (see ch. 3), data collection difficulties, and political views (5,12,14,30,34,35). The percentages cited in the text represent generally accepted estimates.

Box 2-A—The Cost of Mental Disorders

How big a problem do mental disorders present to our Nation? What priority should these disorders receive in the outlay of government funds for research and services? The answers to these questions are often sought in terms of a dollar figure. However, estimating the toll of mental disorders, or any illness, in economic terms is no easy or straightforward task. Everything from the cost of hospitalization, which is relatively easy to estimate, to the cost of reduced productivity, which is more difficult to assess, may be evaluated. And while rarely included in studies, the psychological and social tolls on an individual's life are substantial, though not easily quantified.

During the last 40 years, studies have reported that mental disorders cost the Nation from $3.6 billion to more than $100 billion each year. The variation in estimates reflects changes over time as well as the use of different methods of calculation and sources of data. Dorothy Rice and colleagues have derived the most comprehensive estimate, based on the most recently available survey data. They estimate the total costs of mental disorders—including schizophrenia, major depression, bipolar disorder (manic-depressive illness), anxiety disorders, somatization disorder, antisocial personality disorder, and cognitive impairment—to be $103.7 billion for the year 1985. When adjusted for inflation, this figure reaches $136.1 billion in 1991.

These costs include health-related, or core, costs—that is, the expenditures made and resources lost as a consequence of having a mental disorder. Such costs make up 96 percent of the total estimated costs for 1985, or $99.2 billion. Health-related costs can be broken down further into direct and indirect costs.

Direct health-related costs—$42.5 billion in 1985 and more than $58 billion in 1991—include all expenditures related to the treatment and support of persons with mental disorders. The vast majority of these direct costs—92 percent—are related to treatment and involve expenditures on hospital and nursing home care, physician and other professional services, and drugs (figure 2-1). More than 50 percent of the treatment costs—almost $22 billion in 1985—were spent on care in institutional or hospital settings, such as Department of Veterans Affairs (VA) hospitals, State and county psychiatric hospitals, private psychiatric hospitals, residential treatment centers for emotionally disturbed children, and short-stay (general) hospitals. The costs of care provided by office-based physicians, psychologists, and social workers amounted to approximately $5.7 billion in 1985. Approximately $1.5 billion was spent on prescription drugs, including minor tranquilizers, antidepressants, and antipsychotics. The estimate reached more than $2.2 billion in 1991, when adjusted for inflation. Support costs, which equaled approximately $3.2 billion in 1985, include expenditures for research, physician and nurse training, and program administration (such as health insurance).

Indirect health-related costs estimate the burden of increased morbidity and mortality that accompanies mental disorders. These estimates, which are based on the National Institute of Mental Health's Epidemiologic Catchment Area prevalence data, include the value of lost output caused by decreased productivity, lost work days, or premature death. Rice and colleagues do not include measures of the psychological and social effects of mental disorders on the individual's life. Morbidity and mortality costs were estimated at $47.4 billion and $9.3 billion, respectively, in 1985. For 1991, estimates were $60.0 billion for morbidity costs and $11.7 billion for mortality costs. Thus, according to these data, lost or diminished productivity is the most costly outcome of mental disorders, with morbidity accounting for nearly 50 percent of the total costs of mental disorders. Furthermore, the cost of morbidity is not primarily due to institutionalization. Additional analysis, which considers such factors as the prevalence of mental disorders in various demographic groups, the type of disorder, and income levels, shows that a very large share of the morbidity costs—$44.1 billion in 1985 and $55.8 billion in 1991—derives from noninstitutionalized individuals.

Mental disorders have other, nonhealth-related effects that impose a cost on society. Nonhealth effects lead to public and private expenditures on crime control and social welfare administration, the sum of which was estimated at $1.7 billion by Rice and colleagues. Furthermore, the value of reductions or losses in productivity due to either incarceration for a criminal offense or time spent to care for a family member with a mental disorder exacts a price, estimated at approximately $2.8 billion.

SOURCES: D.P. Rice, S. Kelman, L.S. Miller, et al., *The Economic Costs of Alcohol and Drug Abuse and Mental Illness: 1985*, report submitted to the Office of Financing and Coverage Policy, Alcohol, Drug Abuse, and Mental Health Administration, U.S. Department of Health and Human Services (San Francisco, CA: Institute for Health and Aging, University of California, 1990); The National Foundation for Brain Research, *The Costs of Disorders of the Brain* (Washington, DC: 1992).

The reality of mental disorders—their symptoms, their prevalence, and their costs—commands society's attention, but society's response is incoherent. Despite the fact that Federal, State, and local governments spend more than $20 billion each year on mental health services, the consensus is that mental health policy is fragmented and mental health services often deficient (9,18,26,33,40,43). While a tangle of clinical, economic, social, professional, and legal issues impinges on mental health policy, the answer to the question "What causes mental disorders?" is also important in formulating rational mental health policy. As stated more than a decade ago in the *President's Commission on Mental Health* report:

> Expanding our understanding of the functioning of the mind, the causes of mental and emotional illness, and the efficacy of various treatments is crucial to future progress in mental health (22).

The fundamental causes of most mental disorders are unknown. However, the 1980s witnessed an explosion of biomedical research into the nature of these disorders (3). While a number of factors, including the agenda of some professional groups and the concerns of some consumer advocacy groups,[3] contribute to the emphasis on the biological aspects of mental disorders, the rapid growth and productivity of neuroscience research spearhead this trend. One indicator of the growth in neuroscience is the increased membership of the Society for Neuroscience: Membership in this professional organization grew from 1,100 at its inception in 1970 to more than 17,000 in 1990 (figure 2-2) (28). In 1992, the Society for Neuroscience has more than 19,000 members (29). The 1980s saw a nearly 70 percent increase in the number of papers published in neuroscience and behavioral research (27). Congress captured this enthusiasm for neuroscience in its Decade of the Brain resolution, approved in 1989, to make "the Nation . . . aware of the exciting research advances on the brain. . . ." (Public Law 101-58; see also app. A to this report).

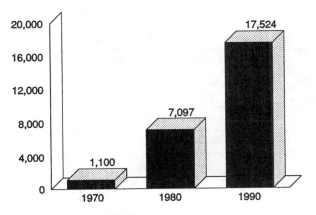

Figure 2-2—Membership in the Society for Neuroscience

Membership in the Society for Neuroscience has grown dramatically since its inception in 1970.
SOURCE: Society for Neuroscience, 1991.

THE MODERN HISTORY OF NEUROSCIENCE

Neuroscience research focuses on how the nervous system works and how it is affected by disease. It is an interdisciplinary field, drawing on expertise from many diverse fields, including anatomy, physiology, physics, electronics, genetics, biochemistry, optics, pharmacology, psychology, neurology, psychiatry, neurosurgery, and computer science. The seeds of modern neuroscience were sown in the late 19th and early 20th centuries, when astute clinical observations and basic technical advances led to such fundamental discoveries as the location of specific functions within the brain and nerve cells. There was palpable enthusiasm about being on the brink of understanding the human mind. As is often observed by today's neuroscientists, even Sigmund Freud, the father of psychoanalysis, entertained the hope of unveiling the brain's relationship to human thought and behavior.

The slow march of progress in neuroscience research proceeded through the subsequent years. The serendipitous discovery of several agents that profoundly affect the symptoms of severe mood

---

[3] For example, the National Alliance for the Mentally Ill (NAMI), a family-based advocacy group with approximately 130,000 members, strongly supports biomedical research into mental disorders, in part to promote the development of better treatments and, ultimately, cures for mental disorders (8). NAMI's staunch support for the biological basis of mental disorders also reflects an anti-stigma stance and a rebuttal to theories blaming the family for causing mental disorders (see ch. 7).

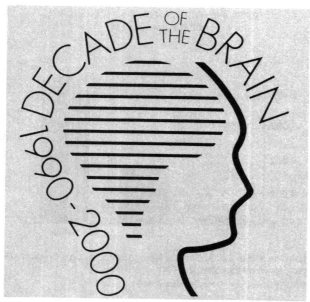

The congressional "Decade of the Brain" resolution, the activities of executive branch agencies, as well as the private efforts of scientists and other advocates all demonstrate enthusiasm for neuroscience research. Pictured is the logo for the National Foundation for Brain Research, a nonprofit organization that promotes brain research.
SOURCE: The National Foundation for Brain Research, 1992.

disorders and schizophrenia ushered in a new age of neuroscience research in the 1950s. The finding that chemical substances can modulate, even control, mental dysfunction was not completely alien to contemporary understanding of the brain, for the chemical nature of nerve cell communication was known. It did, however, precipitate an explosion of research in neurochemistry and psychopharmacology. In the ensuing years, many chemical substances occurring naturally in the brain—neurotransmitters and neuropeptides—were identified.

There was also a quantum leap in understanding how neurotransmitters and neuropeptides influence targeted nerve cells. Receptor molecules—proteins embedded in the surface of nerve cells that bind chemical substances—were identified and isolated. Like a key inserted into a lock, a neurotransmitter fits into a specific receptor, producing a cascade of responses in the receptive neuron (see ch. 4). A single neurotransmitter may activate several different receptors, located in distinct regions of the brain. To date, five different receptors have been found to respond to the brain chemical dopamine alone (31).

The exponential increase in neuroscience research during the last 15 years reflects, in large measure,

technological advances (for review, see 36,41). Dramatically improved methods for staining nerve cells permit researchers to observe the precise location of these cells in the brain. The electrical activity of a single channel in a nerve cell's membrane—which is less than one-trillionth of an inch in diameter—can be measured. Progress in computing and advances in microscopy, especially imaging technology, underlie the spectacular view of living brain tissue—from single nerve cells to the intact human brain. Psychological tests, which analyze and measure the components of complex behaviors and thought processes, make possible analysis of the brain's functions. And molecular biology has revolutionized the study of the brain, resulting in the labeling of specific nerve cells with monoclonal antibodies, the cloning of receptors, and the search for specific genes.

The sophisticated methods and technologies of modern neuroscience research make up the arsenal being used to expose the secrets of mental disorders. The National Institute of Mental Health (NIMH), the primary Federal agency that funds research into mental disorders, has drawn up its battle plan on the basis of developments in neuroscience (41,42). By strongly supporting neuroscience research, NIMH aims to:

. . . understand the workings of the human brain in sufficient detail to effectively treat or prevent the broad variety of behavioral disorders and mental illnesses (41).

A CAUTIONARY NOTE

It is easy to appreciate how excitement about neuroscience might affect the study of mental disorders and foster hope for new treatments. However, the complexity of the brain and behavior, the nature of mental disorders, and the potential repercussions of this research require a note of caution.

Neuroscience research has produced many exciting results, but it has only scratched the surface of understanding how the brain functions. The neuroscientist Wilder Penfield realized earlier in this century that "there was a thrilling undiscovered country to be explored in the mechanisms of the mammalian nervous system" (21). The brain is an immensely complicated organ: It contains 10^{11} nerve cells, and estimates suggest that the number of synapses in the brain, 10^{14}, exceeds the number of stars in our galaxy (13). Mapping the terrain of this still largely "undiscovered country" will require continued research, cross-disciplinary cooperation, and sophisticated management of rapidly accruing information (11).

The complexity of the brain is reflected in its functional output: thought, emotion, and behavior. Thus, mental disorders, which are identified essentially on the basis of psychological and behavioral traits (1) rather than laboratory findings, are perplexing phenomena, difficult to define and classify (see ch. 3 for detailed discussion of the definition of mental disorders). Difficulties in classifying mental disorders can present a serious challenge to biological and behavioral research.

Neuroscience is based on the concept that behavior, thoughts, and emotions are the results of nerve cell interaction (36). Mental disorders, like any other illnesses, however, cannot be understood in biological terms only. As the National Advisory Mental Health Council Report to Congress (41) acknowledged, each mental disorder ". . . represents a complex interaction of biological, psychological, and social variables." While there is overwhelming enthusiasm for biological research into mental disorders, there is also concern that emphasizing biological factors exclusively will shortchange other important areas of research as well as care of the mentally ill.

> With impressive developments in molecular biology, the neurosciences, and imaging technology, psychiatry has moved toward a more biological and medical emphasis. Although these fields hold great promise, efforts must proceed in a balanced way to provide high quality management for those currently ill while seeking more powerful technologies for the future. The history of mental health care attests to how endorsement of organic viewpoints and the professionalization of psychiatry, when it had little specific to offer in any immediate terms, undermined constructive and humane efforts for patient management and rehabilitation (17).

Great hope surrounds neuroscience research in general and biomedical research into mental disorders in particular. Some of the predicted fruits of neuroscience include new and improved treatments for mental, neurological, and substance abuse disorders; reduction, prevention, or reversal of age-related changes in cognition; and development of measures to enhance cognitive performance and productivity (6,36,41).

There can be no doubt that neuroscience research will lead to improved understanding of how the brain works and even to the development of new treatments. There also can be no doubt that improved understanding of the biology of mental disorders will raise new and difficult questions concerning the privacy of genetic information, genetic discrimination, the forcible administration of mind-altering agents, concepts of free will and personal responsibility, the way third-party payers cover mental disorders, and other issues (6,36). Eugenic policies (see ch. 5) and treatment approaches used earlier in this century, which sprang from enthusiasm for (and sometimes misunderstanding of) biological theories of mental disorders, serve as a reminder of the potential misuses of biological advances. Few supporters of neuroscience research mention the potential ethical and legal dilemmas it poses; while the Federal Government has developed a detailed neuroscience research strategy, no official mechanism for considering the possible implications of this research, such as the one organized by the Human Genome Project, has been formalized or even widely discussed.

THE OTA STUDY

Approximately 40 percent of all public funds spent on mental health services—$8 billion each year—derive from Federal sources (33). The Federal Government is also the primary source of support for research into mental disorders and mental health, with NIMH's research budget totaling $497.4 million in 1991 (see ch. 6). The large Federal investment in mental health research—combined with congressional interest in neuroscience research—led the House Committees on Energy and Commerce; Science, Space and Technology; Appropriations; and Veterans Affairs and the Senate Subcommittee on Science, Technology, and Space of the Committee on Commerce, Science, and Transportation to request and Senator Edward M. Kennedy to endorse an Office of Technology Assessment (OTA) report on the status and implications of biological research into mental disorders.

This report reviews the data from research on the biology of several mental disorders, including schizophrenia, bipolar disorder, major depression, obsessive-compulsive disorder, and panic disorder. These disorders—some of the most severe and long-lasting ones that afflict adults—have been subjected to extensive experimental scrutiny aimed at identifying causal factors in the brain.[4] The focus of this report reflects that of recent research—namely, the widely held opinion that biological factors contribute significantly to mental disorders and that medication and other somatic interventions generally form a critical component of the clinical management of these disorders.[5] The causative roles of psychological and social factors (which are important for a comprehensive understanding and treatment of mental disorders) and broad mental health issues are beyond the scope of this report.

In the five chapters that follow, OTA examines: 1) the nature of mental disorders in general and the clinical features of the mental disorders considered in this report; 2) results of research into biological factors that contribute to these disorders; 3) the heritability of these disorders and the clinical implications of genetic research; 4) the support for research into mental disorders and barriers to research; and 5) the impact on public attitudes and policy issues of new knowledge about the biology of mental disorders.

CHAPTER 2 REFERENCES

1. American Psychiatric Association, *Diagnostic and Statistical Manual of Mental Disorders*, 3rd ed., rev. (Washington, DC: American Psychiatric Association, 1987).
2. Anthony, W.A., and Blanch, A., "Supported Employment for Persons Who Are Psychiatrically Disabled: An Historical and Conceptual Perspective," *Psychosocial and Rehabilitation Journal* 11(2):5-23, 1987.
3. Barondes, S.H., "The Biological Approach to Psychiatry: History and Prospects," *Journal of Neuroscience* 10:1701-1710, 1990.
4. Broadhead, W.E., Blazer, D.G., George, L.K., et al., "Depression, Disability Days, and Days Lost From Work in a Prospective Epidemiologic Survey," *Journal of the American Medical Association* 264:2524-2528, 1990.
5. Cohen, C.I., "Crime Among Mental Patients—A Critical Analysis," *Psychiatric Quarterly* 52:100-107, 1980.
6. Downey, M., "Legal Issues in Brain Science Advances," *Courts, Health Science and the Law* 1:471-483, 1991.
7. Eaton, W.W., and Kessler, L.G. (eds.), *Epidemiologic Field Methods in Psychiatry: The NIMH Epidemiologic Catchment Area Program* (Orlando, FL: Academic Press, 1985).
8. Flynn, L., Executive Director, National Alliance for the Mentally Ill, personal communication, Feb. 27, 1992.
9. Frank, R., and Kamlet, M.S., "Direct Costs and Expenditures for Mental Health in the United States, 1980," *Mental Health, United States, 1985*, DHHS Pub. No. (ADM) 87-1518, C.A. Taube and S.A. Barrett (eds.) (Washington, DC: U.S. Government Printing Office, 1985).
10. Institute of Medicine, *Research on Mental Illness and Addictive Disorders: Progress and Prospects* (Washington, DC: National Academy Press, 1984).
11. Institute of Medicine, *Mapping the Brain and Its Functions* (Washington, DC: National Academy Press, 1991).
12. Interagency Council on the Homeless, *Outcasts on Main Street: Report of the Federal Task Force on Homelessness and Severe Mental Illness*, (ADS) 92-1904 (Washington, DC: 1992).
13. Kandel, E.R., Schwartz, J.H., and Jessell, T.M., *Principles of Neural Science*, 3rd ed. (New York, NY: Elsevier Science Publishing, 1991).
14. Levine, I.S., and Haggard, L.K., "Homelessness as a Public Mental Health Problem," *Handbook on Mental Health Policy in the United States*, D.A. Rochefort (ed.) (New York, NY: Greenwood Press, 1989).
15. Manderscheid, R.W., and Barrett, S.A. (eds.), *Mental Health, United States, 1987*, DHHS Pub. No. (ADM) 87-15518 (Washington, DC: U.S. Government Printing Office, 1987).
16. Manderscheid, R.W., and Sonnenschein, M.A. (eds.), *Mental Health, United States, 1990*, DHHS Pub. No. (ADM) 90-1708 (Washington, DC: U.S. Government Printing Office, 1990).
17. Mechanic, D., "Recent Developments in Mental Health: Perspectives and Services," *Annual Review of Public Health* 12:1-15, 1991.
18. Mechanic, D., "Strategies for Integrating Public Mental Health Services," *Hospital and Community Psychiatry* 42:797-801, 1991.

[4] A small but vociferous group of ex-patients, advocates, and others contends that labeling individuals as severely and persistently mentally ill is pejorative (32). Their antipathy stems, in large measure, from an antipsychiatry stance and rejection of involuntary hospitalization and treatment. While many in this group generally accept that individuals diagnosed with what are called mental disorders have undeniable deficits and face terrible problems, they look askance at biological theories of mental disorders because of their association with disparaging labels, forced treatment, and other civil liberty issues. The implications of biological explanations of mental disorders are considered in chapters 3 and 7. A discussion of the important legal, social, and ethical issues that surround involuntary commitment and forced treatment are beyond the scope of this report.

[5] Addictive disorders, Alzheimer's disease, and developmental disorders such as autism have been or are being discussed in other OTA reports and therefore are not considered in any detail in this report (37,38,39).

19. Mental Health Policy Research Center, *Database, Policy in Perspective* (Washington, DC: July 1990).

20. National Foundation for Brain Research, *The Costs of Disorders of the Brain* (Washington, DC: 1992).

21. Penfield, W., *The Mystery of the Mind* (Princeton, NJ: Princeton University Press, 1975).

22. *President's Commission on Mental Health*, vol. I, stock No. 040-000-00390-8 (Washington, DC: U.S. Government Printing Office, 1978).

23. Regier, D.A., Farmer, M.E., Rae, D.S., et al., "Comorbidity of Mental Disorders With Alcohol and Other Drug Abuse: Results From the Epidemiologic Catchment Area (ECA) Study," *Journal of the American Medical Association* 264:2511-2518, 1990.

24. Rice, D.P., Kelman, S., Miller, L.S., et al., *The Economic Costs of Alcohol and Drug Abuse and Mental Illness: 1985*, report submitted to the Office of Financing and Coverage Policy, Alcohol, Drug Abuse, and Mental Health Administration, U.S. Department of Health and Human Services (San Francisco, CA: Institute for Health and Aging, University of California, 1990).

25. Robins, L.N., and Regier, D.A., *Psychiatric Disorders in America: The Epidemiologic Catchment Area Study* (New York, NY: Free Press, 1991).

26. Rochefort, D.A., "Mental Illness and Mental Health as Public Policy Concerns," *Handbook on Mental Health Policy in the United States*, D.A. Rochefort (ed.) (New York, NY: Greenwood Press, 1989), pp. 3-20.

27. *Science Watch*, "Biotechnology, Critical Care, Computing Top List of Lost-Growth Fields in Science," Institute for Scientific Information 9:1-2, 1991.

28. Society for Neuroscience (Washington, DC: 1991).

29. Society for Neuroscience, *Neuroscience Newsletter* 23:1, May 1992.

30. Steadman, H.J., Monahan, J., Duffy, B., et al., "The Impact of State Mental Hospital Deinstitutionalization on United States Prison Populations, 1968-1978," *Journal of Criminal Law and Criminology* 75:474-490, 1984.

31. Sunahara, R.K., Hong-Chang, G., O'Dowd, B.F., et al., "Cloning of the Gene for a Human Dopamine D_5 Receptor With Higher Affinity for Dopamine than D_1," *Nature* 350: 614-619, 1991.

32. Thompson, R., National Association of Psychiatric Survivors, Bethesda, MD, personal communication, 1992.

33. Torrey, E.F., Erdman, K., Wolfe, S.M., et al., "Care of the Seriously Ill: A Rating of State Programs," *Public Citizen Health Research Group and National Alliance for the Mentally Ill*, 3rd ed. (Washington, DC: Public Citizen Health Research Group and National Alliance for the Mentally Ill, 1990).

34. U.S. Congress, General Accounting Office, *Homeless Mentally Ill: Problems and Options in Estimating Numbers and Trends*, GAO/PEMD-88-24 (Washington, DC: August 1988).

35. U.S. Congress, General Accounting Office, *Mentally Ill Inmates*, GAO GGD-91-35 B-242958 (Washington, DC: 1991).

36. U.S. Congress, Office of Technology Assessment, *Impacts of Neuroscience*, background paper, OTA-BP-BA-24 (Washington, DC: U.S. Government Printing Office, March 1984).

37. U.S. Congress, Office of Technology Assessment, *Children's Mental Health: Problems and Services*, background paper, OTA-BP-H33 (Washington, DC: U.S. Government Printing Office, December 1986).

38. U.S. Congress, Office of Technology Assessment, *Losing a Million Minds: Confronting the Tragedy of Alzheimer's Disease and Other Dementias*, OTA-BA-323 (Washington, DC: U.S. Government Printing Office, April 1987).

39. U.S. Congress, Office of Technology Assessment, *Technologies for Understanding the Root Causes of Substance Abuse and Addiction*, in progress.

40. U.S. Department of Health and Human Services, Alcohol, Drug Abuse, and Mental Health Administration, National Institute of Mental Health, *Caring for People With Severe Mental Disorders: A National Plan of Research To Improve Services*, DHHS Pub. No. (ADM) 91-1762 (Washington, DC: 1991).

41. U.S. Department of Health and Human Services, Alcohol, Drug Abuse, and Mental Health Administration, *Approaching the 21st Century: Opportunities for NIMH Neuroscience Research: The National Advisory Mental Health Council Report to Congress on the Decade of the Brain*, DHHS Pub. No. (ADM) 89-1580 (Washington, DC: 1988).

42. U.S. Department of Health and Human Services, Alcohol, Drug Abuse, and Mental Health Administration, *A National Plan for Schizophrenia Research: Panel Recommendations*, DHHS Pub. No. (ADM) 88-1570 (Washington, DC: 1989).

43. U.S. Department of Health and Human Services, Alcohol, Drug Abuse, and Mental Health Administration, *Healthy People 2000: National Health Promotion and Disease Prevention Objectives* (Washington, DC: 1990).

44. Wells, K.B., Stewart, A., and Hays, R.D., "The Functioning and Well-Being of Depressed Patients: Results of the Medical Outcomes Study," *Journal of the American Medical Association* 262:914-919, 1989.

Chapter 3

What Are Mental Disorders?

CONTENTS OF CHAPTER 3

What Are Mental Disorders?

What are mental disorders? For centuries, philosophers, physicians, psychologists, and others have debated this question, variably defining and classifying mental disorders on the basis of presumed causes, observed symptoms, preferred treatment approaches, or social and political values. This lack of agreement has led many to the pessimistic conclusion that:

> [H]istory or experience has not produced a generally accepted definition of mental disorder . . . nor is such a definition likely to be forthcoming in the foreseeable future (17).

The vagaries of definition do not negate the concrete problems mental disorders pose for individuals and society. Rather, society is confronted with the proposition of responding to disorders with important public health, economic, and social implications in the absence of any neat scheme for addressing them. This chapter explores the problems inherent in defining and classifying mental disorders in general and the symptoms, effects, and treatment of the specific disorders considered in this report.

DEFINING MENTAL DISORDERS

Defining a general concept such as mental disorders may seem at first blush to be an abstract, academic pursuit. After all, general concepts of health, disease, and illness evade easy definition, spawning debate over the most useful or appropriate framework for analyzing them (53). Is health simply the absence of disease? How do social values influence decisions about what constitutes disease? The way these general terms are defined influences the boundaries of medicine, professional interest, and perceived social responsibility. A series of recent court decisions on insurance coverage highlights the importance of specifying what mental disorders are. Decisions both to extend and to limit insurance benefits stemmed from the definition of mental disorders accepted by the courts (18,63). This section considers the difficulty of defining mental disorders, the conceptual frameworks that have been erected, and the way mental disorders are classified.

Part of the confusion in defining mental disorders arises from their broad reach and nebulous boundaries. A wide array of behaviors has been classified as symptomatic of mental disorders, ranging from premenstrual syndrome, hostility toward others, or other maladaptive personality traits to full-blown psychosis (3,67). In addition, it is sometimes difficult to delineate where mental health ends and mental illness begins. As observed by Emil Kraepelin, the 19th century patriarch of mental disorder classification:

> Wherever we try to mark out the frontier between mental health and disease, we find a neutral territory, in which the imperceptible change from the realm of normal mental life to that of obvious derangement takes place (36).

While the boundary between physical health and disease can also be indistinct, the lack of clarity between mental health and illness contributes to the impression that mental disorders encompass normal or willful differences in human thought, behavior, and emotion.

The way mental disorders are defined influences issues of research, treatment, social welfare, and public health and safety. Decisions regarding the appropriateness of treatment, research funding priorities, the financing of care by third-party payers, accommodation at the workplace, and criminal responsibility hinge, in part, on expert and popular concepts of mental disorders (85). Furthermore, mental health personnel include many different professionals and paraprofessionals: psychiatrists, psychologists, psychiatric social workers, psychiatric nurses, and other therapists and counselors. Each of these groups has its own area of expertise and professional agenda, and sometimes they conflict (72), creating another obstacle to a unified definition of mental disorders.

The fact that mental disorders affect primarily thought, emotion, and behavior further hinders efforts to arrive at a definition. There is a certain uneasiness about defining as diseased those aspects of the human mind by which we relate to, empathize with, and judge each other. The centuries-old conceptual divide between the mind, as the seat of thought, and the brain, as a biological entity, impairs our ability to classify mental disorders as diseases of the brain. Although an unambiguous link between a biological process and a higher mental function, such as consciousness, has yet to be completely delineated, advances in the neurosciences, psychology, and computer science challenge rigid mind-brain dualism. Clinical medicine is also starting to bridge the mental-physical gap; the influence of mental factors on physical health and disease, as well as that of physical factors on mental disorders, is becoming increasingly apparent (14,26,27,86). Many persons in the mental health field, including professional groups (36,46), the National Institute of Mental Health (97), and other advocates (32), as well as physicians in general (39), assert the importance of biological, psychological, and social factors in understanding and treating health and disease (34).

Unfortunately, the impasse in defining mental disorders and prioritizing mental health needs has a negative impact on public perception and stalls the formulation of public policy. The cause and effect of this deadlock are described by David Rochefort (85), a political scientist and expert in mental health policy:

> Since policy design arises from problem definition, lack of consensus about the nature of the problem being dealt with works counter to a collective sense of purpose and direction in mental health policy making. Although advocates for improved mental health care number many, their influence is often diffused in advancing different priorities for the investment of limited public resources. The situation is exacerbated by specialists' inability to reach agreement upon the boundaries of normal behavior or even the proportion of cases of recognized abnormality severe enough to warrant public intervention.

While it might thwart public policy, the definitional dilemma has not impeded research into and treatment of specific mental disorders. As psychiatrist-researcher Nancy Andreasen (8) observes:

> Mental illness is an abstract concept, with disputable defining characteristics and debatable boundaries. On the other hand, specific illnesses are more easily delineated. There are many different kinds of mental illness that differ in their severity, symptoms, outcome, and effect on the patient's life.

The classification of disorders is the cornerstone of data collection and analysis; it also predicts the outcome for a particular patient and determines the mode of treatment. The last decade saw advances in the classification of specific mental disorders, with the revision of the American Psychiatric Association's *Diagnostic and Statistical Manual of Mental Disorders* (DSM) (3).[1] It is difficult to overestimate the influence of the most recent editions of this manual: DSM-III (2) and DSM-III-R (3). They are the most widely used mental health diagnostic manuals in the world. They provide the framework for studies of mental disorders, and in most cases a DSM-diagnosable disorder is required for third-party reimbursement of treatment costs. Given its widespread use and acceptance, the lexicon of DSM-III-R is used in this report.

DSM-III and DSM-III-R offer several improvements over previous editions of this manual. First, classifications are not founded on unproven notions of what may cause specific disorders.[2] Both editions identify most mental disorders on the basis of expressed mood or thought processes or on observed behaviors. Second, they improve the reliability of diagnosis. The criteria for reaching a diagnosis are explicit, diagnosis is less subjective, and there is greater agreement on diagnosis among clinicians (57).

The revised DSMs are not without critics. Some controversy stemmed from the way specific disorders were selected for inclusion—essentially by consensus of experts who did not represent the full spectrum of mental health professionals. In addition, the detailed criteria for specific disorders make diagnosis formulaic, diminishing the role of clinical judgment. However, the increased reliability of diagnosis is generally considered to outweigh these criticisms. As stated by one researcher, "We are better off having it than not" (42).

While the diagnostic categories listed in DSM-III and DSM-III-R may lead to more reliable diagnoses, the validity of the categories remains uncertain (83). Validity refers to how well the description of a particular disorder reflects the true attributes of a causative factor or disease process—that is, how well it reflects what patients really have and what physicians really see. Mental disorders are classified on the basis of symptoms because there are as yet no

---

[1] The Research Diagnostic Criteria (RDC) was a forerunner of DSM-III (91). It is also used for research purposes.

[2] While DSM-III and III-R are neutral regarding the cause of distinct disorders, they are not strictly atheoretical. They apply a categorical model (36) to diagnosis; that is, their vantage point is one of delimiting categories of disorders in line with the traditional medical approach. Other models for mental disorders are also possible.

biological markers or laboratory tests for them. Such groupings, therefore, may not be completely valid—similar symptoms may result from a variety of causes. The validity of very few diagnostic categories in the DSM has been demonstrated; in fact, methods for evaluating diagnostic validity have been proposed, among them studying the course of symptoms over time and the eventual outcome of the disorder, patients' responsiveness to treatment, the concentration of the disorder within families, and biological and psychological measures (81). Alternative approaches to research, such as evaluating the biology of particular symptoms, are also important in understanding psychopathology. Obviously, pinpointing the causes of mental disorders would go a long way toward specifying their boundaries and validating the way in which they are categorized. As one researcher states:

> Few psychiatric disorders have yet been adequately validated and it is still an open issue whether there are genuine boundaries between the clinical syndromes and normality. In the long run validation depends on the elucidation of etiological process (58).

A DESCRIPTION OF THE MENTAL DISORDERS

Despite the fact that defining mental disorders in general and determining their boundaries specifically are difficult tasks, there is no doubt that the disorders considered in this report—schizophrenia, bipolar disorder, major depression, obsessive-compulsive disorder, and panic disorder—are genuine and often severe. They generally emerge in late adolescence or early adulthood (19). They are chronic and disabling, sometimes ravaging patients over the entire course of their adult lives. The following sections provide an overview of each disorder, summarizing their symptoms, classification, prevalence, course, and most common treatment. Boxes throughout the chapter describe individual experiences with some of the disorders.

Schizophrenia

Schizophrenia "is arguably the worst disease affecting mankind" (74) (box 3-A). It assails thought, perception, emotion, behavior, and movement, distorting an individual's personal experience of life and crippling his or her ability to participate in society.

Table 3-1—The Diagnosis of Schizophrenia

A. Presence of characteristic psychotic symptoms in the active phase: either (1), (2), or (3) for at least 1 week (unless the symptoms are successfully treated):
  1. Two of the following:
     a) delusions;
     b) prominent hallucinations throughout the day for several days or several times a week for several weeks, each hallucinatory experience not being limited to a few brief moments;
     c) incoherence or marked loosening of associations;
     d) catatonic behavior;
     e) flat or grossly inappropriate affect (emotional tone).
  2. Bizarre delusions, i.e., involving a phenomenon that the person's culture would regard as totally implausible (e.g., thought broadcasting, being controlled by a dead person).
  3. Prominent hallucinations [as defined in (1)(b) above] of a voice with content having no apparent relation to depression or elation, or a voice keeping up a running commentary on the person's behavior or thoughts, or two or more voices conversing with each other.

B. During the course of the disturbance, functioning in such areas as work, social relations, and self-care is markedly below the highest level achieved before onset of the disturbance.

C. Schizoaffective disorder (a combination of schizophrenia and mood disorder symptoms) and mood disorder (mania or depression) with psychotic features have been ruled out.

D. Continuous signs of the disturbance are seen for at least 6 months.

E. It cannot be established that an organic factor (brain tumor or trauma, drug intoxication, etc.) initiated and maintained the disturbance.

F. If there is a history of autistic disorder, the additional diagnosis of schizophrenia is made only if prominent delusions or hallucinations are also present.

SOURCE: American Psychiatric Association, *Diagnostic and Statistical Manual of Mental Disorders*, 3rd ed., rev. (Washington, DC: American Psychiatric Association, 1987), as edited by I.I. Gottesman, *Schizophrenia Genesis: The Origins of Madness* (New York, NY: W.H. Freeman and Co., 1991).

Schizophrenia is not split personality, a commonly held misperception (100). Its hallmark is a disturbance of cognition, the processing of information (table 3-1) (9,42,95,97). Components of thought may become dissociated or fragmented, the flow of thought interrupted. Schizophrenia typically impairs the ability to integrate information, to reason, to concentrate, or to focus attention or purpose. The consequence is often an observed vagueness, illogicality, and bizarreness of thinking that, when severe, restricts interpersonal communication.

Individuals with schizophrenia experience delusions and hallucinations. Delusions are beliefs that are clearly implausible but that are compelling and central to an individual's life experience. Persons with this disorder may be suspicious or paranoid in nature. For example, a patient may believe that he or

Box 3-A—One Day in the Life of Sylvia Frumkin

Shortly after midnight on Friday, June 16, 1978, Sylvia Frumkin decided to take a bath. Miss Frumkin, a heavy, ungainly young woman who lived in a two-story yellow brick building in Queens Village, New York, walked from her bedroom on the second floor to the bathroom next door and filled the tub with warm water. A few days earlier, she had had her hair cut and shaped in a bowl style, which she found especially becoming, and her spirits were high. She washed her brown hair with shampoo and also with red mouthwash. Some years earlier, she had tinted her hair red and had liked the way it looked. She had given up wearing her hair red only because she had found coloring it every six weeks too much of a bother. She imagined that the red mouthwash would somehow be absorbed into her scalp and make her hair red permanently. Miss Frumkin felt so cheerful about her new haircut that she suddenly thought she was Lori Lemaris, the mermaid whom Clark Kent had met in college and had fallen in love with in the old "Superman" comics. She blew bubbles into the water.

After a few minutes of contented frolicking, Miss Frumkin stepped out of the tub. She slipped on the bathroom floor—it was wet from her bubble-blowing and splashing—and cut the back of her head as she fell. The cut began to bleed. She attempted to stop the bleeding by applying pressure to the cut, then wrapped her head in a large towel and walked back to her bedroom. On the dresser was a bottle of expensive perfume that an aunt and uncle had given her in May as a thirtieth-birthday present. She poured the contents of the bottle on her cut, partly because she knew that perfume contained alcohol and that alcohol was an antiseptic . . . and partly because she suddenly thought that she was Jesus Christ and that her bleeding cut was the beginning of a crown of thorns. She also thought that she was Mary Magdalene, who had poured ointment on Christ. . . .

Miss Frumkin's head burned when the perfume came in contact with the open cut, and the bleeding subsided but didn't altogether stop. By then, it was after one o'clock. She put on an old nightgown and went downstairs to the office of the building to tell the night supervisor, Dwight Miller, who was on duty from midnight until eight-thirty, what had happened. Miller looked at the cut, told Miss Frumkin to get dressed, and said he would drive her to the emergency room. . . .

As Miller started the car, turned on the car radio, and began to drive toward the hospital, Miss Frumkin seemed to get excited. The radio was playing Paul McCartney's song "The Lovely Linda," and he was singing the words "La, la, la, la, la, the lovely Linda." Unknown to Miller, Miss Frumkin thought that McCartney was singing the lyrics sarcastically, because he had fallen in love with her and was no longer in love with Linda, his wife. Miss Frumkin began to talk fervently to the radio. Miss Frumkin and Miller arrived at the emergency room of L.I.J.-Hillside at two o'clock. Miss Frumkin was first interviewed and examined by a nurse. For a few minutes, she was in sufficient control of herself to let the nurse take her vital signs, test her neurological responses, and look at her cut, and to answer the questions the nurse asked. . . . She became upset while she was waiting to see a doctor and an X-ray technician (she began to speak rapidly, and what she said concerned suffering from hypoglycemia and Wilson's disease and being Cinderella, and didn't make much sense); more upset when the X-ray technician took X rays of her skull and the doctor sewed up the cut (Miss Frumkin was so agitated that the doctor succeeded in putting in only three of five silk sutures he had intended to put in); and still more upset when it turned out that there would be a fairly long wait for the skull X rays to be read. Miss Frumkin got so obstreperous while she and Miller were waiting in the main area of the emergency room that they were shown into one of the small treatment rooms off to one side that the hospital uses to give people privacy, where they were joined by a hospital security guard. In the small treatment room, Miss Frumkin's conduct became increasingly bizarre. She took off all her clothes, accused Miller of kidnapping her and making sexual advances, and then asked Miller and the security guard to have sexual relations with her, saying she hadn't had sex with a man in 5 years. The minute the two men would cover Miss Frumkin with a hospital gown, she would disrobe again.

Around three o'clock, Dr. Conrad Aaronson, a psychiatric resident, came to observe and question Miss Frumkin. . . . His impression of Miss Frumkin's condition was that it was an acute exacerbation of chronic schizophrenia—one of the most common forms of serious mental illness in the world. Dr. Aaronson found that Miss Frumkin was in no shape to return to her room in Queens Village. He wrote in his report, at 4:15 a.m., "Patient removed all her clothing and began chanting and praying on the floor at the conclusion of the interview. . . . Patient is in need of emergency hospitalization as she represents a danger to herself and to others in her present condition."

Miss Frumkin was asked if she would like to be admitted to the psychiatric division of L.I.J.-Hillside. . . . [S]he refused to be admitted there. Instead, she asked to be taken to the Creedmoor Psychiatric Center, in Queens Village—a State mental institution that serves the two million people who live in Queens. . . . She had been a patient there until about two weeks earlier—from May 9, 1978 to May 31, 1978. . . . Miss Frumkin returned to Creedmoor . . . at five-thirty, just as the sun was rising. . . .

It was after eleven o'clock in the morning on Friday, June 16, by the time Miss Frumkin had been screened for admission by Dr. Sun, had changed into State clothes, and had taken a chair in the women's day hall. Soon she was on her feet, hurrying over to the nurse on duty. She demanded to use the telephone. When the nurse told her she would have to wait until another patient had finished making a call, Miss Frumkin screamed at her. The nurse escorted her to the telephone a few minutes later. Miss Frumkin dialed the extension of Dr. Werner, Creedmoor's director. She tried to tell Dr. Werner's secretary her troubles, but became incoherent. The nurse and a therapy aide had to struggle with her to get her to put the telephone down. The nurse, who had been at the admission screening, then led Miss Frumkin to the treatment room and tried to give her the injection of Thorazine that Dr. Sun had ordered that she be given immediately for agitation. Miss Frumkin refused the injection. She said she would take Thorazine orally instead. . . . Between sips of the bad-tasting Thorazine, Miss Frumkin called the nurse a jerk, a slut, and a dodo. After Miss Frumkin's insults became threats and she started to hit the nurse, the nurse went to Dr. Sun, caught him just as he was leaving, and got him to write out a seclusion order, which went into effect at twelve-fifteen. Once Miss Frumkin had been put in the seclusion room, she flopped down on the mattress as if she were relieved to be there. A few minutes later, a therapy aide brought her lunch on a tray. Miss Frumkin, who had been mumbling unintelligibly, took the tray, wolfed down the food, and handed the tray back. She soon lay down and dozed off. When the seclusion order expired, at two-fifteen, the door to the room was opened. Miss Frumkin was asleep. She was left in the room to sleep, with the door open.

Miss Frumkin awakened shortly before four, but she appeared content to stay in the quiet room. Around five o'clock, she felt hungry, got up, and walked into the day hall. When the door to the dining room corridor was opened, she went into the corridor and stood in line with the other patients, whispering to herself. . . .

After shovelling into her mouth three helpings of everything served at dinner on June 16, Miss Frumkin returned to the day hall, settled into an easy chair, and watched television quietly. At nine o'clock, she took the 50 milligrams of Moban that Dr. Khanna had prescribed for her. A therapy aide on the evening shift let her watch TV until ten-thirty before taking her into the dormitory, where the other women were already asleep. She assigned Miss Frumkin an empty bed next to a window. . . . Although Miss Frumkin had had little sleep in the last thirty-six hours, she wasn't tired. She got into bed without taking her clothes off and lay quietly under the sheets and under the bedspread, which the therapy aide had forgotten to remove.

A few minutes after the night shift came on duty, Miss Frumkin got out of bed. She walked hurriedly down the long corridor from the dormitory to the day hall. She then headed back toward the dormitory, but stopped at the employees' lunchroom when she saw a short, stocky black woman named Bernice Parrott sitting there. Miss Frumkin told her that there was some water on the floor of the day hall and asked her if she had a mop. When Mrs. Parrott replied that she didn't, Miss Frumkin warned her that if she didn't mop up the water she would report her to the night supervisor. Mrs. Parrott asked Miss Frumkin to go back to bed, and said she would take care of the water. Mrs. Parrott went into the day hall, found a puddle of urine on the floor, and went to the utility room to get a mop. When she returned to the day hall carrying the mop, she found Miss Frumkin standing a few feet from the puddle. Miss Frumkin ordered Mrs. Parrott, at the top of her voice, to clean up the day hall. Before Mrs. Parrott could clean anything, Miss Frumkin ran over to her and demanded the mop. Mrs. Parrott held on to the mop with all her strength, fearful of what Miss Frumkin would do with it if she got her hands on it. Miss Frumkin grabbed Mrs. Parrott's dress, struck her several times on the head with her fist, kicked her, and tried to bite her, screaming "Nigger, I'll nix you!" as she fought to gain possession of the mop. Mrs. Parrott was in pain, but she whirled around, pinned Miss Frumkin against a wall, pried herself loose, and ran to the nearest telephone, which was in the ward office. She hurled the mop through an open door to the employees' toilet, in the far corner of the office, picked up the telephone, and called the night supervisor, who was in the secretaries' office in the central corridor watching some members of the night shift sign in. Meanwhile, with her free hand Mrs. Parrott continued to fend off Miss Frumkin, who had followed her into the office and was still after the mop. Mrs. Parrott and Miss Frumkin wrestled; Mrs. Parrott succeeded in bringing Miss Frumkin to the floor and was able to hold her until the night supervisor came to her assistance. . . .

Mrs. Parrott and the night supervisor put Miss Frumkin into an empty seclusion room. Miss Frumkin was banging furiously on the door of the seclusion room. The nurse telephoned the doctor on night duty . . . and he gave her a verbal order to put Miss Frumkin in seclusion for two hours. Mrs. Parrott and the night supervisor helped the nurse hold Miss Frumkin down so that the nurse could give her the Thorazine injection for agitation . . . Miss Frumkin remained agitated all night. . . .

SOURCE: Quoted from S. Sheehan, *Is There No Place on Earth for Me?* (Boston, MA: Houghton Mifflin, 1982) Copyright © 1982 by Susan Sheehan. Reprinted by permission of Houghton Mifflin Co.

she is a historical figure or that someone has placed a transmitter in his or her brain. Hallucinations are perceptions without an objective basis. They most commonly take the form of voices or, less frequently, visions, bodily sensations, tastes, or smells. The voices appear to originate from an external source. They tend to be highly personal and may direct the patient to do some act, sometimes commanding self-mutilation or other violent behavior.

Another prominent feature of schizophrenia is impairment of emotional responsiveness. There is a dulling of emotions or an inappropriateness of emotional response. Many individuals with schizophrenia exhibit a "wooden" personality, displaying traits of diminished drive, curiosity, or spontaneity. Schizophrenia may also lead to a disturbance of movement. Patients may grimace involuntarily, walk awkwardly, or suffer impairment of a broad range of subtle movements.

Delusions, hallucinations, and impairments in thought that are marked by incoherence, illogicality, or bizarre behavior together constitute the "positive" symptoms of schizophrenia. These symptoms are typical of psychosis (7); however, schizophrenia and psychosis are not synonymous. Psychosis can accompany other disorders, such as mood disorders, drug-induced reactions, temporal lobe epilepsy, Huntington's disease, encephalitis, and syphilis. There are many pathological features of schizophrenia that are not psychotic, such as the blunting of emotions, apathy, and social withdrawal, all "negative" symptoms of schizophrenia (6,7).

While schizophrenia has been well-characterized as a disorder, symptoms vary widely among patients. Symptoms combine in various ways, and they change over time. This variability has raised questions about how best to conceptualize schizophrenia. Is it a single disorder? A group of disorders? A conglomerate of several disease processes? What is its relationship to other mental disorders?

German psychiatrist Emil Kraepelin was the first to consolidate the diverse manifestations of schizophrenia under a single rubric—dementia praecox, or dementia of the young (62). Eugen Bleuler introduced the term schizophrenia, referring to a split in mental activities, in 1911 (16). This name emphasizes what Bleuler thought was the primary pathology: the dissociation of thoughts, emotion, and behavior. This conception of a single underlying disease process has endured. Those who support this

concept assert that a unified cause or mechanism produces the various symptoms of the disorder. The fact that the varying manifestations of schizophrenia appear to be genetically related (see ch. 5) and that they often respond to similar treatment approaches supports the single-disorder model.

Another model considers schizophrenia to be a clinical syndrome rather than a single disease entity (97). This view holds that although schizophrenia can legitimately be distinguished from other mental disorders (e.g., mood disorders), it has more than one cause. This has led some persons to refer to it as *the* schizophrenia*s*. Because schizophrenia is such a complex disorder and its underlying pathology remains elusive, many expect that more than one cause will eventually be discovered.

Some researchers have proposed that distinct disease processes independently produce some of the symptoms of schizophrenia; that is, no single culprit causes all of the symptoms of schizophrenia. While, certain symptoms do appear to occur semi-independently (20,93,94)—for example, the extent of psychosis is only modestly associated with the extent of social impairment—further study is necessary to test this hypothesis.

Schizophrenia may be related to other mental disorders. Certain personality disorders, typified by eccentric behavior, excessive suspiciousness or paranoia, or extreme indifference to others, are considered part of the schizophrenia spectrum by many researchers, since they resemble schizophrenia and tend to run in families with the disorder (see ch. 5). Some have suggested that mood disorders with psychotic symptoms may also be related to schizophrenia (24,35). Similarly, schizoaffective disorder, which is typified by symptoms of schizophrenia and major mood disorders, has been thought to stem from some of the same causes as schizophrenia. A relationship between mood disorders and schizophrenia is suspected because many persons exhibit symptoms common to both categories of disorders.

Schizophrenia is a common disorder. Approximately 1 of every 100 persons will develop schizophrenia during the course of his or her lifetime (30,55,84). That translates into 1.2 million people with schizophrenia in the United States today. Men and women appear to be at equal risk, although schizophrenia generally strikes men at a younger age

Figure 3-1—The Course of Schizophrenia

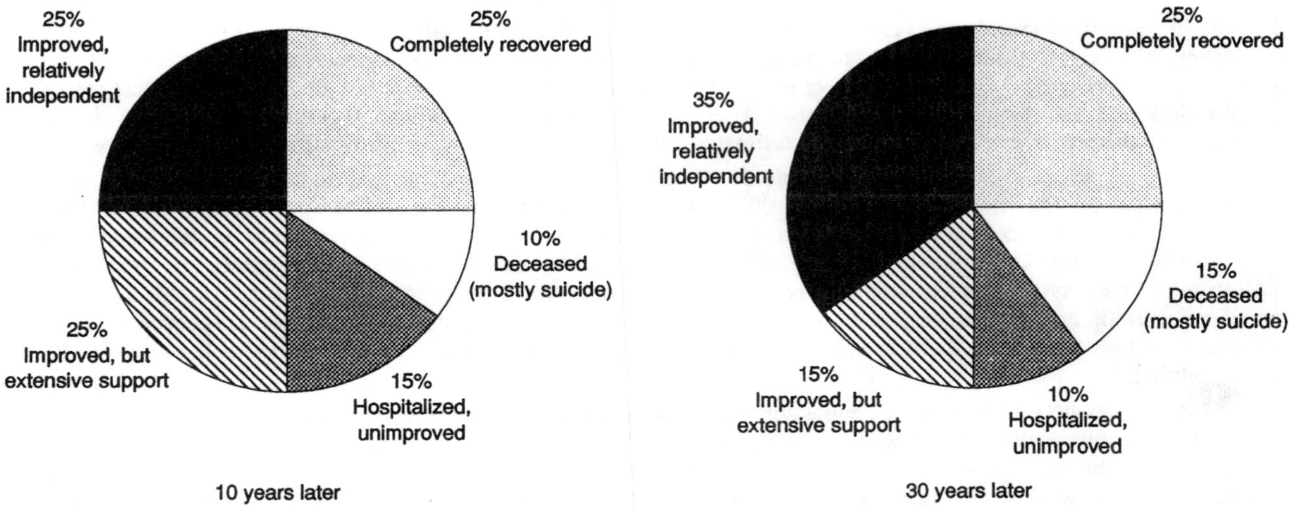

25%
Improved,
relatively
independent

25%
Completely recovered

10%
Deceased
(mostly suicide)

25%
Improved, but
extensive support

15%
Hospitalized,
unimproved

10 years later

25%
Completely recovered

35%
Improved,
relatively
independent

15%
Deceased
(mostly suicide)

15%
Improved, but
extensive support

10%
Hospitalized,
unimproved

30 years later

While schizophrenia does not lead inevitably to lifelong disability, the majority of individuals with this condition suffer long-term consequences.

SOURCE: Adapted with permission from E.F. Torrey, *Surviving Schizophrenia: A Family Manual,* rev. ed. (New York, NY: Harper & Row, 1988).

and women generally have a better long-term prognosis.

Demographic data on schizophrenia paint a picture of considerable social and economic distress (55,95). Individuals who have never been married or who are divorced or separated suffer schizophrenia two to three times as often as their married or widowed counterparts. Compared to the general population, individuals with schizophrenia are less likely to hold a college degree or to be employed. If employed, they are likely to earn less than persons without schizophrenia. Studies have consistently shown that schizophrenia occurs more often among persons in lower socioeconomic groups: It is five times more prevalent among those at the bottom of the socioeconomic ladder than those at the top.[3]

There is a long-standing tendency among both professionals and laypersons to presume that schizophrenia invariably follows a deteriorating course, resulting in an exceptionally poor outcome in most cases. This assumption has always been incorrect. Patients suffering from the disorder have followed a variety of courses over the long term, including some that are relatively benign (figure 3-1). It is true,

however, that there are substantial and enduring consequences for most patients.

One of the hallmarks of schizophrenia is its early onset, usually during the late teens and early 20s (22). Onset of schizophrenia may be sudden, with an unexpected development of psychosis, or it may be insidious, with the earliest signs occurring years before the blatant symptoms of psychosis. Early signs include emotional withdrawal, diminishing social engagement, low energy, and idiosyncratic responses to ordinary events or circumstances. School performance, social interaction, and emotional responsivity may erode gradually, well in advance of the onslaught of hallucinations, delusions, and disorganized thought processes. A more sudden onset usually results in a more favorable outcome.

Psychotic symptoms may persist over an extended period of time, with the patient never achieving full recovery, or they may be episodic, with periods of psychosis followed by relatively complete recovery (96). A substantial number of patients continue to manifest symptoms of schizophrenia throughout their lives. The expressed symp-

---

[3] Two hypotheses have been put forth to explain the higher rates of schizophrenia among persons in lower socioeconomic groups: the breeder hypothesis and the downward drift hypothesis. Simply stated, the breeder hypothesis holds that social stress, such as poverty, causes schizophrenia. The downward drift hypothesis states that the disorder itself leads to downward social mobility (29,42).

Box 3-B—The Final Symptom: Mental Disorders and Suicide

In 1987, 11.7 people in every 100,000—more than 30,000 people—killed themselves in the United States, making it the eighth leading cause of death in the nation. While many factors are associated with suicide, including medical illness, availability of firearms, or stressful events such as a divorce or loss of a job, data indicate that mental disorders are a significant antecedent to many suicides in the United States. About 50 percent of all suicide victims may have suffered a mood disorder, and an estimated 5 to 10 percent of suicide victims suffered from schizophrenia.

Among people with schizophrenia, suicide is the number one cause of premature death, with the estimated age-adjusted suicide rate averaging 90 per 100,000 women with schizophrenia and 210 per 100,000 men with the disorder; 10 to 15 percent of individuals with schizophrenia commit suicide. The higher rate of suicide among men versus women with schizophrenia not only mirrors the suicide statistics in the general population, but also reflects the more severe symptoms that men usually suffer. Some people with schizophrenia may commit suicide as a result of a psychotic episode—in response to a hallucinatory command. More commonly, however, people with this condition take their lives early in the course of the illness during a relatively stable period following a recent hospitalization.

Approximately 15 percent of people with mood disorders will commit suicide, with the suicide rates for men and women with major mood disorders averaging 400 and 180 per 100,000, respectively, 30 times higher than the rate in the general population. The link between mood disorders and suicide is well recognized, with recurrent thoughts of suicide or a suicide attempt being diagnostic criterion for these conditions. Other mental disorders, such as panic disorder, also appear to be correlated with suicide. Although there is little information available concerning the number of people with panic disorder who actually commit suicide, survey data show that approximately 20 percent of people with this condition will attempt suicide during their lifetime.

High rates of suicide among individuals with major mental disorders like schizophrenia or major depression provide chilling evidence of the distressing nature of mental disorders. Furthermore, the strong correlation between mental disorder and suicide indicates that general suicide prevention efforts must include strategies to improve the treatment of mental disorders.

SOURCES: C.B. Caldwell and I.I. Gottesman, "Schizophrenics Kill Themselves Too: A Review of Risk Factors for Suicide," *Schizophrenia Bulletin* 16(4):571-589, 1990; F.K. Goodwin and K.R. Jamison, *Manic-Depressive Illness* (New York, NY: The Oxford University Press, 1990); J. Johnson, M.M. Weissman, and G.L. Klerman, "Panic Disorder, Comorbidity, and Suicide Attempts," *Archives of General Psychiatry* 47:805-808, 1990; E.K. Moscicki, chief, Prevention Research Branch, National Institute of Mental Health, U.S. Department of Health and Human Services, personal communication, Apr. 30, 1991; U.S. Department of Health and Human Services, Public Health Service, National Center for Health Statistics, *Monthly Vital Statistics Report* 40(8 suppl. 2), 1992.

---

toms may combine in various ways, their severity and duration fluctuating over time. Schizophrenia increases the risk of suicide considerably—some 10 to 15 percent of individuals with schizophrenia end their lives, usually within the first 10 years of developing the disorder (box 3-B). With age, the intensity of the psychotic symptoms may diminish, and many patients with long-term impairments regain some degree of social and occupational competence. Although schizophrenia may become easier to manage, the effects of years of dysfunction are rarely overcome.

Currently, there is no way to prevent or cure schizophrenia; however, the symptoms of the disorder can usually be treated. Treatment usually integrates antipsychotic drugs and supportive psycho-therapy. Acutely ill individuals usually require hospitalization; antipsychotic medication, of which there are several chemical classes, is commonly used to manage psychosis (table 3-2) (10,50,65).[4] While not as effective in modulating the negative symptoms of schizophrenia, antipsychotic drugs do diminish the positive symptoms. Furthermore, antipsychotic medications seem to affect the course of the disorder. Data indicate that continued use of these medications prevents the recurrence of psychotic episodes (50), and clinical experience suggests that the earlier antipsychotic medication is administered, the more benign the course of the disorder (108).

Antipsychotic drugs do have some limitations. As mentioned above, they are less effective in controlling the negative symptoms of schizophrenia. Also,

---

[4] In fact, schizophrenia is the most frequently reported diagnosis among individuals hospitalized for mental disorders, especially in State and county mental hospitals and Veterans Administration medical centers (68).

Table 3-2—Traditional Antipsychotic Medications

Chemical family	Generic name	Brand name
Phenothiazines	chlorpromazine	Thorazine and others
	thioridazine	Mellaril, Millazine
	mesoridazine	Serentil
	trifluoperazine	Stelazine, Suprazine
	perphenazine	Trilafon
	fluphenazine	Prolixin, Permitil
	triflupromazine	Vesprin
	prochlorperazine	Compazine
	acetophenazine	Tindal
Butyrophenones	haloperidol	Haldol
	pimozide	Orap
	droperidol	Inapsine
Thioxanthenes	thiothixene	Navane
	chlorprothixene	Taractan
Dibenzoxazepine	loxapine	Loxitane
Dihydroindolone	molindone	Moban

SOURCE: R.J. Baldessarini, "Drugs and the Treatment of Psychiatric Disorders," *The Pharmacological Basis of Therapeutics* (New York, NY: Pergamon Press, 1990).

some patients do not respond to traditional antipsychotic agents. Finally, antipsychotic agents have some side effects, including dry mouth, constipation, blurring of vision, weight gain, restlessness, and tremor. The most serious side effect is tardive dyskinesia, which usually appears after taking the drug for some time. Tardive dyskinesia involves abnormal involuntary movements of the face, tongue, mouth, fingers, upper and lower limbs, and occasionally the entire body. It occurs in at least a mild form in 25 to 40 percent of patients on antipsychotic agents and may be severe or irreversible in 5 to 10 percent of cases (10,50).

A newer drug to treat schizophrenia—clozapine—has claimed the limelight in recent years. It was shown during the 1970s to help patients who were resistant to the therapeutic effects of standard antipsychotic drugs. However, clozapine can cause a potentially lethal blood disorder: 1 to 2 percent of the individuals who take it will develop agranulocytosis, which decreases the number of infection-fighting white blood cells (51,52). A recent large-scale study in the United States demonstrated clozapine's effectiveness in approximately one-third of those patients who were unresponsive to traditional antipsychotic medication (51,73,89). The study also showed that clozapine can be used with relative safety, as long as it is accompanied by careful monitoring for agranulocytosis. A number of new antipsychotic drugs are also being developed (43) (see ch. 4).

Psychosocial treatment is another important aspect of the treatment of schizophrenia (21,66). While individual psychotherapy based on psychodynamic principles has been shown to be ineffective, and perhaps even detrimental (45,59), supportive psychotherapy aimed at helping patients understand their illness, reducing stress, and enhancing coping abilities can reduce the amount of medication necessary and enhance patients' participation in treatment (90). Educating the family about the symptoms and nature of schizophrenia, as well as providing them with tools to deal with stress, is increasingly seen as important in the optimal management of schizophrenia (92).

Rehabilitation attempts to minimize the long-term consequences of schizophrenia rather than to treat the disorder itself. A wide range of rehabilitation programs has been shown to enhance social and occupational outcomes. These programs are adjuncts, but not alternatives, to antipsychotic medication and supportive psychotherapy.

Mood Disorders

Mood disorders, also referred to as affective disorders, are characterized by extreme or prolonged disturbances of mood, such as sadness, apathy, or elation (41,56). DSM-III-R divides mood disorders into two major groups: bipolar disorders and depressive disorders (3). The occurrence of manic symptoms distinguishes bipolar disorders from depressive, or unipolar, disorders.

The most severe depressive disorder is major depression (box 3-C). An episode of major depression is characterized by complete loss of interest or pleasure in activities (table 3-3). Other physical and psychological symptoms often accompany an episode of major depression, including weight gain or loss, insomnia or excessive sleepiness, slowed or agitated movement, diminished energy, intense feelings of guilt or worthlessness, diminished ability to concentrate, and recurrent thoughts of death or suicide. Major depression may entail a single episode or, more commonly, recurrent episodes; it may be chronic or extremely severe. Psychosis sometimes occurs as well. A review of 17 studies concluded that 15 percent of persons suffering from symptoms of depression will commit suicide (44) (see box 3-B).

Bipolar disorder, commonly known as manic depression, is a severe mood disorder characterized

---

Box 3-C—Darkness Visible: A Personal Account of Depression

Depression is a disorder of mood, so mysteriously painful and elusive in the way it becomes known to the self—to the mediating intellect—as to verge close to being beyond description. It thus remains nearly incomprehensible to those who have not experienced it in its extreme mode, although the gloom, 'the blues' which people go through occasionally and associate with the general hassle of everyday existence are of such prevalence that they do give many individuals a hint of the illness in its catastrophic form. But at the time of which I write I had descended far past those familiar, manageable doldrums. . . .

It was not really alarming at first, since the change was subtle, but I did notice that my surroundings took on a different tone at certain times: the shadows of nightfall seemed more somber, my mornings were less buoyant, walks in the woods became less zestful, and there was a moment during my working hours in the late afternoon when a kind of panic and anxiety overtook me, just for a few minutes, accompanied by a visceral queasiness—such a seizure was at least slightly alarming, after all. . . .

I felt a kind of numbness, an enervation, but more particularly an odd fragility—as if my body had actually become frail, hypersensitive and somehow disjointed and clumsy, lacking normal coordination. And soon I was in the throes of a pervasive hypochondria. Nothing felt quite right with my corporeal self; there were twitches and pains, sometimes intermittent, often seemingly constant, that seemed to presage all sorts of dire infirmities. . . .

It was October, and one of the unforgettable features of this stage of my disorder was the way in which my own farmhouse, my beloved home for 30 years, took on for me at that point when my spirits regularly sank to their nadir an almost palpable quality of ominousness. The fading evening light—akin to that famous 'slant of light' of Emily Dickinson's, which spoke to her of death, of chill extinction—had none of its familiar autumnal loveliness, but ensnared me in a suffocating gloom. . . . That fall, as the disorder gradually took full possession of my system, I began to conceive that my mind itself was like one of those outmoded small-town telephone exchanges, being gradually inundated by flood waters: one by one, the normal circuits began to drown, causing some of the functions of the body and nearly all of those of instinct and intellect to slowly disconnect. . . .

What I had begun to discover is that, mysteriously and in ways that are totally remote from normal experience, the gray drizzle of horror induced by depression takes on the quality of physical pain. But it is not an immediately identifiable pain, like that of a broken limb. It may be more accurate to say that despair, owing to some evil trick played upon the sick brain by the inhabiting psyche, comes to resemble the diabolical discomfort of being imprisoned in a fiercely overheated room. And because no breeze stirs this cauldron, because there is no escape from this smothering confinement, it is entirely natural that the victim begins to think ceaselessly of oblivion.

SOURCE: Quoted from W. Styron, *Darkness Visible* (New York, NY: Random House, 1990). Copyright © 1990 by William Styron. Reprinted by permission of Random House, Inc.

---

by one or more full manic episodes and one or more major depressive episodes. During a manic episode, mood is extremely elevated, expansive, or even irritable (table 3-4). Self-esteem is elevated, sometimes to delusional proportions; there is diminished need for sleep; energy abounds and thoughts race; individuals are often extremely talkative and distractible; and individuals indulge in unrestrained buying sprees or sexual and other activity. Psychotic features (i.e., delusions and hallucinations) are not uncommon during a manic episode.

There are several unresolved issues concerning the classification of mood disorders. As mentioned, some observers think that mood disorders, especially in the presence of psychosis, are related to schizophrenia. Individuals often exhibit symptoms of both categories of disorders. Other questions concerning the classification of mood disorders include:

- Is depression a single disorder? A class of disorders?
- How are less severe episodes of depression and other mental disorders related to major depression?
- How is bipolar disorder related to major depression?

A recent report analyzing research on depression in women stated:

The common belief that depression varies along a single continuum from ordinary blues to major depression may be incorrect, because depressions may differ in kind as well as degree. Depression is heterogeneous (5).

Table 3-3—The Diagnosis of Depression

Note: A "Major Depressive Syndrome" is defined as criterion A below.

A. At least five of the following symptoms have been present during the same two-week period and represent a change from previous functioning; at least one of the symptoms is either: 1) depressed mood, or 2) loss of interest or pleasure. (Do not include symptoms that are clearly due to a physical condition, mood-incongruent delusions or hallucinations, incoherence, or marked loosening of associations.)
   1. depressed mood (or can be irritable mood in children and adolescents) most of the day, nearly every day, as indicated either by subjective account or observation by others;
   2. markedly diminished interest or pleasure in all, or almost all, activities most of the day, nearly every day (as indicated either by subjective account or observation by others of apathy most of the time);
   3. significant weight loss or weight gain when not dieting, or decrease or increase in appetite nearly every day;
   4. insomnia or hypersomnia nearly every day;
   5. psychomotor agitation or retardation nearly every day (observable by others, not merely subjective feelings of restlessness or being slowed down);
   6. fatigue or loss of energy nearly every day;
   7. feelings of worthlessness or excessive or inappropriate guilt (which may be delusional) nearly every day (not merely self-reproach or guilt about being sick);
   8. diminished ability to think or concentrate, or indecisiveness, nearly every day (either by subjective account or as observed by others);
   9. recurrent thoughts of death (not just fear of dying), recurrent suicidal ideation without a specific plan, or a suicide attempt or a specific plan for committing suicide.

B. 1. It cannot be established that an organic factor initiated and maintained the disturbance.
   2. The disturbance is not a normal reaction to the death of a loved one (uncomplicated bereavement).

C. At no time during the disturbance have there been delusions or hallucinations for as long as two weeks in the absence of prominent mood symptoms (i.e., before the mood symptoms developed or after they have remitted).

D. Not superimposed on schizophrenia, schizophreniform disorder, and others.

SOURCE: American Psychiatric Association, *Diagnostic and Statistical Manual of Mental Disorders*, 3rd ed., rev. (Washington, DC: American Psychiatric Association, 1987).

Table 3-4—The Diagnosis of Mania

Note: A "Manic Syndrome" is defined as including criteria A, B, and C below.

A. A distinct period of abnormally and persistently elevated, expansive, or irritable mood.

B. During the period of mood disturbance, at least three of the following symptoms have persisted (four if the mood is only irritable) and have been present to a significant degree:
   1. inflated self-esteem or grandiosity;
   2. decreased need for sleep, e.g., feels rested after only three hours of sleep;
   3. more talkative than usual or pressure to keep talking;
   4. flight of ideas or subjective experience that thoughts are racing;
   5. distractibility, i.e., attention too easily drawn to unimportant or irrelevant external stimuli;
   6. increase in goal-directed activity (either socially, at work or school, or sexually) or psychomotor agitation;
   7. excessive involvement in pleasurable activities which have a high potential for painful consequences, e.g., the person engages in unrestrained buying sprees, sexual indiscretions, or foolish business investments.

C. Mood disturbance sufficiently severe to cause marked impairment in occupational functioning or in usual social activities or relationships with others, or to necessitate hospitalization to prevent harm to self or others.

D. At no time during the disturbance have there been delusions or hallucinations for as long as two weeks in the absence of prominent mood symptoms (i.e., before the mood symptoms developed or after they have remitted).

E. Not superimposed on schizophrenia, schizophreniform disorder, and others.

F. It cannot be established that an organic factor initiated and maintained the disturbance.

Note: Somatic antidepressant treatment (e.g., drugs, ECT) that apparently precipitates a mood disturbance should not be considered an etiologic organic factor.

SOURCE: American Psychiatric Association, *Diagnostic and Statistical Manual of Mental Disorders*, 3rd ed., rev. (Washington, DC: American Psychiatric Association, 1987).

There are various ways to conceptualize depression, based on its course, symptoms, association with other disorders, and severity (5). For example, it is known that symptoms of anxiety and depression often occur together (70). The fact that depression may be triggered by, or correlated with, different factors also suggests that depression is heterogeneous. For example, reproductive-related events (e.g., menstruation, pregnancy, childbirth, infertility, abortion, and menopause) are related to some cases of depression among women, who are at greater risk of depressive disorders than men (5). Seasonality has also been observed in depressive episodes—namely,

in seasonal affective disorder, or SAD. In this disorder, individuals have a characteristic onset of depression during the winter months, with remissions or changes from depression to mania during the spring (87). Depression can also appear in a very severe form. Melancholia is a severe form of depression wherein persons take virtually no interest or pleasure in activities and experience such somatic symptoms as early morning waking and weight loss.

While a categorical approach to depression may be convenient for selecting homogeneous groups for research or designing a treatment strategy, it does not preclude the possibility that depression is a single disorder. As stated in a recent psychiatric diagnostic text:

Affective disorders have been divided and subdivided endlessly as investigators endeavor to distinguish 'normal' from 'abnormal' mood . . . after a century there is still no agreement about the most satisfactory classification (40).

Family histories and longitudinal studies provide evidence that depression may constitute a continuum from the blues to medically recognized depression. For example, the immediate family of individuals with a mild mood disorder are more likely than other persons to have major depression (82). Also, many individuals with mild depression go on to suffer full-blown depression (1,105).

The basis for separating bipolar (manic-depressive) and unipolar (depressive) disorders into different categories of illness has been questioned. After a comprehensive review of the literature, however, Goodwin and Jamison conclude that studies evaluating family history, clinical symptoms and course, the response to pharmacological treatment, and other factors strongly support recognition of the distinction between these disorders (41). They also suggest that bipolar disorder and severe cases of recurrent depression may share important features (e.g., response to treatment with lithium) and encourage more research on the cycles in severe mood disorders.

Nearly 8 percent of the U.S. population will develop a mood disorder at some time during their lives (103,104). Bipolar disorder afflicts slightly less than 1 percent of the population (0.8 percent), with men and women being affected equally. Nearly 5 percent (4.9 percent) of the population will develop major depression, which is twice as common in women as men. Substance abuse often coincides with major mood disorders (box 3-D).

Mood disorders appear to be increasing among younger people. Studies show that in this century each succeeding generation has reported an increased lifetime risk and earlier age of onset of major depression (60,101,103,106). Why the rates are increasing is not known. They may reflect an artifact of the data-collecting process, forgetfulness on the part of older individuals when surveyed, or a true increase in depression. Whatever the source of this "cohort effect," it is a significant consideration in certain types of research into depression (e.g., genetic research).

Mood disorders have various social correlates, including marital and employment status (103). Individuals with a mood disorder, especially bipolar disorder, are more likely never to have married or to have been divorced. Major mood disorders and socioeconomic status are not directly related (103). While schizophrenia is highly concentrated in the lower socioeconomic classes, bipolar disorder and major depression afflict individuals in every class and occupation. In fact, many highly successful and creative individuals have suffered a major mood disorder, suggesting a link between the disorder and creativity (49).

The onset of major depression typically occurs in the late 20s, although it can emerge at any time (56,103). Over 50 percent of patients will have more than one bout of major depression, the mean number being five or six episodes in a lifetime (64). The highest rate of relapse occurs during the months immediately following recovery from a previous episode (78).

Bipolar disorder typically begins in the mid-20s (41). Episodes of mania or depression emerge every several months to a year or more, with periods of recovery separating the mood swings. Some individuals exhibit rapid cycling, with multiple episodes in a single year. Manic episodes tend to begin rather abruptly, with mild symptoms quickly developing into a full-blown state of mania, sometimes with accompanying psychosis. Depressive episodes tend to begin more slowly. If untreated, episodes last 4 to 13 months, with depressive episodes generally outlasting manic ones. External events may trigger an episode, especially in the early phase of the disorder; with time, episodes of depression and mania emerge independent of outside events. Bipolar disorder is chronic, with the cycles of mania and depression, separated by periods of recovery, continuing throughout an individual's lifetime.

It is useful to conceptualize the treatment of mood disorders in three phases: treatment of acute episodes, continued treatment, and long-term maintenance, or prophylactic treatment (41,64). Acute treatment lasts from the beginning of a depressive or manic episode until its remission. This phase of treatment usually involves medication or electroconvulsive therapy (see later discussion) and psy-

Box 3-D—*Alcohol, Drugs, and Mental Disorders*

While alcohol and drug problems in society may not be attributable primarily to mental disorders, they are apparently exacerbated among people with mental disorders. Regier and colleagues (1990), in the most comprehensive study to date, found a high prevalence of comorbid (that is, occurring at the same time) mental disorders and alcohol or other drug disorders—including both abuse and dependence syndromes, as defined in the DSM-III-R (figure 3-2). They used data from NIMH's Epidemiologic Catchment Area (ECA) survey of 20,291 adults in the community and in various institutional settings (prisons, mental hospitals, nursing homes, and specialized treatment centers).

The study assessed the prevalence of comorbid alcohol, other drug, and mental disorders from the perspective of three categories of primary disorder: mental disorders, alcohol disorders, and other drug disorders. Schizophrenia, mood disorders, and anxiety disorders were among those studied. Specific drugs studied, in addition to alcohol, include marijuana, cocaine, opiates, barbiturates, amphetamines, and hallucinogens.

An estimated 13.5 percent of all adults in the United States will have a diagnosis of alcohol abuse or dependence: Of this number, 36.6 percent will have at least one mental disorder and 21.5 percent another

Figure 3-2—Substance Abuse and Mental Disorders

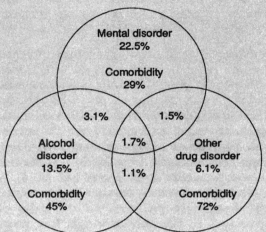

Epidemiological data suggest that there is a high degree of comorbidity for mental and addictive disorders in the United States. For example, 29 percent of individuals with a mental disorder will also have an addictive disorder.

SOURCE: D.A. Regier, M.E. Farmer, D.S. Rae, et al., "Comorbidity of Mental Disorders With Alcohol and Other Drug Abuse: Results From the Epidemiologic Catchment Area (ECA) Study," *Journal of the American Medical Association* 264: 2511-2518, 1990.

drug disorder in their lifetime. Specific comorbid mental disorders found in people with alcohol abuse-dependence disorder include anxiety disorders (19.4 percent), mood disorders (13.4 percent), and schizophrenia (3.8 percent). Some 6.1 percent of the total adult population will have abused or been dependent on drugs other than alcohol at some time in their lives: Of this number, 53.1 percent will have a mental disorder and 47.3 percent will have an alcohol abuse-dependence disorder. Of people with comorbid mental disorders, 28.3 percent will have an anxiety disorder, 26.4 percent will have a mood disorder, and 6.8 percent will have schizophrenia.

At some time in their lives, 22.5 percent of all adults in the United States will have a diagnosis of mental disorder: Of this number, 22.3 percent will also have an alcohol abuse or dependence disorder, 14.7 percent will have a drug abuse-dependence disorder, and 28.9 percent will have either alcohol or drug disorders. Compared to individuals with no history of mental disorder, people with a diagnosis of mental disorder face twice the odds of having alcohol abuse-dependence and over four times the odds of drug abuse-dependence.

Comorbid alcohol and other drug abuse or dependence disorders occur frequently in people with the specific subtypes of mental disorders included in this study. Of those who develop schizophrenia and related disorders during their lifetime (approximately 1.0 percent of the U.S. population), 47 percent will abuse or be dependent on alcohol or other drugs, or both. Thirty-two percent of people with mood disorders (8.3 percent of the total adult population) will abuse or become dependent on alcohol, other drugs, or both. Within this group, over 60 percent of people with bipolar disorder will abuse or become dependent on alcohol, other drugs, or both. About 27 percent of people with major depression will have an alcohol or other drug disorder, or both, odds almost two times greater than those for people without major depression. The anxiety disorders, as a group, occur at some time in the lives of 14.6 percent of the population and are highly likely to be associated with an alcohol or other drug abuse or dependence disorder. For example, 35.8 percent of people with panic disorder and 32.8 percent of people with obsessive-compulsive disorder will have some form of alcohol or other drug abuse or dependence disorder.

SOURCES: R.E. Drake, F.C. Osher, and M.A. Wallach, "Alcohol Use and Abuse in Schizophrenia: A Prospective Community Study," *Journal of Nervous and Mental Disease* 177:408-414, 1989; F.K. Goodwin and K.R. Jamison, *Manic-Depressive Illness* (New York, NY: The Oxford University Press, 1990); D.A. Regier, M.E. Farmer, D.S. Rae, et al., "Comorbidity of Mental Disorders With Alcohol and Other Drug Abuse: Results From the Epidemiologic Catchment Area (ECA) Study," *Journal of the American Medical Association* 264:2511-2518, 1990.

chotherapy; it may involve hospitalization.[5] Continued treatment consists of those interventions maintained from the time of a remission until a second episode would be expected to occur. Long-term maintenance is intended to prevent or attenuate future episodes.

The depressive and manic symptoms of mood disorders are generally well managed with a wide array of medications. Significant advances have occurred in the pharmacological treatment of major depression during the last decade (10). Traditional antidepressant medications include tricyclic antidepressants, monoamine oxidase inhibitors (MAOIs), and newer antidepressant drugs (table 3-5). Various other agents are under development (see ch. 4). A therapeutic response usually requires days to weeks; a good response is predicted on the basis of symptoms such as insomnia or weight loss, more severe symptoms, past episodes of depression, or a family history of mood disorders.

Antidepressant agents have varying side effects. Tricyclic antidepressants may lead to such side effects as a dry mouth, constipation, sedation, nervousness, weight gain, increased appetite, or diminished sexual drive. MAOIs, which are generally used for patients who fail to respond to tricyclic antidepressants, can interact with certain foods and medications, producing potentially fatal bouts of hypertension. Fluoxetine, or Prozac, is a newer antidepressant that produces fewer of these side effects, making it the most widely prescribed antidepressant agent in the United States in 1989. Prozac often facilitates weight loss. Its side effects include nausea, tremor, insomnia, and nervousness. A minority of patients may suffer from agitation or anxiety when using Prozac.[6]

Psychotherapy, either alone or as an adjunct to medication, is important in treating depression (37,38). Various psychotherapeutic approaches are used, including supportive psychotherapy, behavioral therapy, psychodynamic psychotherapy, cognitive therapy, interpersonal psychotherapy, and others (table 3-6). While studies have generally found psychotherapy to be an effective intervention in

Table 3-5—Medications for the Treatment of Depression

Class of medication	Generic name	Brand name
Tricyclic antidepressants	amitriptyline	Elavil, Endep
	nortriptyline	Aventyl, Pamelor
	protriptyline	Vivactil
	desipramine	Norpramin, Pertrofran
	doxepin	Adapin, Sinequan
	imipramine	Tofranil, Imavate
Inhibitors	tranylcypromine	Parnate
	phenelzine	Nardil
Newer antidepressants	fluoxetine	Prozac
	sertraline	Zoloft

SOURCE: Adapted from American Psychological Association, *Women and Depression: Risk Factors and Treatment Issues* (Washington, DC: American Psychological Association, 1990).

depression, positive outcomes have not been linked to any particular approach (5,33,80,109). This suggests that some element or elements common to all forms of psychotherapy produce the positive effects.

In cases of severe depression, or when an individual is suicidal, hospitalization may be required. Electroconvulsive therapy (ECT) may also be used in these instances (4,15,88). ECT generally relieves symptoms of depression rapidly, but it results in memory loss for an indeterminate period of time following the procedure. In the case of SAD, phototherapy can be applied (87). This treatment involves exposure to bright artificial light in the early morning, in the evening, or at both times. It is generally effective in relieving the symptoms of depression in SAD, with few, if any, side effects.

The symptoms of bipolar disorder are treated with medication (41). Depressive episodes are treated with antidepressant drugs, as described above. Severe cases of mania require hospitalization. When psychosis accompanies bouts of mania, antipsychotic medication is indicated. Lithium carbonate is crucial in the treatment of bipolar disorder. It is used to diminish manic symptoms and to prevent new episodes from occurring. However, lithium does produce side effects, such as increased thirst and urination, memory problems, tremor, and weight gain, that may cause patients not to comply with treatment. Long-term treatment with lithium, which

---

[5] Mood disorders account for the second most frequent diagnosis in inpatient facilities and for the largest percentage of patients in private psychiatric hospitals and nonfederal general hospitals (68).

[6] Prozac has been under siege as a factor in suicide and other violent acts. The U.S. Food and Drug Administration has ruled that there is insufficient evidence indicting the drug.

Table 3-6—Psychotherapy and Depression

Modality	Definition
Behavioral therapy	A form of psychotherapy that focuses on modifying faulty behavior rather than basic changes in the personality. Instead of probing the unconscious or exploring the patient's thoughts and feelings, behavior therapists seek to eliminate symptoms and to modify ineffective or maladaptive patterns by applying basic learning techniques and other methods. (Examples: relaxation therapy, self-control therapy, social skills training.)
Cognitive therapy	A psychotherapeutic approach based on the concept that emotional problems are the result of faulty ways of thinking and distorted attitudes toward oneself and others. The therapist takes the role of an active guide who helps the patient correct and revise his or her perceptions and attitudes by citing evidence to the contrary or eliciting it from the patient. The therapist uses cognitive and behavioral techniques to correct distortions of thinking associated with depression, that is, pessimism about oneself, the world, and the future. Brief treatment.
Interpersonal psychotherapy	A form of psychotherapy in which the therapist seeks to help the patient to identify and better understand his or her interpersonal problems and conflicts and to develop more adaptive ways of relating to others. The therapist focuses on client's current interpersonal relationships. Helps clients learn more effective ways of relating to others and coping with conflicts in relationships. Brief, focused treatment.
Psychodynamic psychotherapy	Any form or technique of psychotherapy that focuses on the underlying, often unconscious factors (drives and experiences) that determine behavior and adjustment.

SOURCE: Adapted from American Psychological Association, *Women and Depression: Risk Factors and Treatment Issues* (Washington, DC: American Psychological Association, 1990).

is generally necessary, can have toxic effects on the thyroid gland, the kidney, and the nervous system. Lithium can also cause abnormalities in the fetuses of women taking the drug. The anticonvulsive drug carbamazepine is an alternative for persons who do not respond to lithium or are intolerant of its side effects. In addition to drug therapy, supportive psychotherapy is generally required to help patients understand and deal with symptoms of bipolar disorder.

Anxiety Disorders

In this age of crowding, traffic jams, time pressures, and media bombardment of our minds with horrific tragedies, it is no wonder that some people consider this the Age of Anxiety, as Leonard Bernstein entitled his symphony. Everyone experiences anxiety at some time—that diffuse feeling of unease or apprehension, usually of a vague or unknown threat. The manifestations of anxiety vary from individual to individual and may include a racing heartbeat, butterflies in the stomach, or a headache. It is different from fear, which is an immediate, strong response to sudden and imminent danger, such as a car approaching rapidly as one crosses the street. Anxiety may produce a paradoxical effect—bringing about that which the person fears most. For example, a person who is anxious about public speaking may find himself or herself muted by anxiety. However, anxiety can serve a positive function—it can prompt actions that ward off potential threats to well-being. For example, anxiety about an upcoming exam may lead to increased study.

Anxiety can be pathological. According to the DSM-III-R, pathological anxiety can be separated into what are called anxiety disorders, including panic disorder, phobias, obsessive-compulsive disorder, posttraumatic stress disorder, and generalized anxiety disorder (3). Pathological symptoms of anxiety are often present in other disorders, notably depression (13,40,56,70). Although anxiety disorders are grouped together by their symptoms, they are quite different in how they are best treated, and they appear to have quite different causes. We concentrate on panic disorder and obsessive-compulsive disorder because the role of biological factors in causing them has been more fully explored and is considered by many to be paramount.

Box 3-E—The Auto Accident That Never Was

I'm driving down the highway doing 55 MPH. I'm on my way to take a final exam. My seat belt is buckled and I'm vigilantly following all the rules of the road. No one is on the highway—not a living soul.

Out of nowhere an Obsessive-Compulsive Disorder (OCD) attack strikes. It's almost magical the way it distorts my perception of reality. While in reality no one is on the road, I'm intruded with the heinous thought that I *might* have hit someone . . . a human being! God knows where such a fantasy comes from.

I think about this for a second and then say to myself, "That's ridiculous. I didn't hit anybody." Nonetheless, a gnawing anxiety is born. An anxiety I will ultimately not be able to put away until an enormous emotional price has been paid.

I try to make reality chase away this fantasy. I reason, "Well, if I hit someone while driving, I would have *felt* it." This brief trip into reality helps the pain dissipate . . . but only for a second. Why? Because the gnawing anxiety that I really did commit the illusionary accident is growing larger—so is the pain.

The pain is a terrible guilt that I have committed an unthinkable, negligent act. At one level, I know this is ridiculous, but there's a terrible pain in my stomach telling me something quite different.

Again, I try putting to rest this insane thought and that ugly feeling of guilt. "Come on," I think to myself, "this is *really* insane!"

But the awful feeling persists. The anxious pain says to me, "*You Really Did Hit Someone.*" The attack is now in full control. Reality no longer has meaning. My sensory system is distorted. I have to get rid of the pain. Checking out this fantasy is the only way I know how.

I start ruminating, "Maybe I did hit someone and didn't realize it. . . . Oh my God! I might have killed somebody! I have to go back and check." Checking is the only way to calm the anxiety. It brings me closer to truth somehow. I can't live with the thought that I actually may have killed someone—I have to check it out. . . .

I think to myself, "Rush to check it out. Get rid of the hurt by checking it out. Hurry back to check it out. God, I'll be late for my final exam if I check it out. But I have no choice. Someone could be lying on the road, bloody, close to death." Fantasy is now my only reality. So is my pain.

I've driven five miles farther down the road since the attack's onset. I turn the car around and head back to the scene of the mythical mishap. I return to the spot on the road where I "think" it "might" have occurred. Naturally, nothing is there. No police car and no bloodied body. Relieved, I turn around again to get to my exam on time.

Feeling better, I drive for about twenty seconds and then the lingering thoughts and pain start gnawing away again. Only this time they're even more intense. I think, "Maybe I should have pulled *off* the road and checked the side brush where the injured body was thrown and now lies? Maybe I didn't go *far enough* back on the road and the accident occurred a mile farther back."

The pain of my possibly having hurt somebody is now so intense that I have no choice—I really see it this way.

I turn the car around a second time and head an extra mile farther down the road to find the corpse. I drive by quickly. Assured that this time I've gone far enough I head back to school to take my exam. But I'm not through yet.

"My God," my attack relentlessly continues, "I didn't get out of the car to actually *look* on the side of the road!"

Obsessive-Compulsive Disorder

Obsessive-compulsive disorder (OCD) is characterized by recurrent and persistent thoughts, images, or ideas that are experienced as intrusive and senseless (obsessions) and stereotypic, repetitive, and purposeful actions perceived as unnecessary (compulsions) (box 3-E) (79) (table 3-7). Individuals with OCD cannot resist these persistent ideas or impulses, although they view them as irrational and unwanted. One common manifestation of this disorder is the obsessive feeling of being dirty or contaminated, which leads to the compulsion of repeated hand-washing (table 3-8). Hand-washing may be so frequent that the skin is rubbed raw. Another common obsession is excessive doubt, which leads to compulsive checking. For example, an individual fears that he or she has left the stove on or the door unlocked, resulting in his or her checking and rechecking the stove or door. The doubts often reflect concern for a dangerous outcome or a

So I turn back a third time. I drive to the part of the highway where I think the accident happened. I park the car on the highway's shoulder. I get out and begin rummaging around in the brush. A police car comes up. I feel like I'm going out of my mind.

The policeman, seeing me thrash through the brush, asks, "What are you doing? Maybe I can help you?"

Well, I'm in a dilemma. I can't say, "Officer, please don't worry. You see, I've got obsessive-compulsive disorder, along with 4 million Americans. I'm simply acting out a compulsion with obsessive qualities." I can't even say, "I'm really sick. Please help me." The disease is so insidious and embarrassing that it cannot be admitted to anyone. Anyway, so few really understand it, including myself.

So I tell the officer I was nervous about my exam and pulled off to the roadside to throw up. The policeman gives me a sincere and knowing smile and wishes me well.

But I start thinking again. "Maybe an accident did happen and the body has been cleared off the road. The policeman's here to see if I came back to the scene of the crime. God, maybe I really did hit someone . . . why else would a police car be in the area?" Then I realize he would have asked me about it. But would he, if he was trying to catch me?

I'm so caught up in the anxiety and these awful thoughts that I momentarily forget why I am standing on the side of the road. I'm back on the road again. The anxiety is peaking. Maybe the policeman didn't know about the accident? I should go back and conduct my search more *thoroughly*.

I want to go back and check more . . . but I can't. You see, the police car is tailing me on the highway. I'm now close to hysteria because I honestly believe someone is lying in the brush bleeding to death. Yes . . . the pain makes me believe this. "After all," I reason, "why would the pain be there in the first place?"

I arrive at school late for the exam. I have trouble taking the exam because I can't stop obsessing on the fantasy. The thoughts of the mystical accident keep intruding. Somehow I get through it.

The moment I get out of the exam I'm back on the road checking again. But now I'm checking two things. First that I didn't kill or maim someone and second, that the policeman doesn't catch me checking. After all, if I should be spotted on the roadside rummaging around the brush a second time, how in the world can I possibly explain such an incriminating and aimless action? I'm totally exhausted, but that awful anxiety keeps me checking, though a part of my psyche keeps telling me that this checking behavior is ridiculous, that it serves absolutely no purpose. But, with OCD, there is no other way.

Finally, after repeated checks, I'm able to break the ritual. I head home, dead tired. I know that if I can sleep it off, I'll feel better. Sometimes the pain dissipates through an escape into sleep.

I manage to lie down on my bed—hoping for sleep. But the incident has not totally left me—nor has the anxiety. I think, "If I really did hit someone, there would be a dent in the car's fender."

What I now do is no mystery to anyone. I haul myself up from bed and run out to the garage to check the fenders on the car. First I check the front two fenders, see no damage, and head back to bed. But. . . *did I check it well enough?*

I get up from bed again and now find myself checking the *whole body* of the car. I know this is absurd, but I can't help myself. Finally . . . finally, I disengage and head off to my room to sleep. Before I nod off, my last thought is, "I wonder what I'll check next?"

SOURCE: Description of OCD by a 36-year-old male professional who has the disorder, in J.L. Rapoport, *The Boy Who Couldn't Stop Washing* (New York, NY: American Library, 1989). Reprinted by permission of Dr. Rapoport.

gnawing sense of guilt. Another common obsession is with symmetry or order, leading to the compulsion of repeatedly going in and out of a door or ordering and arranging various items.

Less frequently, an individual may be plagued only by obsessional thoughts, without any compulsions, such as a preoccupation with sexual or aggressive acts that are abhorrent to the individual. And finally, individuals may express what is called "an obsessional slowness." In this manifestation, an individual takes hours to eat a single meal or to brush his or her teeth in a ritualistic fashion.

Many individuals with OCD also have another diagnosis, the most common being depression (54,79). In fact, OCD was once posited to be a type of mood disorder because of the intimate link between its symptoms and those of depression. Other problems that may be associated with OCD include other anxiety disorders, eating disorders, alcohol abuse, Tourette's syndrome, and psychosis. The comorbid-

Table 3-7—The Diagnosis of Obsessive-Compulsive Disorder

A. Either obsessions or compulsions:
Obsessions: (1), (2), (3), and (4):
1. recurrent and persistent ideas, thoughts, impulses, or images that are experienced, at least initially, as intrusive and senseless, e.g., a parent's having repeated impulses to kill a loved child, a religious person's having recurrent blasphemous thoughts;
2. the person attempts to ignore or suppress such thoughts or impulses or to neutralize them with some other thought or action;
3. the person recognizes that the obsessions are the product of his or her own mind, not imposed from without (as in thought insertion);
4. if another Axis I disorder is present, the content of the obsession is unrelated to it, e.g., the ideas, thoughts, impulses, or images are not about food in the presence of an eating disorder, about drugs in the presence of a psychoactive substance use disorder, or guilty thoughts in the presence of a major depression.

Compulsions: (1), (2), and (3):
1. repetitive, purposeful, and intentional behaviors that are performed in response to an obsession, or according to certain rules or in a stereotyped fashion;
2. the behavior is designed to neutralize or to prevent discomfort or some dreaded event or situation; however, either the activity is not connected in a realistic way with what it is designed to neutralize or prevent, or it is clearly excessive;
3. the person recognizes that his or her behavior is excessive or unreasonable (this may not be true for young children; it may no longer be true for people whose obsessions have evolved into overvalued ideas).

B. The obsessions or compulsions cause marked distress, are time-consuming (take more than an hour a day), or significantly interfere with the person's normal routine, occupational functioning, or usual social activities or relationships with others.

SOURCE: American Psychiatric Association, *Diagnostic and Statistical Manual of Mental Disorders*, 3rd ed., rev. (Washington, DC: American Psychiatric Association, 1987).

ity of OCD and neurological disorders such as Tourette's syndrome suggests that they have the same anatomical basis (see ch. 4).

Recent epidemiological data indicate that OCD, once thought to be quite rare, afflicts approximately 2.6 percent of the U.S. population at some time during their lives (54). Men and women appear to be afflicted equally, although OCD may be slightly more common among women. The symptoms begin in childhood or adolescence in one-third to one-half of the individuals who develop the disorder; the average age of onset is 20. While the symptoms of OCD usually seem to be unprovoked, stressful life events may precipitate or exacerbate them. Sometimes symptoms recede completely with time, but most often patients suffer chronic OCD, with symptoms waxing and waning. Some patients,

however, suffer a continuous or deteriorating course; their symptoms may become so extreme that hospitalization is necessary. Followup studies of individuals who have been treated clinically show that the disorder is chronic and recurrent; at least 50 percent of those treated with psychotherapy or older drug therapies suffered from the disease for 7 to 20 years.

OCD was long thought to be resistant to treatment, with antidepressant drugs being prescribed to relieve the accompanying symptoms of depression (28). Currently there are two primary treatments for OCD that may be effective: behavioral therapy and/or medication (28,47,48,76). Behavioral therapy entails repeated exposure of the patient to the stimulus that sets off a ritualistic act. For example, if a patient has a compulsion to wash his or her hands 20 to 30 times a day, the patient's hands may be deliberately dirtied and the patient prevented from washing them. This approach seems to be more effective in treating compulsions than in treating obsessions. Medications acting on the brain chemical serotonin (see ch. 4) have proven quite effective, with the drug clomipramine (Anafranil) commonly used to treat OCD. The therapeutic effects of this drug may take days or weeks to manifest themselves, and this drug too may be more effective in treating compulsions than obsessions. The side effects of clomipramine are those typical of tricyclic antidepressants (see earlier discussion).

Panic Disorder

The hallmark symptom of panic disorder is a sudden, inexplicable attack of intense fear that is associated with powerful physical symptoms. A panic attack typically unfolds quite rapidly: In just a few minutes, an extreme sense of fear overtakes an individual, his or her heart begins racing, he or she starts to perspire—sometimes profusely—and he or she has trouble breathing (table 3-9). A single attack is short-lived, lasting 20 minutes to an hour on average. These symptoms often leave a patient believing that he or she is suffering from a heart attack or is losing his or her mind. Some patients go to the emergency room in the belief that they are about to die from a heart attack. In fact, many individuals with panic disorder seek general medical professional care at an increased rate (69). Individuals with panic disorder may receive repeated and extensive diagnostic testing for cardiac or neurological problems (61).

Table 3-8—Obsessions and Compulsions

Obsessions	Reported symptom at initial interview[a]	
	(no.)	(%)
Concern with dirt, germs, or environmental toxins	28	(40)
Something terrible happening (fire, death, or illness of self or loved one)	17	(24)
Symmetry, order, or exactness	12	(17)
Scrupulosity (religious obsessions)	9	(13)
Concern or disgust with bodily wastes or secretions (urine, stool, saliva)	6	(8)
Lucky or unlucky numbers	6	(8)
Forbidden, aggressive, or perverse sexual thoughts, images, or impulses	3	(4)
Fear might harm others or oneself	3	(4)
Concern with household items	2	(3)
Intrusive nonsense sounds, words, or music	1	(1)

Compulsions	Reported symptom at initial interview	
	(no.)	(%)
Excessive or ritualized hand-washing, showering, bathing, tooth-brushing, or grooming	60	(85)
Repeating rituals (going in or out of a door, up or down from a chair)	36	(51)
Checking (doors, locks, stove, appliances, emergency brake on car, paper route, homework)	32	(46)
Rituals to remove contact with contaminants	16	(23)
Touching	14	(20)
Measures to prevent harm to self or others	11	(16)
Ordering or arranging	12	(17)
Counting	13	(18)
Hoarding or collecting rituals	8	(11)
Rituals of cleaning household or inanimate objects	4	(6)
Miscellaneous rituals (such as writing, moving, speaking) ...	18	(26)

[a]The most frequent obsessions and compulsions among 70 children and adolescents who were diagnosed as having OCD by the author and her colleagues at the National Institute of Mental Health (NIMH). The proportions total more than 100 percent because many sufferers have more than one symptom.

SOURCE: J.L. Rapoport, "The Biology of Obsessions and Compulsions," *Scientific American* 260(3):83-89, 1990.

Panic attacks occur about two times a week, although the frequency varies considerably among patients. One person's panic attack may be rare, having little effect on his or her functioning, while another's panic attacks and accompanying anxiety may be so intense that he or she remains completely sequestered at home (99). Individuals with panic disorder often exhibit other disorders. They may develop a fear of being in public places (agoraphobia), especially because they may be embarrassed or unable to leave a situation quickly. In fact, the majority of individuals diagnosed with agoraphobia are thought to have panic attacks, and approximately one-third of individuals with panic disorders also have agoraphobia (107). Depression and substance abuse are common among individuals with panic disorder (box 3-D), and these persons may experience other disorders more frequently also, including mitral valve prolapse, irritable bowel syndrome, asthma, and migraine headaches.

Data show that approximately one to two persons in 100 will develop panic disorder during their lifetime, with women being twice as likely to develop it as men (31,102). While panic attacks have been described in children and adolescents, the average age of onset is 24. Forty percent of patients experience the onset of panic disorder before the age of 30 (71).

A panic attack usually emerges unprovoked, although a stressful life event may precipitate it. As attacks continue to occur, they preoccupy the patient, and the patient may become generally anxious or depressed. Further research is needed to determine the long-term course of panic disorder; however, data suggest that many patients suffer chronic panic attacks, with the severity of symptoms waxing and waning over time (77).

Panic disorder is treated with medication or psychotherapy or both (12,25,75). Antidepressant

Table 3-9—The Diagnosis of Panic Disorder

A. At some time during the disturbance, one or more panic attacks (discrete periods of intense fear or discomfort) have occurred that were: 1) unexpected, i.e., did not occur immediately before or on exposure to a situation that almost always caused anxiety, and 2) not triggered by situations in which the person was the focus of others' attention.

B. Either four attacks, as defined in criterion A, have occurred within a 4-week period, or one or more attacks have been followed by a period of at least a month of persistent fear of having another attack.

C. At least four of the following symptoms developed during at least one of the attacks:
1. shortness of breath (dyspnea) or smothering sensations;
2. dizziness, unsteady feelings, or faintness;
3. palpitations or accelerated heart rate (tachycardia);
4. trembling or shaking;
5. sweating;
6. choking;
7. nausea or abdominal distress;
8. depersonalization or derealization;
9. numbness or tingling sensations (paresthesias);
10. flushes (hot flashes) or chills;
11. chest pain or discomfort;
12. fear of dying;
13. fear of going crazy or of doing something uncontrolled.

Note: Attacks involving four or more symptoms are panic attacks; attacks involving fewer than four symptoms are limited symptom attacks.

D. During at least some of the attacks, at least four of the C symptoms developed suddenly and increased in intensity within ten minutes of the beginning of the first C symptom noticed in the attack.

E. It cannot be established that an organic factor initiated and maintained the disturbance, e.g., amphetamine or caffeine intoxication, hyperthyroidism.

Note: Mitral valve prolapse may be an associated condition, but does not preclude a diagnosis of panic disorder.

SOURCE: American Psychiatric Association, *Diagnostic and Statistical Manual of Mental Disorders,* 3rd ed., rev. (Washington, DC: American Psychiatric Association, 1987).

drugs (see earlier discussion), including tricyclics (such as imipramine) and MAOIs (such as phenelzine), and antianxiety agents (such as the benzodiazepine alprazolam) are somewhat effective (11,71,107). The antidepressants generally require several weeks of administration before they become effective. Their side effects were discussed previously. Antianxiety agents act quickly and are therefore useful in acute situations. These medications may pose a risk of dependence, however, and thus may not be appropriate for long-term use (23). Behavioral therapy aimed at reducing phobic avoidance and anticipatory anxiety may help diminish panic attacks and the anxiety associated with them. Relaxation techniques may also be useful. Cognitive therapy, aimed at helping individuals restructure their think-ing and develop a different way of looking at that which they fear, is also used. Cognitive and behavioral therapy usually diminish the severity and frequency of panic attacks. There is not enough information available to compare the effectiveness of psychotherapeutic and pharmacological approaches. Further information concerning the optimal duration of treatment is also necessary.

CHAPTER 3 REFERENCES

1. Akiskal, H.S., ''The Milder Spectrum of Bipolar Disorders: Diagnostic, Characteristic, and Pharmacologic,'' *Psychiatry Annals* 17:32-37, 1987.
2. American Psychiatric Association, *Diagnostic and Statistical Manual of Mental Disorders,* 3rd ed. (Washington, DC: American Psychiatric Association, 1980).
3. American Psychiatric Association, *Diagnostic and Statistical Manual of Mental Disorders,* 3rd ed., rev. (Washington, DC: American Psychiatric Association, 1987).
4. American Psychiatric Association, *The Practice of Electroconvulsive Therapy: Recommendations for Treatment, Training, and Privileging. A Task Force Report of the American Psychiatric Association* (Washington, DC: American Psychiatric Association, 1990).
5. American Psychological Association, *Women and Depression: Risk Factors and Treatment Issues,* E. McGrath, G.P. Keita, B.R. Strickland, and N.F. Russo (eds.) (Washington, DC: American Psychological Association, 1990).
6. Andreasen, N.C., ''Negative Symptoms in Schizophrenia: Definition and Reliability,'' *Archives of General Psychiatry* 39:784-788, 1982.
7. Andreasen, N.C., ''Negative Versus Positive Schizophrenia: Definition and Validation,'' *Archives of General Psychiatry* 39:789-794, 1982.
8. Andreasen, N.C., *The Broken Brain: The Biological Revolution in Psychiatry* (New York, NY: Harper & Row, 1984).
9. Andreasen, N.C., ''The Diagnosis of Schizophrenia,'' *Schizophrenia Bulletin* 13:9-22, 1987.
10. Baldessarini, R.J., ''Drugs and the Treatment of Psychiatric Disorders,'' *The Pharmacological Basis of Therapeutics,* 8th ed., A. Goodman Gilman, T.W. Rall, A.S. Nies, and P. Taylor (eds.) (New York, NY: Pergamon Press, 1990).
11. Ballenger, J.C., ''Long-Term Pharmacologic Treatment of Panic Disorder,'' *Journal of Clinical Psychiatry* 52(suppl.):18-23, 1991.
12. Barlow, D.H., ''Long-Term Outcome for Patients With Panic Disorder Treated With Cognitive-Behavioral Therapy,'' *Journal of Clinical Psychiatry* A51(suppl.):17-23, 1990.

13. Barlow, D.H., DiNardo, P.A., Vermilyea, B.B., et al., "Co-Morbidity and Depression Among the Anxiety Disorders," *Journal of Nervous and Mental Diseases* 174:63-72, 1986.
14. Berkman, L.F., Berkman, C.S., Kasl, S., et al., "Depressive Symptoms in Relation to Physical Health and Functioning in the Elderly," *American Journal of Epidemiology* 124:372-388, 1986.
15. Black, D.W., Winokur, G., and Nasrallah, A., "ECT in Unipolar and Bipolar Disorders: A Naturalistic Evaluation of 460 Patients," *Convulsive Therapy* 2:231-237, 1986.
16. Bleuler, E., *Dementia Praecox or the Group of Schizophrenias*, J. Zinken (trans.) (New York, NY: International Universities Press, 1950).
17. Brakel, S.J., Parry, J., and Weiner, B.A., *The Mentally Disabled and the Law*, 3rd ed. (Chicago, IL: American Bar Foundation, 1985).
18. *Brewer* v. *Lincoln Nation*, 8th Circuit Court, No. 90-1227EM.
19. Burke, K.C., Burke, J.D., and Regier, D.A., et al., "Age at Onset of Selected Mental Disorders in Five Community Populations," *Archives of General Psychiatry* 47:511-518, 1990.
20. Carpenter, W.T., and Buchanan, R.W., "Domains of Psychopathology Relevant to the Study of Etiology and Treatment of Schizophrenia," *Schizophrenia: Scientific Progress*, S.C. Schulz and C.T. Tamminga (eds.) (New York, NY: Oxford University Press, 1989).
21. Carpenter, W.T., and Keith, S.J., "Integrating Treatments in Schizophrenia," *Psychiatric Clinics of North America*, vol. 9 (Philadelphia, PA: W.B. Saunders, 1986).
22. Carpenter, W.T., and Kirkpatrick, B.W., "The Heterogeneity of the Long-Term Course of Schizophrenia," *Schizophrenia Bulletin* 14:645-652, 1988.
23. Coryell, W., and Winokur, G. (eds.), *The Clinical Management of Anxiety Disorders* (New York, NY: Oxford University Press, 1991).
24. Crowe, T.J., "The Continuum of Psychosis and Its Implications for the Structure of the Gene," *British Journal of Psychiatry* 149:419-429, 1986.
25. Davidson, J.R.T., "Continuation Treatment of Panic Disorder With High-Potency Benzodiazepines," *Journal of Clinical Psychiatry* A51(suppl.):31-37, 1990.
26. Deanfield, J.E., Shea, M., Kensett, M., et al., "Silent Myocardial Ischaemia Due to Mental Stress," *Lancet* 2:1001-1005, 1984.
27. Dembroski, T.M., MacDougall, J.M., Costa, P.T., et al., "Components of Hostility as Predictors of Sudden Death and Myocardial Infarction in the Multiple Risk Factor Intervention Trial," *Psychosomatic Medicine* 51:514-522, 1989.
28. DeVeaugh-Geiss, J., "Pharmacologic Treatment of Obsessive-Compulsive Disorder," *The Psychobiology of Obsessive-Compulsive Disorder*, J. Zohar, T. Insel, and S. Rasmussen (eds.) (New York, NY: Springer Publishing, 1991).
29. Dohrenwend, B.P., Levav, I., Shrout, P.E., et al., "Socioeconomic Status and Psychiatric Disorders: The Causation-Selection Issue," *Science* 255:946-952, 1992.
30. Eaton, W.W., "Epidemiology of Schizophrenia," *Epidemiological Review* 7:105-126, 1985.
31. Eaton, W.W., Dryman, A., and Weissman, M.N., "Panic and Phobia," *Psychiatric Disorders in America: The Epidemiologic Catchment Area Study*, L.N. Robins and D.A. Regier (eds.) (New York, NY: Free Press, 1991).
32. Eisenberg, L., "Treating Depression and Anxiety in Primary Care: Closing the Gap Between Knowledge and Practice," *New England Journal of Medicine* 326: 1080-1084, 1992.
33. Elkin, I., Shea, T., Watkins, J.T., et al., "National Institute of Mental Health Treatment of Depression Collaborative Research Program: General Effectiveness of Treatments," *Archives of General Psychiatry* 46:971-982, 1989.
34. Engel, G.L., "The Clinical Application of the Biopsychosocial Model," *American Journal of Psychiatry* 137:535-544, 1980.
35. Farmer, A.E., McGuffin, P., and Gottesman, I.I., "Twin Concordance for DSM-III Schizophrenia: Scrutinizing the Validity of the Definition," *Archives of General Psychiatry* 44:634-641, 1987.
36. Frances, A., Pincus, H.A., Widiger, T.A., et al., "DSM-IV: Work in Progress," *American Journal of Psychiatry* 147:1439-1448, 1990.
37. Frank, E., Kupfer, D.J., Peret, J.M., et al., "Three-Year Outcomes for Maintenance Therapies in Recurrent Depression," *Archives of General Psychiatry* 47:1093-1099, 1990.
38. Frank, E., Kupfer, D.J., Wagner, E.F., et al., "Efficacy of Interpersonal Psychotherapy as a Maintenance Treatment of Recurrent Depression With Contributing Factors," *Archives of General Psychiatry* 48:1053-1059, 1991.
39. Goodman, A., "Organic Unity Theory: The Mind-Body Problem Revisited," *American Journal of Psychiatry* 148:553-563, 1991.
40. Goodwin, D.W., and Guze, S.B., *Psychiatric Diagnosis*, 4th ed. (New York, NY: Oxford University Press, 1989).
41. Goodwin, F.K., and Jamison, K.R., *Manic-Depressive Illness* (New York, NY: Oxford University Press, 1990).
42. Gottesman, I.I., *Schizophrenia Genesis: The Origins of Madness* (New York, NY: W.H. Freeman, 1991).

43. Gurlach, J., "New Antipsychotic Classification, Efficacy, and Adverse Effects," *Schizophrenia Bulletin* 17:247-261, 1991.

44. Guze, S.B., and Robins, E., "Suicide and Primary Affective Disorders," *British Journal of Psychiatry* 117:437-438, 1970.

45. Hadley, S.W., and Strupp, H.H., "Contemporary Views of Negative Effects in Psychotherapy," *Archives of General Psychiatry* 33:1291-1302, 1976.

46. Hartmann, L., "Response to the Presidential Address: Humane Values and Biopsychosocial Integration," *American Journal of Psychiatry* 148:1130-1134, 1991.

47. Insel, T.R., and Murphy, D.L., "The Psychopharmacological Treatment of Obsessive-Compulsive Disorder: A Review," *Journal of Clinical Psychopharmacology* 1:304-311, 1981.

48. Insel, T.R., Mueller, E.A., Gillin, J.C., et al., "Tricyclic Response in Obsessive-Compulsive Disorder," *Progress in Neuropsychopharmacology and Biological Psychiatry* 9:25-31, 1985.

49. Jamison, K.R., "Mood Disorders and Seasonal Patterns in British Writers and Artists," *Psychiatry* 52:125-134, 1989.

50. Kane, J.M., "Schizophrenia: Somatic Treatment," *Comprehensive Textbook of Psychiatry*, 5th ed., vol. 1 (Baltimore, MD: Williams & Wilkins, 1989).

51. Kane, J.M., "New Developments in the Pharmacologic Treatment of Schizophrenia," *Schizophrenia Bulletin* 17:193-195, 1991.

52. Kane, J.M., Honigfeld, G., Singer, J., et al., "Clozapine for the Treatment-Resistant Schizophrenic—A Double Blind Comparison With Chlorpromazine," *Archives of General Psychiatry* 45:89-796, 1988.

53. Kaplan, A.L., "The Concepts of Health and Disease," *Medical Ethics*, R.M. Veatch (ed.) (Boston, MA: Jones and Bartlett, 1989).

54. Karno, M., and Golding, J.M., "Obsessive Compulsive Disorder," *Psychiatric Disorders in America: The Epidemiologic Catchment Area Study*, L.N. Robins and D.A. Regier (eds.) (New York, NY: Free Press, 1991).

55. Keith, S.J., Regier, D.A., and Rae, D.S., "Schizophrenic Disorders," *Psychiatric Disorders in America: The Epidemiologic Catchment Area Study*, L.N. Robins and D.A. Regier (eds.) (New York, NY: Free Press, 1991).

56. Keller, M.B., Beardslee, W., Lavori, P.W., et al., "Course of Major Depression in Non-referred Adolescents: A Retrospective Study," *Journal of Affective Disorders* 15:235-243, 1988.

57. Keller, M.B., Lavori, P.W., McDonald-Scott, P., et al., "Reliability of Lifetime Diagnosis and Symptoms in Patients With a Current Psychiatric Disorder," *Journal of Psychiatric Research* 4:229-240, 1981.

58. Kendell, R.E., "Clinical Validity," *The Validity of Psychiatric Diagnosis*, L.N. Robins and J.E. Barrett (eds.) (New York, NY: Raven Press, 1989).

59. Klerman, G.L., "Ideology and Science in the Psychotherapy of Schizophrenia," *Schizophrenia Bulletin* 10:608-612, 1984.

60. Klerman, G.L., Lavori, P.W., Rice, J., et al., "Birth-Cohort Trends in Rates of Major Depressive Disorder Among Relatives of Patients With Affective Disorder," *Archives of General Psychiatry* 42:689-693, 1985.

61. Klerman, G.L., Weissman, M.M., Ouellette, R., et al., "Panic Attacks in the Community: Social Morbidity and Health Care Utilization," *Journal of the American Medical Association* 265:742-746, 1991.

62. Kraepelin, E., *Dementia Praecox and Paraphrenia*, R.M. Barclay and G.M. Robertson (trans.) (Edinburgh, Scotland: E&S Livingstone, 1919).

63. *Kunin v. Benefit Trust Life Insurance Company*.

64. Kupfer, D.J., "Long-Term Treatment of Depression," *Journal of Clinical Psychiatry* 52(suppl.):28-34, 1991.

65. Levinson, D.F., "Pharmacologic Treatment of Schizophrenia," *Clinical Therapeutics* 13:326-352, 1991.

66. Liberman, R.P., Corrigan, P.W., and Schade, H.L., "Drugs and Psychosocial Treatment Interactions in Schizophrenia," *International Review of Psychiatry* 1:283-294, 1989.

67. McHugh, P.R., and Slavney, P.R., *The Perspectives of Psychiatry* (Baltimore, MD: Johns Hopkins University Press, 1983).

68. Manderscheid, R.N., and Sonnenschein, M.A., (eds.) *Mental Health, United States, 1990*, U.S. Department of Health and Human Services, Pub. No. (ADM) 90-1708 (Washington, DC: U.S. Government Printing Office, 1990).

69. Markowitz, J.S., Weissman, M.M., Ouellette, R., et al., "Quality of Life in Panic Disorder," *Archives of General Psychiatry* 46:984-992, 1989.

70. Maser, J.D., and Cloninger, C.R. (eds.), *Comorbidity of Mood and Anxiety Disorders* (Washington, DC: American Psychiatric Press, 1990).

71. Matuzas, W., and Jack, E., "The Drug Treatment of Panic Disorder," *Psychiatric Medicine* 9:215-243, 1991.

72. Mechanic, D., "Recent Developments in Mental Health: Perspectives and Services," *Annual Review of Public Health* 12:1-15, 1991.

73. Melzer, H.Y., Matsubara, S., and Lee, J., "The Ratios of Serotonin and Dopamine-2 Affinities Differentiate Atypical and Typical Antipsychotic

Drugs," *Psychopharmacology Bulletin* 25:390-392, 1989.

74. *Nature*, "Editorial," 336:95, 1988.

75. Noyes, R., and Perry, P., "Maintenance Treatment With Antidepressants in Panic Disorder," *Journal of Clinical Psychiatry* A51(suppl.):24-30, 1990.

76. Perse, T., "Obsessive-Compulsive Disorder: A Treatment Review," *Journal of Clinical Psychiatry* 49:48-55, 1988.

77. Pollack, M.H., Otto, M.W., Rosenbaum, J.F., et al., "Longitudinal Course of Panic Disorder: Findings From the Massachusetts General Hospital Naturalistic Study," *Journal of Clinical Psychiatry* A51(suppl.): 12-16, 1990.

78. Potter, W.Z., Rudorfer, M.V., and Manji, H., "The Pharmacologic Treatment of Depression," *New England Journal of Medicine* 325:633-642, 1991.

79. Rasmussen, S.A., and Eisen, J.L., "Phenomenology of OCD: Clinical Subtypes, Heterogeneity, and Coexistence," *The Psychobiology of Obsessive-Compulsive Disorder*, J. Zohar, T. Insel, and S. Rasmussen (eds.) (New York, NY: Springer Publishing, 1991).

80. Rehm, L.P., "Psychotherapies for Depression," paper presented at the meeting of the Boulder Symposium on Clinical Psychology: Depression, Boulder, CO, April 1989.

81. Robins, E., and Guze, S.B., "Establishment of Diagnostic Validity in Psychiatric Illness: Its Application to Schizophenia," *American Journal of Psychiatry* 126:983-987, 1970.

82. Robins, E., and Guze, S.B., "Classification of Affective Disorders: The Primary-Secondary, the Endogenous-Reactive, and the Neurotic-Psychotic Concepts," *Recent Advances in the Psychobiology of the Depressive Illnesses*, T.A. Williams, M.M. Katz, J.A. Shield, Jr. (eds.) (Washington, DC: U.S. Government Printing Office, 1972).

83. Robins, L.N., and Barrett, J.E., *The Validity of Psychiatric Diagnosis* (New York, NY: Raven Press, 1989).

84. Robins, L.N., and Regier, D.A. (eds.), *Psychiatric Disorders in America: The Epidemiologic Catchment Area Study* (New York, NY: Free Press, 1990).

85. Rochefort, D.A., "Mental Illness and Mental Health as Public Policy Concerns," *Handbook on Mental Health Policy in the United States*, D.A. Rochefort (ed.) (New York, NY: Greenwood Press, 1989).

86. Rodin, G., and Voshart, K., "Depressive Symptoms and Functional Impairment in the Medically Ill," *General Hospital Psychiatry* 9:251-258, 1987.

87. Rosenthal, N.E., and Blehar, M.C. (eds.), *Seasonal Affective Disorders and Phototherapy* (New York, NY: Guilford Press, 1989).

88. Runck, B., "Consensus Panel Backs Cautious Use of ECT for Severe Disorders," *Hospital and Community Psychiatry* 36:943-946, 1985.

89. Safferman, A., Lieberman, J.A., Kane, J.M., et al., "Update on the Clinical Efficacy and Side Effects of Clozapine," *Schizophrenia Bulletin* 17:289-309, 1991.

90. Schooler, N.R., and Keith, S.J., "Role of Medication in Psychosocial Treatment," *Handbook of Schizophrenia, Psychosocial Treatment of Schizophrenia*, vol. 4 (New York, NY: Elsevier Science Publishing, 1990).

91. Spitzer, R.L., Endicott, J., and Robins, E., "Research Diagnostic Criteria: Rationale and Reliability," *Archives of General Psychiatry* 35:773-782, 1978.

92. Stachan, A.M., "Family Intervention for the Rehabilitation of Schizophrenia: Toward Protection and Coping," *Schizophrenia Bulletin* 12:678-698, 1986.

93. Strauss, J.S., and Carpenter, W.T., "The Prediction of Outcome in Schizophrenia. I. Characteristics of Outcome," *Archives of General Psychiatry* 27:739-746, 1972.

94. Strauss, J.S., and Carpenter, W.T., "The Prediction of Outcome in Schizophrenia. II. Relationships Between Predictor and Outcome Variables: A Report From the International Pilot Study of Schizophrenia," *Archives of General Psychiatry* 31:37-42, 1974.

95. Torrey, E.F., *Surviving Schizophrenia*, rev. ed. (New York, NY: Harper & Row, 1988).

96. Tsuang, M.T., Woolson, R.F., and Fleming, J.A., "Long-Term Outcome of Major Psychoses, I: Schizophrenia and Affective Disorder Compared With Psychiatrically Symptom-Free Surgical Conditions," *Archives of General Psychiatry* 36:1295-1306, 1979.

97. U.S. Department of Health and Human Services, Alcohol, Drug Abuse, and Mental Health Administration, *A National Plan for Schizophrenia Research: Panel Recommendations*, Pub. No. (ADM) 88-1570 (Washington, DC: U.S. Government Printing Office, 1988).

98. U.S. Department of Health and Human Services, National Institutes of Health, Consensus Development Conference Statement: Electroconvulsive Therapy, U.S. Government Printing Office #491 242 21264, 1985.

99. U.S. Department of Health and Human Services, National Institutes of Health, Consensus Development Conference Statement: Treatment of Panic Disorder, Sept. 25-27, 1991.

100. Wahl, O.F., "Public Versus Professional Conceptions of Schizophrenia," *Journal of Community Psychology* 15:285-291, 1987.

101. Warshaw, M.G., Klerman, G.L., and Lavori, P.W., "Are Secular Trends in Major Depression an

Artifact of Recall?'' *Journal of Psychiatric Research* 25:141-151, 1991.

102. Weissman, M.M., ''The Epidemiology of Panic Disorder and Agoraphobia,'' *Review of Psychiatry*, R.E. Hales and A.J. Frances (eds.) (Washington, DC: American Psychiatric Press, 1988).

103. Weissman, M.M., Bruce, M.L., Leaf, P.J., et al., ''Affective Disorders,'' *Psychiatric Disorders in America: The Epidemiologic Catchment Area Study*, L.N. Robins and D.A. Regier (eds.) (New York, NY: Free Press, 1991).

104. Weissman, M.M., and Klerman, G.L., ''Gender and Depression,'' *Trends in Neuroscience* 8:416-420, 1985.

105. Weissman, M.M., Meyers, J., Thompson, W., et al., ''Depressive Symptoms as a Risk Factor for Mortality and for Major Depression,'' *Life Span Research on the Predictors of Psychopathology*, L. Erlenmayer-Kimling and N. Miller (eds.) (Hillsdale, NJ: Erlbaum, 1986).

106. Wickramratne, P.J., Weissman, M.M., Leaf, P.J., et al., ''Age, Period and Cohort Effects on the Risk of Major Depression: Results From Five United States Communities,'' *Journal of Clinical Epidemiology* 42:333-343, 1989.

107. Wood, W.G., ''The Diagnosis and Management of Panic Disorder,'' *Psychiatric Medicine* 8:197-209, 1990.

108. Wyatt, R.J., ''Neuroleptics and the Natural Course of Schizophrenia,'' *Schizophrenia Bulletin* 17:325-351, 1991.

109. Zeiss, A.M., Lewinsohn, P.M., and Munoz, R.F., ''Nonspecific Improvement Effects in Depression Using Interpersonal Skills Training, Pleasant Activity Schedules, or Cognitive Training,'' *Journal of Consulting and Clinical Psychology* 47:427-439, 1979.

Chapter 4
Mental Disorders and the Brain

CONTENTS OF CHAPTER 4

Mental Disorders and the Brain

Studying the factors that play a role in mental disorders is like putting together a jigsaw puzzle. The pieces of the puzzle are bits of information about the workings of the human brain. This chapter considers the chemistry, structure, and function of the human brain in mental disorders. Another key piece in the puzzle is the heritability of these disorders, which is discussed in chapter 5.

The nature and amount of information available about the biology of mental disorders reflects the course of neuroscience research over the years. During the 1960s and 1970s there were advances in the methods used to study the chemistry of the brain and a resulting increase in knowledge about brain pharmacology and biochemistry. Many scientists therefore focused their work on the roles of natural chemicals and pharmaceuticals in mental disorders. The following decade, the 1980s, saw advances in molecular biology and imaging technologies, which in turn led to study of brain anatomy and activity and the molecules involved. The pace and extent of research into the biological components of mental disorders mirror these developments, with the body of knowledge concerning the chemistry of the brain being much larger than the growing database about other factors. Currently, some of the most active research involves techniques that enable investigators to study the activity of the brain in living subjects. These advances and the expectation of future discoveries have infused researchers in the area of mental disorders with optimism that further studies will pay off in a greater knowledge of the brain, a better understanding of disorders, and the development of new treatments for them.

Scientists examine the activity of the brain to determine its normal functioning and to see whether biological factors are associated with a given mental disorder. When a factor is identified, an important distinction must be made as to whether it is correlated with the disorder or in fact causes it. A correlated factor is one that is linked to the disorder and may result in some of its symptoms. For example, a perturbation of the chemical functioning of an area of the brain may be correlated with symptoms characteristic of a disorder. Understanding the perturbation can explain how the symptoms occur—that is, what the biological underpinnings

are—but it does not explain what caused the chemical disturbance. Thus, a correlated factor—in this case the chemical perturbation—is secondary to the underlying cause of the disorder. The consistent association of either a causative or correlative factor with a disorder can provide a biological marker to aid in the diagnosis of the disorder, which in turn can be critical to research and treatment. The identification of factors that are associated with a disorder can also provide an understanding of the mechanisms underlying symptoms; this is crucial to the development of rational therapeutic interventions. Most basic of all is the identification of specific causes of mental disorders. To date, research into the biology of the mental disorders considered here has identified several factors that are associated with their symptoms; there is much less evidence regarding the causes of these disorders.

To solve the puzzle of what causes and contributes to mental disorders, all of the pieces have to be studied and fit together. It is important to note that not all of them will necessarily be biological. Although beyond the scope of this report, psychological and social factors also contribute. Thus, when a biological factor is identified, research must point out how it interacts with psychological and social factors that may produce, modify, or determine how mental disorders are expressed. For example, it may be that biological factors create a predisposition to certain disorders. The psychological and social experiences of an individual, such as exposure to stress or a negative life event, may then shape the likelihood that that factor will manifest itself as the clinical condition.

METHODS USED TO STUDY MENTAL DISORDERS

To understand the involvement of biological factors in mental disorders, researchers conduct experiments in animals, analyze biological samples from patients, and study patients' biochemistry, brain anatomy, behavior, and mental activities. In general, basic mechanisms of the brain's physiology, chemistry, and anatomy are studied in either animal models that approximate aspects of a disorder or in tissue samples from living persons and brain samples from deceased ones. Patient populations are examined to learn more about symptoms and characteristics associated with disorders. Understanding mental disorders depends on connecting information from these diverse observations. Ultimately, the most comprehensive information is derived from studies and techniques that permit direct measurements in humans, both those with and those without mental disorders. Although it is very difficult to study the working brain in humans, new techniques enable investigators to observe some physiological processes in living subjects. Refinement of these techniques, and the development of additional ones, will most likely enhance the understanding of mental disorders.

It is often difficult to put disparate biological pieces together into a unified hypothesis about the biological underpinnings of a mental disorder. Many times, results from studies contradict each other or are inconsistent, which further complicates this process. A number of factors contribute to these contradictions and inconsistencies. A better understanding of the workings of the healthy brain is essential to understanding what might go wrong in mental disorders. As a result, there is still much to be learned. Also, some older research techniques provide only crude measures of brain activity, producing less precise findings. Finally, the difficulty of distinguishing specific mental disorders may result in a heterogeneous research population, which can then produce difficult-to-interpret results. To some

extent, the explosion in neuroscience research in recent years and the development of new, sophisticated techniques and methodologies for more precise, complex analysis have reduced, and will continue to alleviate, many of these problems.

Biochemistry

Study of the biochemistry of the brain involves examining the many chemicals involved in communication and processing of information in the brain. Neurotransmitters are chemicals released by nerve cells, or neurons, to communicate with each other. Neurons are the cells that process information in the brain. A neuron consists of a cell body with long extensions, much like the branches of a tree, called dendrites (figure 4-1). Also projecting out of the cell body is a single fiber called the axon, which can extend a great distance (figure 4-1). When a neuron is activated, it releases a neurotransmitter into the synapse, the gap between two neurons (figure 4-2). The molecules of the neurotransmitter move across the synapse and attach themselves, or bind, to proteins, called receptors, in the outer wall of an adjacent cell (figure 4-2). Usually, the axon terminal is the part of the cell that releases neurotransmitters into the synapse, and the dendrites and cell body are the areas of the neuron which contain receptors that form synapses with the axons of other neurons.

Once the neurotransmitter has activated a receptor, it unbinds from the receptor. It then has to be

Figure 4-1—Neurons

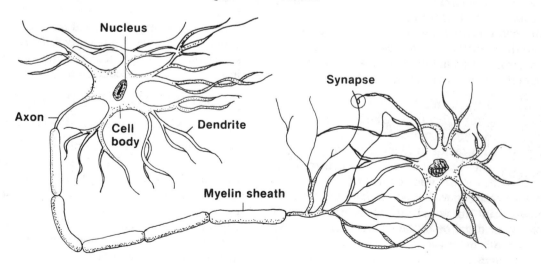

Two neurons in synaptic contact.
SOURCE: R. Restak, *The Brain* (New York, NY: Bantam Books, 1984).

Figure 4-2—The Synapse

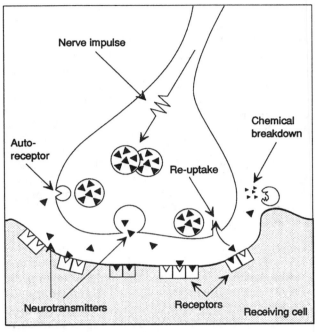

The synapse and associated structures.
SOURCE: Office of Technology Assessment, 1992.

removed from the synapse so the synapse will be available for a new message. This is done either by the neurotransmitter's being taken back up into the neuron that released it (a process called reuptake) or by it being broken down chemically into compounds called metabolites (figure 4-2).

For each neurotransmitter in the brain, there are specific receptors to which it can attach. Binding by the neurotransmitter activates the receptor, which can have different effects, depending on the receptor. Receptors can be linked to a variety of biochemical and cellular mechanisms that are turned on or off by the activation of the receptor. A neuron can have thousands of receptors for many different neurotransmitters. Some neurotransmitters activate neurons (excitatory neurotransmitters), while others decrease the activity of neurons (inhibitory neurotransmitters).

When a neuron is activated, changes occur in its membrane, resulting in a shift in the balance of ions (electrically charged molecules) between the inside and outside of the neuron. This change in ionic balance triggers an electrical impulse inside the neuron. The electrical impulse travels from the cell body, down the axon, to the axon terminal. At the

axon terminal, the impulse causes the release of neurotransmitter from the neuron into the synapse.

Sometimes a receptor for one neurotransmitter can affect a receptor for another neurotransmitter. In such cases, the receptors are biochemically coupled: The activation of one modulates the functioning of the other, either increasing or decreasing its activity. A neuron can also have receptors for the neurotransmitter it releases; these are usually located near the site where the neurotransmitter is released into the synapse (figure 4-2). Such receptors are acted on by the neuron's own neurotransmitter to regulate the release of the neurotransmitter. Thus, these autoreceptors, as they are called, act as a feedback mechanism to regulate a neuron's activity. The activity of a neuron will be determined by the cumulative activity of all its various receptors.

While receptors are specific for a neurotransmitter, there may be a variety of receptor subtypes, linked to different cellular mechanisms, that all respond to the same neurotransmitter. In this way, one neurotransmitter can have diverse effects in various areas of the brain. Also, the number of receptors in the brain is not static. In response to increased production of a neurotransmitter, the number of receptors for that neurotransmitter will decrease; conversely, depletion of a neurotransmitter will result in an increase in the number of receptors for that neurotransmitter. This mechanism allows the brain to compensate for changes in neurotransmitter levels. Such receptor changes are important in therapeutics; some drugs mimic neurotransmitters by stimulating increases or decreases in receptor numbers. In some cases, these changes may be directly related to the drug's therapeutic effect.

Many chemicals have been identified as neurotransmitters, among them acetylcholine, the catecholamines (norepinephrine, epinephrine, dopamine), serotonin, various amino acids, and peptides, including certain hormones. Various chemicals in the brain other than neurotransmitters and their receptors are necessary for brain function. They may be associated with the biochemical mechanisms activated by neurotransmitter-receptor interactions, involved with the production and breakdown of neurotransmitters, or responsible for carrying out metabolic activity.

Abnormalities in any of these chemicals, their receptors, or the cellular mechanisms that are turned on or off by the receptors could contribute to mental disorders. For example, there may be too much or too little of a neurotransmitter, or the receptors for a neurotransmitter may not function properly. Mechanisms activated by receptors may be defective, or the systems responsible for deactivating neurotransmitters may be faulty. Also, breakdowns in the chemical systems responsible for the normal functioning of cells in the nervous system may play a role in mental disorders. Such alterations in neurotransmitter systems have been implicated in the symptoms of certain mental disorders (see later discussions).

Scientists use a variety of tools and methods to study these factors. Biochemical assays are available to measure receptor number and activity, concentrations of neurotransmitters, and many other biochemical parameters of brain function. The majority of these assays are used with tissue from animals or from patients (i.e., postmortem brain samples or tissue samples from living patients). For example, information about concentrations of neurotransmitters is derived from measuring these compounds or their metabolites in samples of blood or cerebrospinal fluid (i.e., fluid inside and surrounding the brain and spinal cord). Nevertheless, such samples provide only an indirect measure of what is occurring in the brain. The inability to observe and measure the chemical activity of the brain directly has hampered investigators' understanding of how these processes may go awry in mental disorders. One new technique that enables scientists to study biochemistry in the living brain is positron emission tomography (PET) (see later discussion). In particular, it can be used to assay some biochemical measures, such as distribution and number of receptors, in living human subjects.

The last decade has also seen the application of molecular biological techniques to study the brain. Genetic information about the brain and its components is studied and manipulated to understand the cellular and molecular workings of the brain. While these new techniques are just beginning to have an impact on the study of mental disorders, they have already provided valuable information about receptor subtypes (box 4-A) and other aspects of the biochemistry of the brain.

Information about underlying biochemical abnormalities is also often derived from studying the actions of therapeutically effective drugs (i.e., psychopharmacology). In fact, many initial advances in understanding the biochemistry of mental disorders came from studies of drug actions in the brain. If a drug is found to be effective in treating a disorder, examination of that drug's chemical action in the brain may lead to the discovery of an intrinsic pathology. For example, the finding that effective antidepressant drugs act on catecholamines led to the study of these neurotransmitters in depression (see later discussion). Conversely, drug development may be guided by previously acquired knowledge about a disorder, which directs research efforts to create compounds that will act on an already identified pathology. If a specific neurotransmitter system is identified as being aberrant in a disorder, drugs can be designed to interact with some aspect of that system, such as the receptors, to try to reverse the abnormality.

Anatomy and Activity

Abnormalities in the structure of the brain or in its activity in specific locations can contribute to mental disorders. In the brain, neurons that share the same anatomical region, and to varying degrees the same function, are assembled into groups called nuclei. The brain is made up of hundreds of nuclei. Some consist of neurons that produce many different neurotransmitters, while others are predominantly of one type. Axons extending from nuclei convey information between and among them. Thus, the brain comprises many nuclei, which are connected by pathways of axons that contain various neurotransmitters. Information is conveyed and processed via networks made up of interconnected nuclei.

Some networks of nuclei are particularly relevant to mental disorders (figure 4-3). In general, these are networks that control cognitive (i.e., perception, recognition, reasoning, judgment, imagination), behavioral, and emotional functions. Disruptions of these areas are likely to be involved in the thinking and mood disturbances characteristic of severe mental disorders. The cerebral cortex (the portion of the brain that is critical in decisionmaking) is important in this regard, especially the frontal lobes, which are considered to be the seat of higher-order thinking and which enables humans to reason abstractly. The limbic system, a network of structures (e.g., hippocampus, amygdala, parts of the temporal lobe of the cortex) located in the upper part of the brain (figure 4-3) and involved in control of emotional behavior, is also important in mental disorders. Additional areas of the brain implicated in mental disorders are the basal ganglia, a group of

Box 4-A—Cloning Dopamine Receptors

Advances in the ability to manipulate and express genetic information provide an important new means of studying the brain. One area in which the tools of the molecular biologist have contributed significantly is the identification of receptor subtypes for neurotransmitters. These techniques have permitted the cloning of genes for specific receptors and have provided a detailed characterization of the receptor's three-dimensional structure. Not only is this information important for understanding better how the brain works, but it also aids the development of drugs specifically designed to act only on certain receptors. This specificity can increase the efficacy of a drug while decreasing the side effects it causes. The recent identification of several receptor subtypes for the neurotransmitter dopamine is an example of the contribution molecular biology is making to understanding the brain.

Previous to the use of molecular biological techniques, two dopamine receptors had been characterized, based on the ability of various drugs to bind to them. For example, drugs that are effective in treating schizophrenia (called typical antipsychotic drugs) all bind to the same dopamine receptor—the D_2 receptor. In addition, another receptor that binds dopamine, but not typical antipsychotic drugs, was identified and called the D_1 receptor. Other evidence, derived using pharmacological techniques, suggested that there might be additional dopamine receptors, but it was not until the gene for each of the dopamine receptor subtypes was identified that their existence was confirmed.

Currently, six dopamine receptor subtypes have been identified and cloned using molecular biological techniques. Although all of these receptors are acted on by dopamine, they all have slightly different molecular structures. In addition, there are some differences in their location in the brain, the cellular mechanisms that they turn on when they are activated, and their ability to bind typical antipsychotic drugs. Both the D_1 and D_5 receptors are linked to the same cellular mechanism, are located in the hippocampus and cortex, and do not readily bind typical antipsychotic drugs. They differ in their ability to bind dopamine and dopamine-like drugs. There are two types of D_2 receptors: Both bind typical antipsychotic drugs, and both are found in parts of the limbic system, basal ganglia, and cortex. They differ in that each is linked to a different cellular mechanism, and one is a dopamine autoreceptor—a receptor that lies on the dopamine neuron itself, regulating the cell's activity (see text). The D_3 and D_4 receptors are found predominantly in the limbic system. While it is unclear what cellular mechanisms are activated by these receptors, the D_3 receptor is thought to be an autoreceptor. Neither binds typical antipsychotic drugs as effectively as D_2 receptors, and the D_4 receptor readily binds a new atypical antipsychotic drug, clozapine (see text).

The identification of these dopamine receptor subtypes has provided new insights into how more efficacious antipsychotic medications can be designed. Since clozapine is a highly effective antipsychotic drug but produces fewer side effects than typical antipsychotics, it is thought that its mixture of strong binding to D_4 receptors and weak binding to D_2 receptors accounts for its action. Currently there is great interest in understanding the various dopamine receptor subtypes to determine their role in schizophrenia and how drugs can be designed to target them.

The complexity of the dopamine receptor system indicates the many ways that a single neurotransmitter can have myriad effects in the brain. Molecular biological techniques provide an important tool for clarifying these basic brain mechanisms, providing new information about how they may be disturbed in mental disorders and leading the way for the development of more efficacious medications.

SOURCES: E. Kandel, J. Schwartz, and T. Jessell (eds.), *Principles of Neuroscience* (New York, NY: Elsevier Science Publishing, 1991); P. Sokoloff, B. Giros, M. Martres, et al., "Molecular Cloning and Characterization of a Novel Dopamine Receptor (D3) as a Target for Neuroleptics," *Nature* 347:146-151, 1990; R. Sunahara, H. Guan, B. O'Dowd, et al., "Cloning of the Gene for a Human Dopamine D5 Receptor With Higher Affinity for Dopamine Than D1," *Nature* 350:614-619, 1991; H. van Tol, J. Bunzow, H. Guan, et al., "Cloning of the Gene for a Human Dopamine D4 Receptor With High Affinity for the Antipsychotic Clozapine," *Nature* 350:610-614, 1991.

nuclei just below the cerebral cortex, some of which coordinate movement and others of which are part of the limbic system; the hypothalamus, a collection of nuclei at the base of the brain (figure 4-3) that regulate hormones and behaviors such as eating, drinking, and sex; the locus ceruleus, a nucleus in the brainstem (figure 4-3) made up of norepinephrine neurons that are intimately involved in the body's response to stressful situations (i.e., the fight-or-flight response); and the raphe nuclei, also found in the brainstem (figure 4-3), made up of serotonin neurons that regulate sleep, are involved with behavior and mood, and are connected to the limbic system. It must be kept in mind, however, that if any of these, or other brain structures, are impaired in a mental disorder, it is unlikely that only the function of that structure will be affected. Since the brain is organized as networks of nuclei, any structural or

Figure 4-3—Brain Structures Involved in Mental Disorders

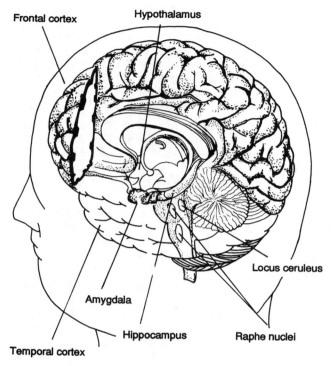

Three-dimensional drawing of the human brain.

SOURCE: Adapted from Lewis E. Calver, University of Texas, Southwestern Medical Center, Dallas, TX, 1992.

functional impairment in part of a network can create a disturbance throughout the network.

Structural changes associated with mental disorders can include anatomical abnormalities in the structure of the brain or irregularities in the individual cells within a region of the brain. The classical techniques for gathering information about brain structure—the macroscopic and microscopic post-mortem examination of normal brains and brains from individuals who have had mental disorders—have been augmented with a number of newer techniques and machines that make possible the study of the structure of the brain in living persons (table 4-1). Computerized axial tomography (CAT), which uses computers to combine a series of x-rays, provides clearer pictures of the brain than x-rays alone. Remarkably clear and detailed images of brain structure are obtained using magnetic resonance imaging (MRI) scans, which detect molecular

changes in the brain that occur when an individual is exposed to a strong magnetic field. Abnormalities that can be detected by either CAT or MRI scans include structural brain abnormalities, changes in the volume of brain tissue, and enlargement of the cerebral ventricles.[1] Decreases in the volume of brain tissue and enlargement of the cerebral ventricles indicate either atrophy or underdevelopment of a brain region.

The activity of the brain can also be studied to determine damage or malfunctioning in a region of the brain. Neuropsychological testing seeks to determine brain damage by measuring deficits in a person's performance on various tasks. For example, deficits on tests that measure language performance imply damage to the regions of the brain that subserve language skills, while poor performance on certain types of puzzles indicates abnormalities in regions devoted to various kinds of cognitive and sensory information processing. While neuropsychological testing is helpful in identifying areas of brain pathology, the measures used are indirect, and exact locations of involved regions can only be inferred. However, when combined with more direct methods of looking at the brain, they provide a powerful tool for studying brain function and anatomy.

Measurement of electrical activity in the brain using the electroencephalograph (EEG) provides a more direct indication of brain function, and combining the EEG with computer analysis provides an even more detailed measure. Electrical activity can be measured while subjects are resting or engaging in some sort of sensory or cognitive task. By examining the electrical patterns of the brain, investigators can observe changes in normal brain responses and where they occur. A shortcoming of these measures is that they reflect the cumulative activity of broad areas of the brain, usually near the surface. This makes it more difficult to locate areas of possible pathology.

PET scanning and single-photon-emission computed tomography (SPECT) are imaging techniques that reveal brain activity. They do so by creating computerized images of the distribution of radioactively labeled materials in the brain. Researchers administer labeled materials to a subject either by injection or inhalation. Subsequent distribution of

---

[1] The cerebral ventricles are spaces in the brain that are filled with cerebrospinal fluid.

Table 4-1—Techniques for Imaging the Brain

Technique	How it works	What it images
Computerized axial tomography (CAT)	Computer construction of x-ray images	Structure
Magnetic resonance imaging (MRI)	Images molecular changes in brain cells when exposed to a strong magnetic field	Structure and activity (when used in conjunction with a magnetically active substance)
Computer analysis of electroencephalogram (EEG)	Creates maps of brain electrical activity by computer analysis of EEG	Activity
Single-photon-emission computed tomography (SPECT)	Creates images of the distribution of radioactively labeled substances in the brain following either injection into the blood or inhalation	Activity (regional cerebral blood flow)
Positron emission tomography (PET)	Creates images of the distribution of radioactively labeled substances following injection into the blood	Activity (regional cerebral blood flow, glucose utilization) and neurochemical activity (receptor number and distribution)

SOURCE: Office of Technology Assessment, 1992.

these materials reflects the activity of the brain. Recently, MRI scanning has also been adapted for this function. PET, SPECT, and MRI enable researchers to measure the utilization of glucose or the amount of blood flowing in a region of the brain (i.e., regional cerebral blood flow). Both glucose utilization and regional cerebral blood flow are indicators of brain activity: The more active a region is, the more blood will flow through it and the more glucose it will use. Abnormal activity levels in specific brain regions, in the whole brain, or in the normal asymmetry of activity between the two sides of the brain can be discerned with these techniques. Also, as previously mentioned, PET scanning can be done following the injection of labeled drugs that attach to specific receptors, making it possible to visualize the number and distribution of receptor populations. As with EEG measures, these scanning techniques can be done either while the subject is at rest or doing a task. While the imaging techniques now being used to study mental disorders will undoubtedly be refined, they provide for the first time a window through which to view the human brain at work.

SCHIZOPHRENIA

The symptoms of schizophrenia reflect a broad range of cognitive and emotional dysfunctions that are commonly categorized as either positive or negative symptoms (see ch. 3). Positive symptoms include hallucinations and delusions, paranoid psychosis, as well as bizarre behaviors and thought

disorder. Negative symptoms include emotional flattening (i.e., flat affect), loss of motivation, general loss of interest, and social withdrawal. In some cases, specific alterations in the biochemistry or anatomy of the brain have been associated with either positive or negative symptoms. As with other severe mental disorders, there are many clues available regarding schizophrenia, and a number of hypotheses have been put forward in an attempt to unify this information into an explanation of the underlying pathology.

Biochemistry

Dopamine

The most prominent and enduring theory regarding the biochemistry of schizophrenia concerns the role of the neurotransmitter dopamine. This theory is based on two sets of observations about drug action. First, drugs that increase dopamine activity, such as amphetamine, L-dopa, cocaine, and methylphenidate, sometimes induce a paranoid psychosis in normal individuals that is similar to some aspects of schizophrenia. The same drugs, when administered to patients with schizophrenia, sometimes induce a transitory worsening of symptoms, particularly increasing psychosis and disturbance of thought. Second, and in contrast, drugs that block certain dopamine receptors often ease the symptoms, in particular the positive symptoms, of schizophrenia. In general, there is a close correlation between how well these drugs block dopamine receptors and their antipsychotic effect. The therapeutic effectiveness of dopamine-blocking drugs and the ability of dopamine-enhancing drugs to worsen the symptoms of schizophrenia provide evidence for the role of excessive concentrations or transmission of dopamine in at least some aspects of the disorder. Nevertheless, studies that have tried to measure dopamine activity in schizophrenia are less conclusive (81).

The concentrations of certain chemicals (e.g., homovanillic acid, a metabolite of dopamine) can be measured by scientists to provide information about dopamine activity. A number of investigators have measured these chemicals in the tissue and fluids of persons with and without schizophrenia. If higher concentrations of dopamine are associated with schizophrenia, then higher concentrations of these chemicals would be expected in persons with schizophrenia. The results are inconclusive. A review of this research (12) shows that in some studies higher dopamine concentrations were found in persons with schizophrenia; in others no such association was found. Conflicting results have also been found in studies of dopamine receptors, although one subtype of dopamine receptor (the D_2 receptor) may be increased in schizophrenia (12).

Thus, regardless of the index of dopamine activity examined in studies, results are variable. Data supporting the dopamine-excess hypothesis are usually contradicted by data that fail to find differences between persons with schizophrenia and controls. Part of this variability is undoubtedly due to the imprecision of some of the measures used. The use of newer, more sophisticated techniques may resolve some of these contradictions. For example, as previously described, there are a number of dopamine receptor subtypes (see box 4-A). As the ability to study these receptor subtypes improves, alterations in a specific receptor population may become evident. Part of the variability in results may also be due to differences in the characteristics of the patients with schizophrenia studied. Factors such as how long an individual has had the disorder and his or her age when it first appeared can affect findings.

There also is some evidence that dopamine activity may be associated with specific symptoms of schizophrenia. For example, when changes reflecting increased dopamine function are observed, they often occur in patients with prominent positive symptoms, particularly psychosis (12). Other studies support the proposition that dopamine deficiency is associated with the negative symptoms of schizophrenia. For example, a correlation between low levels of dopamine chemicals in cerebrospinal fluid and negative symptoms has been reported (59). In addition, dopamine-blocking drugs used to treat the positive symptoms of schizophrenia produce behaviors suggestive of the negative symptoms in animals and humans free of mental disorders (81,88). Thus, the contradictions between dopamine excess and dopamine deficiency as explanations for schizophrenia can be reconciled by proposing that each is associated with different symptoms of the disease—that is, positive and negative symptoms, respectively (12,60,88)—and that each involves different neural networks (see later discussion). However, these hypotheses are controversial and it is possible that one or both are incorrect. Nonetheless, most scientists agree that dopamine plays some role in schizophrenia.

Other Neurotransmitters

Alterations in the amount or function of other neurotransmitters in persons with schizophrenia have also been examined by researchers. Both increased and decreased levels of serotonin have been postulated as being associated with schizophrenia. The decreased-level hypothesis was based on the effects of LSD (lysergic acid diethylamide), which blocks serotonin activity in the brain and causes effects that are similar to some of the positive symptoms (e.g., hallucinations) seen in patients with schizophrenia (21). These observations were not supported by other data; in particular, they were contradicted by evidence that some drugs effective against schizophrenia reduce serotonin activity. Also, as with the dopamine hypothesis, measures of serotonin in the blood, cerebrospinal fluid, and postmortem brain tissue do not provide clear answers. Both increased and decreased measures of serotonin and its metabolites in blood and cerebrospinal fluid have been observed, and results from measures in postmortem brain tissue have been inconclusive (53). Thus, while there is some indication that serotonin activity may be altered in schizophrenia, the exact nature of its involvement is unclear.

Both an excess and a deficiency in the activity of the neurotransmitter norepinephrine have been associated with schizophrenia, although data indicate that an excess of norepinephrine is more likely to produce symptoms (80,90). Increased norepinephrine has been observed in the cerebrospinal fluid and blood of patients with schizophrenia (21,82). Since dopamine and norepinephrine have complex interactions, namely, that disturbances in one affect the other, it is unclear whether any observed increase in norepinephrine is primary to schizophrenia or secondary to changes in the dopamine system (53).

These neurotransmitters interact with and modulate the activity of many other neurotransmitter and neuropeptide systems; awareness of this fact has led to the study of these chemicals in schizophrenia. The opiate peptides are thought to affect dopamine neurons, and naloxone, a drug that blocks opiate receptors, may have antipsychotic properties (53). In addition, there have been findings relating other peptides to schizophrenia (53). Since alterations in such neuropeptides could facilitate, inhibit, or otherwise alter the pattern of activity of other nerve cells, further study of the status of peptides in schizophrenia is warranted.

Finally, a more specific neurotransmitter hypothesis involves the action of the drug phencyclidine (PCP) (31). PCP can produce symptoms that resemble both the positive and the negative symptoms of schizophrenia and can exacerbate these symptoms in people with the disorder. It is thought that PCP produces these dual effects by acting at different sites in the brain (21). PCP inhibits the activity of the excitatory neurotransmitter glutamate by interfering with the receptor for glutamate. From that observation, it has been speculated that inhibition of the glutamate receptor in the hippocampus results in the negative symptoms associated with schizophrenia (21). PCP also weakly blocks the reuptake of dopamine, and in other areas of the limbic system there is some evidence that PCP inhibition of glutamate secondarily causes an increase in dopamine activity. These effects on dopamine could result in the positive symptoms of schizophrenia. In both instances, there is implicit involvement of glutamate in the onset of symptoms of schizophrenia. While there is currently little experimental evidence to support this hypothesis, it represents a new avenue of investigation in schizophrenia research.

Thus, while it is likely that dopamine plays some role in schizophrenia, the involvement of other neurotransmitters is unclear. Since brain neurotransmitter systems interact with each other, it is often difficult to isolate a cause-effect relationship. The

modulatory action that neurotransmitters exert suggests that there may be complex interactions in schizophrenia between dopamine systems and these other brain chemicals.

Anatomy and Activity

Alterations in a number of brain structures, notably the frontal cortex and limbic system, have been implicated in schizophrenia. In particular, ventricular enlargement and evidence of changes in the size of various brain regions have been observed in imaging studies and postmortem examinations (figure 4-4). Limbic structures, such as the hippocampus and parts of the temporal lobes, are most affected. However, the specificity of these findings for schizophrenia has been questioned because they also occur in normal aging and in a variety of other neurological and psychiatric conditions (10, 21).

Attempts to replicate these findings have yielded contradictory results. In some cases, evidence of changes in the volume of the frontal cortex and temporal lobes has been observed, but the data are not conclusive and additional studies are needed to confirm the results (10). Some PET studies have examined brain metabolism in schizophrenia and have observed decreased activity in the frontal cortex and limbic structures, as well as increased

Figure 4-4—MRI Scan of an Individual With Schizophrenia

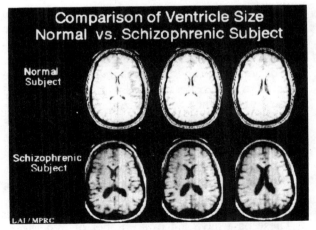

Brain structure shown of individual who does not have schizophrenia (top) and a person who does (bottom). The ventricles are enlarged in schizophrenia (black areas).

SOURCE: W. Carpenter, Maryland Psychiatric Research Center, and H. Loats, Loats Associates, Inc.

Figure 4-5—PET Scan of an Individual With Schizophrenia

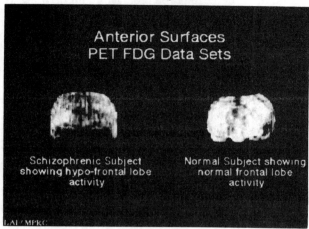

Brain activity in an individual who does not have schizophrenia (right) and a person who does (left). The frontal cortex shows more activity in schizophrenia (white areas).

SOURCE: W. Carpenter, Maryland Psychiatric Research Center, and H. Loats, Loats Associates, Inc.

activity in the basal ganglia (10,21) (figure 4-5). In general, these studies indicate that decreased frontal cortex activity is associated with the negative symptoms of schizophrenia. This coincides with data from animal studies, which indicate that damage to the frontal lobes produces behaviors similar to the negative symptoms.

EEG studies that show a higher incidence of abnormal electrical activity in the brain of patients with schizophrenia than in normal subjects provide further evidence of the involvement of the frontal cortex. These abnormalities often appear in the temporal lobe as well. Impairments on neuropsychological tests, such as problem-solving and attention deficits, also indicate that these structures are affected in schizophrenia (34,39). For example, 65 percent of patients with schizophrenia often have difficulty visually following a moving object, compared to 8 percent of subjects who do not have schizophrenia (21) (see ch. 5). It is thought that defects in maintaining attention, as a result of a dysfunction in the frontal lobes and limbic system, contribute to these visual task defects.

These data have led to a number of hypotheses that attempt to unify the information regarding brain structures implicated in schizophrenia. In particular, these theories assign important functions to the limbic system and frontal cortex. The limbic system is integral to motivation, gratification, memory, and many other emotions and thought-processes whose disturbance is associated with psychosis and the other positive symptoms of schizophrenia. The frontal cortex has been implicated in the negative symptoms of schizophrenia. The proposed theories differ as to whether the two sets of dysfunctions should be viewed as dependent or independent and in the specific structures presumed to be involved.

One theory postulates that they are dependent and that an insult during the development of the brain that affected the functioning of the frontal cortex (see later discussion) can lead to negative symptoms (84). Since the frontal cortex and limbic system are interconnected, with the frontal cortex inhibiting activity in the limbic system, this theory posits that the dysfunction of the frontal cortex reduces the inhibition on the limbic system, leading to the positive symptoms.

Another theory suggests that positive and negative symptoms are mediated by two different networks within the frontal cortex and limbic system and that dysfunction in one of these networks is separate from dysfunction in the other (9). This coincides with data from PET studies which show that negative symptoms are only correlated with decreased activity in the frontal cortex.

A third theory implicates a disruption in the activity of the basal ganglia and its interaction with other brain structures (16,17). This theory is based on three experimental findings: First, there is increased metabolic activity in the basal ganglia of patients with schizophrenia; second, patients with schizophrenia have difficulty performing visual attention tasks, which are mediated by areas of the cortex; and third, animals with lesions in dopamine-containing areas of the brain that project to the basal ganglia display some of the behavioral impairments seen in schizophrenia. This evidence has led to the hypothesis that schizophrenia is related to impaired activity in a network composed of the basal ganglia, certain cortical areas, and other brain structures and that the impairment is secondary to decreased dopamine activity.

These hypotheses attempt to find a basis for the disturbed behaviors observed in schizophrenia; they are overlapping and not always mutually exclusive. The available data point to networks involving certain limbic structures in psychosis and networks involving the frontal cortex in negative symptoms.

The precise interaction between these networks and the possible involvement of other brain structures and areas still need to be clarified. Based on these theories, predictions (which can themselves be tested with additional studies) can be made about the involvement of various areas of the brain in schizophrenia.

Other Factors

Immune and Viral Factors

Viral theories for the cause of schizophrenia are derived from reports that a number of viral and immune indices, such as the number and function of immune system cells, are deviant in patients with the disorder (13,32,83). Also, there is some epidemiological evidence to support a viral hypothesis. Schizophrenia may have a north-to-south prevalence gradient, may be endemic in a few areas (e.g., northern Sweden), and occurs somewhat more often in persons born in the winter. It has also been observed that fetuses in the second trimester of gestation during an influenza epidemic have an increased risk of developing schizophrenia as adults. However, it has been difficult to conduct definitive studies, since any potential marker of an immune or viral process associated with schizophrenia is applicable in only some cases and is subject to interpretation as secondary to conditions associated with the disease (e.g., crowding of hospitalized patients, exposure of individuals living in low socioeconomic circumstances, and poor health habits).

Developmental Factors

The observed changes in brain volume of persons with schizophrenia, and the cellular alterations that accompany these changes, are thought to be irreversible but not progressive (54). Current information suggests that the magnitude and nature of anatomical and morphological changes in schizophrenia are present at the onset of the disorder and do not vary over the lifetime of an individual. A possibility is that these abnormalities reflect changes that occurred very early in life or in utero, either as the result of some specific damage or a pathological alteration in the normal development of the brain.

Evidence that developmental factors may play a role derives from the observation that infants born after a complicated pregnancy or labor are at increased risk for developing schizophrenia as adults (41,42). One mechanism by which gestational or birth complications may alter brain development is diminished oxygen supply (i.e., hypoxia). This theory is attractive for two reasons. First, many pregnancy and birth complications are associated with temporary hypoxia. Second, limbic structures, especially the hippocampus, are among the most sensitive areas in the developing brain to the adverse consequences of hypoxia. Also, subtle deviations in neurological and psychological functioning have been observed from infancy in children who are at high risk of developing schizophrenia (11). Although far from established, it is possible that early, adverse gestational influences on the developing brain create a risk of both birth complications and, later, schizophrenia. A corollary to this proposition is that a pathological influence operating early in gestation alters the development of the brain to create subsequent vulnerability to schizophrenia. An intriguing possible instance of this proposition is the relationship, discussed earlier, between pregnancy during influenza epidemics and the development of schizophrenia.

What specific alterations in the brain may result from such insults is unknown; however, it is clear that subtle deviations in the development of the brain could create dysfunctions associated with specific behaviors. Furthermore, it is possible that such subtle brain abnormalities are not manifest until much later in life, when new demands are placed on the brain systems during adolescence and adulthood. Postmortem findings of abnormalities in the number and organization of some nerve cells (1,37) suggest that the developmental process of cell migration, by which the cells in the brain become organized into the normal pattern of neuronal networks, may have gone awry in schizophrenia. Altered cell migration could be a genetic result, might be caused by gestational insults, or might involve an interaction of both. Another process that might be involved is the pruning of nerve cells that occurs as the brain develops (18). During early development, the brain has more neurons than it needs; the fine-tuning necessary for efficient functioning involves eliminating certain nerve cells and many of the synapses connecting cells. Failure to prune nerve cells and synapses adequately, or an error in selecting which ones to prune, could underlie dysfunctions that lead to the manifestation of the symptoms of schizophrenia. Whatever developmental processes play a role in schizophrenia is still an open question.

Synthesis

Although various alterations in the biochemistry, anatomy, and activity of the brain have been observed in schizophrenia, there are several important points regarding these data (21). The high variability among patients on any one of the biological factors and the lack of agreement among studies about many of them suggest that schizophrenia is a heterogeneous disorder, with patients exhibiting different clusters of symptoms. This variability could also reflect the effects of other factors, such as psychosocial variables, on the biological components. The fact that some of the biological abnormalities observed in schizophrenia are also seen in other conditions calls into question their specificity to, and their role in, schizophrenia.

Despite the equivocal nature of the research findings, conclusions can still be drawn from them. Dopamine plays a role in at least some of the symptoms of schizophrenia; however, the characteristics of that involvement are unclear, and dopamine's precise relationship to the positive and negative symptoms of schizophrenia remains to be elucidated. The role of other neurotransmitters in schizophrenia, and if and how they interact with dopamine systems, needs to be clarified. Given the cognitive and emotional functions governed by the frontal cortex and limbic system, it is not surprising that alterations in these regions have been implicated in schizophrenia. Abnormal functioning of the frontal lobes has been one of the most consistent findings in schizophrenia, and, while less well documented, there does seem to be a relationship between decreased frontal cortex activity and negative symptoms. Positive symptoms appear to be associated with increased metabolic activity in the limbic system.

While completed studies furnish valuable information regarding what might be wrong in the brain of a person with schizophrenia, the question of why schizophrenia occurs remains unanswered. The role of abnormal brain development or an injury to the brain, either during development or early in life, is an important avenue of investigation. As with other factors associated with schizophrenia, the precise mechanisms that may be involved are subject to speculation. The interaction of such a precipitating event with genetic factors (see ch. 5) is another plausible cause.

MOOD DISORDERS

Mood disorders include major depression and bipolar disorder. As the name indicates, major depression is marked by a deep depression that can be unremitting. Bipolar disorders are characterized by periods of depression alternating with manic episodes. Sadness is a normal human emotion in response to various life events, but depression that has no known cause or unremitting depression that interferes with normal activity is pathological. Available data regarding the role of biological factors in major depression and bipolar disorder often overlap. This reflects the fact that these disorders may be closely linked. The depressed state may be mediated by the same brain regions in both conditions. However, different brain mechanisms may be involved in the manic state and the swing from depression to mania that is characteristic of bipolar disorder.

Biochemistry

Neurotransmitter Systems

Prominent hypotheses concerning depression have focused on altered function of the group of neurotransmitters called monoamines (i.e., norepinephrine, epinephrine, serotonin, dopamine), particularly norepinephrine (NE) and serotonin (25,51,70). Evidence that monoamines are involved comes from the knowledge of the mechanism of action of the two classes of clinically effective antidepressant medications—tricyclic antidepressants and monoamine oxidase inhibitors (MAOIs). Tricyclic antidepressants block the reuptake of neurotransmitters, and MAOIs block the action of monoamine oxidase, the enzyme involved in the chemical breakdown of the monoamine transmitters once they are released into the synapse. The net effect of both of these types of drugs is to prolong the activity of these neurotransmitters in the synapse.

In the 1960s, the clinical observation that patients who were taking a norepinephrine-blocking drug for high blood pressure developed depression led to the hypothesis that depression was the result of low concentrations of monoamines, in particular NE (25). Some experiments have shown that patients with bipolar disorder have decreased NE metabolites during depression and increased amounts during mania, which supports the NE imbalance hypothesis; other studies, however, have shown that patients

---

Box 4-B—Serotonin and Suicide

More than 30,000 Americans commit suicide each year, making it the eighth leading cause of death in the Nation. It is the second leading cause of death among adolescents. Changes in a number of indices of serotonin activity are correlated with suicide attempts and suicide completions. Suicidal behavior is associated with decreased concentrations of serotonin and its metabolites in cerebrospinal fluid and the brain. Among successful suicides, decreased concentrations are usually found in the brainstem, where the raphe nuclei, the major serotonin-containing nuclei in the brain, are located. Also, increased numbers of serotonin receptors have been observed in the brains of suicide victims, usually in the frontal cortex. Since certain frontal cortex neurons receive connections from those of the raphe nuclei, it is possible that the receptor increase is a compensatory response to decreased serotonin activity in the raphe neurons. A decrease in the number of serotonin autoreceptors in suicide victims has been reported in some studies. Finally, suicide attempters, as compared to nonattempters, show decreased release of the hormone prolactin following administration of a serotonin-stimulating drug. This blunted prolactin response is indicative of a low level of serotonin activity. These data indicate that a net decrease in serotonin activity in the brain is associated with suicidal behavior.

These data do not mean that decreased serotonin causes a person to commit suicide. First of all, not every suicide victim exhibits decreased serotonin. For example, serotonin metabolite concentrations are not reduced in individuals with bipolar disorder who attempt suicide, compared to individuals with bipolar disorder who do not attempt suicide. Also, there is some evidence that among suicide attempters, measures of decreased serotonin activity correlate with the lethality of the method used; that is, the more violent the attempted suicide method (e.g., cutting arteries v. drug overdose), the more depressed the serotonin activity. In addition, some of these same measures of serotonin activity, such as low levels of serotonin metabolites in the cerebrospinal fluid and blunted response to prolactin, can be observed in individuals who exhibit impulsive and aggressive behavior. This suggests that, rather than causing suicide, decreased serotonin activity is correlated with a behavioral predisposition that can lead to suicide. If individuals who are burdened with feelings of despondency also have depressed serotonin activity, the propensity for aggression may be directed internally, tragically resulting in a successful suicide attempt.

SOURCES: E.F. Coccaro and J.L. Astill, "Central Serotonergic Function in Parasuicide," *Progress in Neuro-Psychopharmacology & Biological Psychiatry* 14:663-674, 1990; K.Y. Little and D.L. Sparks, "Brain Markers and Suicide: Can a Relationship Be Found?" *Journal of Forensic Sciences* 35:1393-1403, 1990; J.J. Mann, V. Arango, M.D. Underwood, et al., "Neurochemical Correlates of Suicidal Behavior: Involvement of Serotonergic and Non-Serotonergic Systems," *Pharmacology and Toxicology* 3:37-60, 1990; J.J. Mann, V. Arango, and M.D. Underwood, "Serotonin and Behavior," *Annals of the New York Academy of Sciences* 600:476-484, 1990; L.C. Ricci and M.M. Wellman, "Monoamines: Biochemical Markers of Suicide?" *Journal of Clinical Psychology* 46:106-116, 1990.

---

with major depression exhibit increased concentrations of NE metabolites (51,70).

As more information has been gathered, it has become clear that the chemistry of depression is more complex and that other neurotransmitters, especially serotonin, may be involved. For example, fluoxetine, a highly effective antidepressant drug that is widely prescribed, acts exclusively on serotonin.

Although the results from studies of serotonin metabolites are not conclusive, there is some indication that concentrations of serotonin are decreased in mood disorders (25). Also, low concentrations of serotonin metabolites have been observed in people who commit suicide (box 4-B). As a result of these findings, it has been hypothesized that decreased serotonin plays a role in mood disorders (25,46). In

addition, decreased dopamine metabolites have been observed in some, but not all, studies of depression.

One fact that argues against the monoamine imbalance hypothesis is the time lag between administration of antidepressant medications and their clinical effect. These medications increase neurotransmitter levels almost immediately upon administration, but their therapeutic effects often do not appear until 2 or 3 weeks after initiation of drug therapy. This time lag has led to the suggestion that the receptors for monoamines may be involved— specifically, that the clinical effects of these drugs are due to reductions in the number of receptors to compensate for the drug-induced increased levels of monoamine neurotransmitters. It would take weeks for such compensatory changes to come about.

One hypothesis related to drug-induced changes in receptors involves a receptor for NE (25). There are a number of NE receptor subtypes. One is an autoreceptor that decreases the release of NE into the synapse when it is activated. It has been hypothesized that these NE autoreceptors are overly active in depression. The therapeutic effects of antidepressant drugs are the result of exposing the autoreceptors to higher concentrations of neurotransmitter, which decreases their number, ultimately increasing the activity of the NE-containing neurons. While this hypothesis would explain the delayed appearance of clinical effects of antidepressant drugs, studies of the NE autoreceptor in depression have found no specific evidence of an abnormality to date.

Currently, no clear evidence links abnormal serotonin receptor activity in the brain to depression (51). Increased receptors for serotonin have been observed in the brains of suicide victims (box 4-B), but there are conflicting results from studies that have examined serotonin receptors in depressed persons (25). Changes in serotonin receptor activity have been measured indirectly in mood disorders, notably bipolar disorder, using blood platelets (a type of cell found in the blood) which also contain serotonin and are used to investigate mechanisms related to serotonin and its receptors (46). Both increased numbers of a subtype of serotonin receptor and decreased sites for the reuptake of serotonin into the platelets have been seen in the platelets of persons with depression (46). However, it is unclear how these changes relate to serotonin activity in the brain of persons with major depression and bipolar disorder.

While there is sufficient evidence to support the notion that abnormalities in monoamine systems are an important component of depression, the data currently available do not provide consistent evidence either for altered neurotransmitter levels or for disruption of normal receptor activity. This has led to a dysregulation hypothesis, which states that there is a more general perturbation in the mechanisms that regulate the activity of the monoamine neurotransmitters and that clinically effective drugs restore efficient regulation (70). Linked to this hypothesis is the fact that the monoamine systems interact with each other—the activity of one affects and modulates the activity of another. Based on available data, it has been proposed that decreased activity within the NE-serotonin component of the system is associated with depression, while increased activity of the NE-dopamine component tends to promote mania (25).

Complicating the picture is the fact that other neurotransmitters have been implicated in bipolar disorder. Based on evidence that agents which activate acetylcholine systems can induce depression and that agents which block such activity have some ability to alleviate depression (51), it has been postulated that increased acetylcholine activity induces depression and decreased activity induces mania (15,25,30,70). Furthermore, a number of investigators have proposed that the salient mechanism may be the balance between NE and acetylcholine systems, with a predominance of acetylcholine activity associated with depression and a predominance of NE activity associated with mania (25,28,51,70). A role for the inhibitory neurotransmitter gamma-aminobutyric acid (GABA) has also been put forth, based on the paradoxical finding that increased GABA activity has both an antidepressant and an antimanic effect (25,40,51). Given that GABA is a ubiquitous inhibitory neurotransmitter, it is possible that increasing its activity can result in the modulation of a number of other neurotransmitter systems, which could explain its broad range of effects. Finally, there is evidence that some neuropeptides may also be involved in mood disorders (6,23,25). In particular, decreased levels of somatostatin and increased levels of corticotropin-releasing factor are associated with depression.

Thus, a number of neurotransmitters have been implicated in mood disorders, with NE and serotonin being the most prominent. Lithium is the most effective drug for the treatment of mania and for controlling the mood swings between depression and mania that characterize bipolar disorder. It is not known how lithium affects the activity of neurons, but like many other chemicals that are important to normal brain functioning, lithium is an ion—that is, a molecule that has an electrical charge. It is thought that, whatever its action on neurons, lithium has many different effects in the brain (8). It increases serotonin activity, decreases acetylcholine activity, affects the activity of both norepinephrine and dopamine, and inhibits some of the intracellular mechanisms that are initiated by activation of receptors. Since lithium has such a broad range of actions that can affect the neurotransmitter systems implicated in mood disorders, its therapeutic effect may be due to its capacity to correct the neurotransmitter abnormalities associated with mania and depression, and to prevent the changes in neurochemical balance that are thought to be responsible for the mood swings of bipolar disorder.

Neuroendocrine Systems

Abnormalities in hormone regulation are common in depression (7,25,70,71), perhaps because regulation of hormones and the glands that secrete them is under the control of the same neurotransmitters in the brain that are thought to be dysfunctional in depression. In particular, the activities of the pituitary, adrenal, and pineal glands are affected. Many of the symptoms associated with depression (e.g., changes in appetite, sleep, and sex drive) may be related to these hormonal changes, which means that the hormonal abnormalities may be secondary to the neurotransmitter alterations of the disorder (7). Nonetheless, there is great interest in studying these changes in hopes of discovering a biological marker and developing diagnostic tests for depression.

A number of hormones have been studied to determine if depressed persons consistently exhibit abnormal concentrations of them or show an abnormal release of them in response to some sort of pharmacological challenge. Current information indicates that while some of these hormones are altered in depression, variability in baselines and pharmacological response, as well as the possibility of changes due to other causes, makes them unreliable markers for depression (7,70,71).

Depressed persons often have elevated concentrations of the hormone cortisol (7,25,70,71), which results from increased concentrations of corticotropin-releasing factor. In healthy individuals, administration of the drug dexamethasone suppresses the concentration of cortisol in the blood. The dexamethasone-suppression test (DST), developed as a test of hormone functioning, has been studied as a possible diagnostic tool in depression. Approximately 40 to 50 percent of persons diagnosed with major depression have an abnormal DST in that they do not suppress cortisol in response to dexamethasone (70). In very severe cases, particularly psychotically depressed patients, the percentage ranges from 60 to 80. It is not known why only some patients show an abnormal DST. Whether this reflects variability in response to DST or a subpopulation of depressed patients has yet to be resolved. Therefore, there are several problems with using the DST as a diagnostic tool (7,25,70,71). Aside from the fact that not all depressed patients show an abnormal DST, a number of other clinical (e.g., Alzheimer's disease,

anorexia nervosa) and nonclinical conditions (e.g., fasting, ingestion of caffeine) can result in abnormal DSTs. Although its effectiveness as a diagnostic tool is limited, the test may be useful in predicting which patients are likely to relapse following cessation of drug therapy: If DST results remain abnormal during therapy, the patient is more likely to relapse once the antidepressant is withdrawn (7).

Another aspect of endocrine function related to depression is the association between depression and reproduction-related events in women (2). Hormonal alterations related to menstruation, pregnancy, childbirth, and menopause can affect neurotransmitters that regulate mood and behavior. The evidence regarding the relationship between these hormonal fluctuations and the occurrence of depression is mixed. Nevertheless, the clear association of mood alterations with these reproductive events in some women suggests an area for additional investigation. Understanding these biochemical interactions could provide new insights into the pathology of depression.

Anatomy and Activity

It is unclear which areas of the brain may be involved in mood disorders. The data regarding anatomical defects and activity in the brain of persons with mood disorders are equivocal. Given that few studies have been conducted and that their results have varied, it is impossible to come to any conclusions regarding relationships between the data and the cause and symptoms of mood disorders. Overall, the data suggest an association between mood disorders and abnormalities of large regions of the brain, especially the frontal and temporal lobes; they also imply an abnormal difference between the left and right sides of the brain. Normally, the left and right sides of the brain are involved in different, although overlapping, functions. For example, the left is usually more specialized for language and logical thinking, while the right is more involved with spatial processing. As a result of these different functions, the two halves of the brain often exhibit different levels of activity. In mood disorders, some of the normal differences in activity level between the right and left sides of the brain appear to be altered.

Few postmortem studies have investigated anatomical alterations in the brains of persons with mood disorders, although a number of studies have examined depression and mania that are secondary to other insults to the brain (e.g., tumors, stroke, wounds) (25). Often, the trauma-induced alteration in mood occurs as a single episode of either depression or mania; there are only a few reports of bipolar disorder occurring as a result of brain damage. Although the secondary nature of the disorders severely limits the usefulness of these studies, some anatomical patterns can be discerned. In general, depression and mania are associated with damage to the frontal and temporal lobes of the brain, while bipolar disorders are associated with diverse areas of the brain. Depression tends to be associated with damage to the left side of the brain and mania with damage to the right (25).

Additional information has been derived from studies using CAT and MRI scans (25). While not conclusive, data from CAT scans indicate that patients with mood disorders, especially bipolar disorder, have decreased cortical volume. The clinical features most frequently correlated with decreased cortical volume are psychotic symptoms and poor response to treatment. The few MRI studies of persons with bipolar disorder indicate that there may be some structural abnormalities present, especially in the frontal and temporal lobes (25).

Studies measuring cerebral blood flow and glucose utilization have also produced some evidence of abnormal activity in mood disorders (25,85) (figure 4-6). The available data suggest that persons with bipolar disorder, as well as persons with major depression, show decreased activity in a specific portion of the frontal lobes called the prefrontal cortex; persons with bipolar disorder also show a more general decrease in activity involving the whole cortex and the left frontal lobes (25). Thus, these studies implicate the left side of the brain. However, results of studies using neuropsychological testing and observations of electrical activity in the brain caused by performing a task implicate a deficit in the right side (25,74,86). Neuropsychological testing consistently finds deficits in tasks related to right-hemisphere functioning, such as spatial learning and memory, among persons with mood disorders (25). The imaging data, which are consistent with the postmortem studies, are from studies of the brain in its resting state, whereas the neuropsychological testing and electrophysiological studies measured the active functioning of the brain in response to a task. It is unclear whether the divergence in observations represents discrete ab-

Figure 4-6—PET Scans of an Individual With Bipolar Disorder

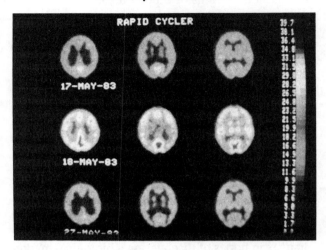

Brain activity in a person when depressed (top and bottom rows) and when in the manic state (middle row).

SOURCE: L. Baxter, M. Phelps, J. Mazziotta, et al., "Cerebral Metabolic Rates for Glucose in Mood Disorders: Studies With Positron Emission Tomography and Fluorodeoxyglucose F18," *Archives of General Psychiatry* 42:441-447, 1985 (copyright 1985 © American Medical Association).

normalities that are detected selectively by the different methods. Additional data need to be collected, using imaging techniques in conjunction with performance tasks, to clarify this issue and to determine the significance of these differences in activity on the two sides of the brain.

Other Factors

Sleep and Biological Rhythms

Sleep disturbances are common in persons with major depression (25,38,68,70) and, like the alterations in endocrine function discussed earlier, are likely to be secondary to a primary pathology. Sleep consists of rapid eye movement (REM) sleep (the time during which dreaming takes place) and non-REM sleep. Both REM and non-REM sleep can be monitored with the EEG. In the course of a night, REM and non-REM sleep cycle approximately every 90 minutes. In depression, the first REM period occurs earlier than normal after sleep begins, the time spent in REM sleep is increased, and the length of non-REM sleep decreases. In 80 to 85 percent of depressed persons, sleep is broken by frequent awakenings, while the remaining percentage show features of hypersomnia. It has been suggested that depressed persons can be differentiated from other individuals on the basis of the abnormalities in REM sleep (70). The early occurrence of REM sleep has been repeatedly demonstrated in depression. Based on these observations, it has been suggested that shortened REM latency, and possibly other REM sleep measures, can be used to diagnose depression (70); others question the specificity of these changes to depression (25).

The sleep of persons with bipolar disorder is often disturbed and varies with clinical state, severity, and stage of the disorder (25). When depressed, bipolar patients may sleep excessively, and when manic, may sleep little or not at all. Sleep can also influence the switch from one phase to another. Sleep loss often precedes, and may trigger, a manic episode. Also, one or two nights of sleep deprivation can have a short-term antidepressant effect (25,79). This evidence indicates that in some cases mania can be prevented and depression treated by appropriate manipulation of the sleep-wake cycle (25).

The sleep cycles previously described are an example of a biological rhythm. The preceding report in the Office of Technology Assessment's neuroscience series (79) describes and discusses biological rhythms—the changes in various physiological and behavioral functions that repeat at regular intervals and provide a framework of temporal organization for those functions—and their effects and consequences. While sleep stages are measured in minutes, many biological rhythms (e.g., body temperature, secretion of hormones, sleep-wake cycle, alertness, memory) have a 24-hour cycle and are called circadian rhythms. For example, body temperature fluctuates over 24 hours, with peak body temperature occurring during the day and lowest body temperature occurring at night.

The cyclic pattern of bipolar disorder and the fact that people with depression exhibit daily and seasonal fluctuations in mood suggest a link between mood disorders and biological rhythms. Whether that link is causative or correlative is unknown (79). Changes in biological rhythms have been observed in some persons with mood disorders (25,72). The fact that animal studies have indicated that some antidepressant medications have an effect on the organization of circadian rhythms provides a further link between mood disorders and biological rhythms. Finally, a seasonal variation in the occurrence of depression has been observed. A specific syndrome of winter depression, which remits during the summer, has been identified and named seasonal affective disorder (SAD). Although it is not clear whether SAD is associated with altered biological rhythms, it is related to changes in the length of daylight across the seasons. Exposure to additional light during the winter is an effective treatment for SAD.

Kindling and Sensitization

Recurrences of mania and depression in bipolar disorder tend to increase in frequency over time. The neurobiological phenomena of electrical kindling and behavioral sensitization observed in animals may provide clues to the physiological mechanisms underlying this pattern of cycling (25). Repeated administration of low-level electrical stimulation to an area of the brain results in kindling, or increased responsiveness to electrical stimulus that leads to the development of seizures. If the stimulation is repeated frequently enough, the area becomes so sensitive that seizures will occur spontaneously. Similarly, behavioral sensitization refers to the increasing behavioral response that results from repeated administration of the same dose of a stimulant drug.

While these phenomena are not directly analogous to the mood disturbances of bipolar disorder, they do share certain characteristics (62). For example, in each, early episodes require a precipitating event, while later ones can occur spontaneously. Also, repeated exposure to precipitating events leads to more frequent occurrence of episodes. These characteristics coincide with the concept that early episodes of mania or depression result from some sort of psychosocial stress but later episodes can occur in the absence of such a stimulus, and with the observation that episodes tend to occur with a shorter and shorter cycle.

Thus, the same or similar brain mechanisms controlling kindling and sensitization could play a role in the cycling of bipolar disorder. Some evidence for this is seen in the fact that serotonin, norepinephrine, and GABA, neurotransmitters implicated in mood disorders, all inhibit the kindling phenomenon (25). Also, lithium, which is efficacious in treating bipolar disorder, blocks behavioral sensitization, while carbamazepine, an antiseizure medication that is also effective in bipolar disorder, blocks kindling.

Immune and Viral Factors

Results from some studies have raised the possibility that mood disorders may be associated with abnormalities in the body's immune system or with viral infection (25). For example, some studies indicate that persons with major depression may have a compromised immune system, as indicated by their diminished response to infectious challenges. Also, some studies have found increased antibodies to certain viruses that infect the nervous system (i.e., cytomegalovirus, herpes, and Borna disease virus) in some persons with mood disorders. Thus, there is limited evidence that immune system dysfunction or viral infection may be associated with mood disorders in some persons, although the available data are far from conclusive. If such associations exist, it is unclear what relationship they may have to the onset and symptoms of the disorder.

Synthesis

There are many disparate pieces to the puzzle of mood disorders, and fitting the available ones together is difficult. Early theories that depression and bipolar disorder are the result of a simple imbalance in norepinephrine or that a specific anatomical locus could be identified are now recognized as simplistic. Clinically effective drugs have shown that adjusting the activity in monoamine-containing regions of the brain has an antidepressant effect. Whether this indicates there is a primary dysfunction in these regions in depression has yet to be proved. The implications of the other factors described in this section are also unclear.

An approach that encompasses the diversity of experimental data and is at the same time harmonious with the clinical profile of the disorders is needed in order to construct a meaningful hypothesis. As discussed in chapter 3, it is unclear whether depression is a single disorder or a collection of disorders. This possible heterogeneity complicates attempts to delineate biological factors that might be involved. It is likely that the same regions of the brain mediate depression in both major depression and bipolar disorder. If separate subtypes of depression exist, this same network of structures is likely to be involved; what differentiates the disorders may be the factors that disrupt the network. This idea coincides with information suggesting that mood disorders occur because integrated control systems

in the brain are disrupted, rather than because of defects in specific regions. The explanations that there is an overall dysregulation in the balance between the different monoamine neurotransmitter systems and that the brain mechanisms which control biological rhythms may be involved in mood disorders are examples of hypotheses involving disruptions of integrated control systems. As more information is gathered about these and other systems, researchers will gain a clearer understanding of how they may be disrupted in mood disorders.

ANXIETY DISORDERS

Anxiety is a normal human emotion that can help people cope with certain situations. It is only when anxiety or its manifestations become excessive and interfere with normal performance or health that they are considered pathological and termed a disorder (see ch. 3). Anxiety disorders include generalized anxiety disorder, panic disorder, obsessive-compulsive disorder (OCD), social and simple phobias, and posttraumatic stress disorder (PTSD). This discussion will be limited to the disorders in which biological factors have been most extensively studied, namely, OCD and panic disorder.

Obsessive-Compulsive Disorder

Idiosyncratic daily rituals and odd personal habits are ubiquitous. It is only when obsessions or compulsions, or both, cause marked distress, occupy more than 1 hour a day, and cause significant social or occupational dysfunction that the diagnosis of OCD is made (63) (see ch. 3). OCD is commonly accompanied by depression. Symptoms include recurrent obsessions with fears of contamination, harming others, and worries that doors are not locked or lights have not been turned off. Compulsions such as washing, checking, counting, and rearranging are common. Though most patients know that these thoughts and behaviors are irrational, they cannot put them out of their mind. The involuntary, repetitive nature of the cognitive or motor behaviors associated with OCD, coupled with recent experimental findings, suggests a role for biological factors in OCD.

Biochemistry

Drugs that are effective in treating OCD act by blocking the reuptake of serotonin into the neuron from which it was released (49,50,87). Not all persons with OCD respond to these drugs (91), however, and it is unclear whether these persons represent a subgroup of patients with OCD (91). The potency of drugs that block serotonin reuptake suggests that persons who do respond may have abnormal serotonin functioning, but supporting evidence is meager. Like other neurotransmitter systems, the serotonin system is complex. Serotonin is found in a number of specific areas of the brain, and several receptor subtypes have been identified. While a few studies have shown that drugs that block serotonin receptors can exacerbate OCD symptoms, no abnormalities in the synthesis, release, reuptake, metabolism, or receptors of serotonin in patients with OCD have been identified in other studies (87). Also, while the reuptake-blocking effects of drugs occur immediately, the therapeutic response usually does not develop until after several weeks of treatment (24,87). This delay suggests that the clinical effect could be the result of adaptive changes in the serotonin or other neurotransmitter systems in response to the changes in serotonin levels induced by the drugs (87). Thus, it is not certain whether these drugs act directly on a primary defect of the disorder or whether they act indirectly, via the serotonin system, to counteract the effects of a primary defect.

It has also been proposed that dopamine systems play a role in OCD (24). Symptoms of OCD sometimes result from damage to the basal ganglia, which have high concentrations of dopamine. Tourette's syndrome, a disorder characterized by motor and vocal tics, and often symptoms of OCD as well, is thought to result from a dysfunction of the dopamine system in the basal ganglia. Based on observations that serotonin can inhibit the activity of dopamine systems and that the basal ganglia receive input from serotonin-containing neurons, a hypothesis has been put forward that an alteration in the normal interaction of these neurotransmitter systems in the basal ganglia may be involved in OCD (24). There are some preliminary findings that drugs that act on dopamine may have an effect on OCD (24), and data from anatomical studies also indicate a role for the basal ganglia in OCD. This hypothesis is considered in greater detail in the next section, which describes the basal ganglia and some of their anatomical connections.

Anatomy and Activity

Persons with OCD exhibit a variety of abnormalities on neuropsychological tests (91). In general,

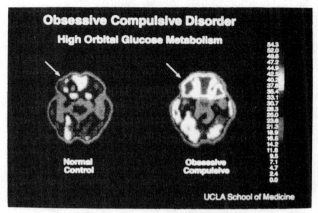

Figure 4-7—PET Scan of an Individual With Obsessive-Compulsive Disorder

Brain activity in the brain of a person with OCD (right) and the brain of a person without OCD (left). In OCD, there is increased activity in the frontal cortex.
SOURCE: L. Baxter, UCLA Center for Health Sciences, Los Angeles, CA.

these tests point to dysfunctions in the frontal lobes, basal ganglia, and hippocampus. For example, persons with OCD often perform poorly on tests that measure memory and attention. PET studies of glucose utilization have shown greater than normal activity in parts of the basal ganglia and an area of the frontal cortex, the orbital cortex, in OCD (4,5,91) (figure 4-7). Data from the few CAT studies that have been done indicate that the only difference between the brains of OCD patients and controls is a decrease in the size of various regions in the basal ganglia (64,91). These data, coupled with those previously discussed, lead to the hypothesis that OCD is the result of an abnormal interaction between the basal ganglia and other areas of the brain, principally the orbital cortex (4,5,35,64,91). These areas work together to coordinate movement in response to thought. If the basal ganglia are damaged, involuntary movements such as tics occur.

The thoughts and impulses that often make up obsessions (e.g., those related to aggression, hygiene, sex, and danger) are thought to be generated in the frontal cortex. In normal individuals, the basal ganglia-orbital system filters these impulses, putting them aside so that they are not acted upon. According to this theory of OCD, the filtering effect that keeps an individual from acting on thoughts or impulses does not work properly. As a result, a thought occurs and the person takes action. Again, the association with Tourette's syndrome is striking. Individuals with this disorder exhibit not only motor tics, but involuntary vocalizations, often of an obscene or socially unacceptable nature (such as racial epithets). The basal ganglia-orbital cortex hypothesis posits a dysfunction in the normal control of thoughts (obsessions), which can lead to reactive motor activity (compulsions).

Panic Disorder

Panic disorder is marked by recurrent periods of intense fear that last for several minutes. The attacks are not triggered by anxiety-provoking situations, and patients often report that they occur ''out of the blue.'' Many persons with panic disorder experience varying degrees of anxiety between attacks in anticipation of the next panic attack (57). This ''fear of fear'' often results in patients with panic disorder developing agoraphobia, the fear of being in public places.

Several theories have been postulated to explain panic disorder (57). One views panic as the result of hyperactivity of the physiological mechanisms that are normally activated in stressful situations (i.e., the sympathetic nervous system). Another posits that individuals have an increased psychological sensitivity to normal fluctuations in physiological responses. This theory suggests that patients may misinterpret normal physiological changes as dangerous, inducing more anxiety and precipitating a panic attack. Another theory suggests that there is a primary defect in brain mechanisms related to the neurotransmitter norepinephrine, which is associated with the sympathetic response. A role for sensitivity to the chemicals lactate and carbon dioxide, for hyperventilation, and for dysfunction in the temporal lobe of the brain have also been proposed. There is experimental evidence to support, or in some cases refute, these various theories. Thus, while there are a lot of puzzle pieces, there is currently no unified theory of panic disorder.

Biochemistry

Information about the pharmacology associated with panic disorder can be derived both from drugs that are effective in treating the disorder and from agents that induce a panic attack when given to a patient. The most effective drugs for treating anxiety are the benzodiazepines. In high doses, these drugs are also effective in controlling panic disorder. Benzodiazepines exert their antianxiety effects indirectly, by increasing the action of the inhibitory

neurotransmitter GABA. The discovery that there are specific receptors in the brain for benzodiazepines indicates that there must be a chemical produced by the brain that would normally attach to these receptors (although such a chemical has yet to be discovered). Benzodiazepine receptors are coupled to GABA receptors, and activation of the former accentuates the effects of GABA, which turns off overly active brain cells (14,76).

Unlike GABA and its receptors, which are found throughout the brain, benzodiazepine receptors are located in only a few brain structures. Thus, not all GABA receptors are coupled with benzodiazepine receptors. The GABA receptors that are coupled to benzodiazepine receptors and that respond to the drug are known as $GABA_A$ receptors. The areas of the brain that contain both benzodiazepine and $GABA_A$ receptors include the hippocampus and the amygdala, both limbic system structures (76). As described previously, the limbic system plays a role in controlling emotional behavior. Thus, it is thought that the antianxiety effect of benzodiazepines results from their action on $GABA_A$ receptors in the hippocampus and amygdala.

Another compound, buspirone, is effective for treating general anxiety, but instead of affecting GABA, it acts on other chemical systems in the brain. Buspirone decreases the activity of the neurotransmitter serotonin in some areas of the brain and activates receptors for the neurotransmitter dopamine in other areas (76). Buspirone acts on serotonin systems through a complex interaction with a number of different subtypes of serotonin receptors. This action, coupled with other experimental findings, has led to the speculation that increased activity in serotonin-containing areas, particularly the raphe nuclei, may be involved in anxiety (55). It is thought that the raphe nuclei, via their connections with the limbic system, may be involved in mediating anxious behavior and that activation would cause anxiety.

The most effective drugs for treating panic disorder are the drugs used to treat depression, although they exert a therapeutic action in panic that is different from that in depression (76). The efficacy of these drugs has led to the theory that panic results from overactivity of the norepinephrine systems in the brain that mediate the fight-or-flight response, principally the locus ceruleus (3,43,55,65). It should be kept in mind, however, that the neurons in the locus ceruleus make connections with neurons in the limbic system and can affect their activity. The hypothesis is that a panic attack is the result of inappropriate activation of the norepinephrine system in the locus ceruleus. Studies have shown that panic attacks can be caused by drugs that increase either the activity of cells in the locus ceruleus or the release of norepinephrine from them, whereas the antidepressants used to treat panic decrease the activity of the locus ceruleus (29,55,61,76).

Any number of agents can provoke panic attacks in persons who suffer from panic disorder, including the chemical lactate (administered intravenously) and carbon dioxide (inhaled). At a high enough concentration, carbon dioxide will also induce panic in controls. The mechanism by which these agents cause panic attacks is unknown (22,27,73,76). Lactate has complex actions in the brain, including effects on serotonin, norepinephrine, and other transmitter systems, as well as areas of the brain that respond to changes in blood chemistry and regulate respiration (73). Inhalation of carbon dioxide upsets the balance of oxygen in the blood and can affect its acidity (27). The areas of the brain that monitor and control functions such as respiration and the cardiovascular system are connected with the locus ceruleus as part of the fight-or-flight response. One theory holds that the norepinephrine system in the locus ceruleus is unusually sensitive in persons with panic disorder. Thus, according to this theory, lactate and carbon dioxide cause changes in either the body or the brain that indirectly activate the norepinephrine system in the locus ceruleus, precipitating a panic attack (27,55,73,92). Lactate induces a panic attack in about 80 percent of persons with panic disorder (55). This high correlation has led to the suggestion that lactate response can be considered a diagnostic marker for the disorder (20), although variability in the characteristics of the response among patients has called this into question (55).

While it seems likely that the locus ceruleus is involved in panic disorder, other experimental evidence raises the question as to whether that role is primary or secondary to the cause of the disorder and whether other brain systems are also involved (76). For example, serotonin has also been implicated in the genesis of panic attacks (55,58,76). Serotonin connections to the locus ceruleus inhibit

the activity of locus ceruleus cells, and drugs that potentiate the action of serotonin suppress panic attacks (76). It has been postulated that a primary decrease in activity in this serotonin-inhibiting system may play a role in inducing panic attacks (58) and that the role of the locus ceruleus is secondary to this effect. In addition, the action of caffeine indicates that other brain systems besides the locus ceruleus may be involved. Caffeine can precipitate a panic attack in persons with panic disorder (55,76,77). As a result, people who suffer from panic attacks often learn, on their own, to avoid caffeine-laden products such as coffee and chocolate. Caffeine's principal action in the brain is to block the receptors for the inhibitory neurotransmitter adenosine. However, caffeine also has some effect on norepinephrine, dopamine, and benzodiazepine systems. It is not known whether caffeine produces panic by inhibiting adenosine activity, some other action, or a combination of these (77). It is also unclear how or whether caffeine's panic-inducing action relates to the occurrence of panic disorder.

Anatomy and Activity

The few CAT and MRI studies that have examined the brain structure of persons with panic disorder provide evidence of brain atrophy or underdevelopment, particularly in the frontal and temporal lobes (33). However, given the limited number of studies that have been done, the significance of these results is unclear and must be considered preliminary (33).

Abnormal activity has also been observed in the brains of persons with panic disorder (26,44,45,67). At rest, panic disorder patients who are sensitive to lactate exhibited increased cerebral blood flow to the parahippocampal gyrus (PHG), an area of the cerebral cortex that is associated with the limbic system (figure 4-8). Normal controls or lactate-insensitive panic patients did not show these changes. Based on these results, it was proposed that a PHG abnormality was involved in a predisposition to panic, and it was further hypothesized that activation of a norepinephrine pathway to the PHG initiates an attack (67). However, this hypothesis is based on limited data, and confirmation will require additional studies. Furthermore, it does not explain what mechanism might be present in lactate-insensitive panic disorder patients. Other studies have demon-

Figure 4-8—PET Scan of an Individual With Panic Disorder

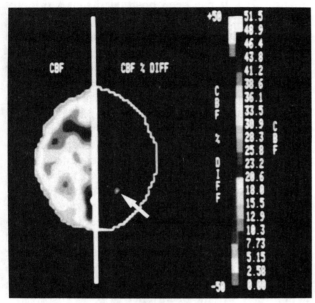

Whole brain activity (left side) and abnormal activity in the parahippocampal gyrus (right side) in the brain of a person with panic disorder in the nonpanic state.
SOURCE: E. Reiman, Good Samaritan Hospital, Phoenix, AZ.

strated that there is an increase in cerebral blood flow during lactate-induced panic attacks (67).

Synthesis

There is evidence that a number of different biological factors play a role in OCD and panic disorder. The possible role of the basal ganglia-orbital cortex system in OCD is an intriguing theory, coupling areas of the brain involved in cognitive and motor activity. Further examination of these brain regions, the role of dopamine mechanisms, and their interactions with serotonin systems are important areas for future research related to OCD. Both limbic structures and the locus ceruleus are implicated in panic disorder. Data suggest that the limbic structures mediate generalized feelings of anxiety, influenced by the activity of GABA, while the locus ceruleus controls an active response to anxiety-provoking stimuli (i.e., panic attacks). The anatomical connections between these two regions of the brain suggest that there might be some interaction of these systems in panic disorder, but additional study of these systems and their interaction is necessary.

IMPLICATIONS FOR TREATMENT

One of the greatest promises of research into the biology of mental disorders is the development of more efficacious treatments—particularly drugs. At the same time, effective treatment of a mental disorder must take into consideration all aspects of the disorder—biological, psychological, and social. Thus, developments related to biological factors associated with a disorder contribute to the total therapeutic protocol available to treat patients.

The antipsychotic drug chlorpromazine, used to treat persons with schizophrenia, provides an example of the development of a biological treatment. The discovery that chlorpromazine was an antipsychotic drug was serendipitous (36). The drug was originally developed in the search for an effective antihistamine; the chance clinical observation that it had an antipsychotic effect led to its use in schizophrenia. Once chlorpromazine's effect was established, research into its mechanism of action led to the finding that it exerted its effect by blocking the D_2 dopamine receptor subtype (see earlier discussion). This led in turn to the development of additional antipsychotic drugs, called typical antipsychotics, that also act by blocking D_2 dopamine receptors.

The chlorpromazine story also illustrates the point that most therapeutic advances in psychopharmacology have occurred by chance. A drug discovered to be efficacious was then examined further, to advance researchers' understanding of the biological mechanisms underlying a disorder (36).

The impetus for developing new drugs comes from the fact that current drugs are imperfect (89). Side effects are common, and not all patients respond to a given drug. In general, these problems result from existing drugs' inability to act selectively on the symptoms of a disorder. For example, while typical antipsychotic drugs act by blocking D_2 receptors in areas of the brain involved with schizophrenia symptoms, they also block D_2 receptors in other areas of the brain, which produces the movement side effects characteristic of these drugs. Another example is the side effects associated with antidepressant drugs, which result when the antidepressants act on other neurotransmitter systems besides the monoamine systems thought to be involved with depression.

Beyond the need for more efficacious drugs with fewer side effects, the financial impact that more effective treatments can have is another factor driving the search for new drugs. Improved treatments can decrease total treatment costs by reducing the need for hospitalization; they can decrease other financial effects as well, such as lost wages due to disability. For example, a study conducted in 1980 estimated that the introduction of lithium in 1969, for the treatment of bipolar disorder, resulted in an average yearly savings in treatment costs of $290 million in the United States (66). It was also estimated that in the first year following the introduction of lithium, $92 million in lost wages was regained (66).

By attaining a better understanding of what neurochemical systems are affected in a disorder and how those systems interact with others, more effective drugs can be developed to treat the symptoms of a disorder while minimizing side effects. The recent strides that have been made in basic neuroscience research, particularly advances in molecular and cellular neurobiology, will facilitate this process (75,78). The ability to clone receptor subtypes and identify precisely the molecular structure of receptors and other biochemical constituents of the brain will enable scientists to construct drugs that act more precisely. Thus, the development of drugs for mental disorders is entering a new phase in which both clinical and basic research findings will be applied to the design of more efficacious medications.

The antipsychotic drug clozapine and the antidepressant fluoxetine are examples of this new generation of drugs. Clozapine, a so-called atypical antipsychotic drug, not only blocks D_2 receptors but also acts on other dopamine receptors (see box 4-A) and on serotonin receptors to create different effects on these systems in different areas of the brain (47). Clozapine is thought to block sufficient dopamine in appropriate areas of the brain to control psychosis, while acting on other areas of the brain to avert the blanket D_2 blockade that produces side effects. Unlike traditional antidepressants, which have a broad effect on catecholamine and other neurotransmitter systems, fluoxetine (Prozac) was designed specifically to block serotonin reuptake (69). As a result, it has an antidepressant action equivalent to that of older drugs, but without many of their side effects.

Table 4-2—Drugs in Development for Mental Disorders

Disorder	United States	Other countries
Schizophrenia	76	42
Mood disorders	83	61
Anxiety disorders	91	46

SOURCE: PJB Publications, *Pharmaprojects* (Surrey, England: PJB Publications, 1992).

Both of these drugs are improvements on older medications, but neither is totally without problems. Although clozapine does not produce the movement side effects associated with typical antipsychotic drugs, it is associated with an even more dangerous side effect. About 2 percent of persons taking clozapine develop a potentially deadly blood disease, agranulocytosis. As a result, anyone taking the drug must be tested regularly; if there is any indication of the disease, treatment must be stopped. The need for constant monitoring makes administration of clozapine costly, ranging between $6,000 and $9,000 a year (19). While fluoxetine has many fewer side effects than older antidepressants, it is associated with such adverse reactions as nausea, nervousness, insomnia, and headache (56).

Despite these problems, the advantages of these drugs make them highly popular. For example, in spite of the costs associated with clozapine, results from a study demonstrated that over a 2-year period there was a savings of approximately $16,000 per patient, per year, as a result of decreased hospitalization among 37 patients who had taken the drug (48). Total U.S. sales of clozapine in 1991 were estimated to be $60 million (19), while 1990 sales for fluoxetine were put at $500 million (52). Currently, a number of other drugs, which may represent further improvements on the medications that have been used in the past to treat mental disorders, are being developed and tested (table 4-2). These new drugs represent the latest efforts to apply information derived from the study of the biology of mental disorders to treatment of patients.

SUMMARY AND CONCLUSIONS

Evidence exists for the activity of a variety of biological factors in each disorder reviewed in this report. However, it is difficult to put the strands of evidence together in a unified hypothesis about the role of biological factors in a given disorder.

Most of the biological factors that have been identified relate to changes in the brain that are correlated with a disorder. These include alterations in neurotransmitter systems, such as the association of increased or decreased levels of dopamine with the various symptoms of schizophrenia and the role of monoamines in mood disorders. Disruptions in brain activity are associated with disorders as well, such as the decreased activity found in the frontal lobes of persons with schizophrenia and the increased activity in the basal ganglia of persons with OCD. These factors, and the others discussed in this chapter, provide insights into the mechanisms underlying the symptoms displayed by patients. A better understanding of such mechanisms should enable scientists to develop more effective treatments.

Less is known about the causes of mental disorders. The influence of various factors, such as developmental and viral factors, has been hypothesized, but as yet there is no definitive explanation for any of these disorders. To understand what leads to the onset of mental disorders, researchers must consider the role of psychological and social factors and how they may interact with a pathological biological condition. For example, the alterations in the limbic system and locus ceruleus associated with panic disorder may represent a biological predisposition that is shaped by an individual's experiences to determine whether and how the disorder is manifested, while the kindling-sensitization model of bipolar disorder suggests that life events can modify abnormal brain activity.

It is essential to learn how the healthy brain works. Research in the basic neurosciences provides the foundation for research on the biology of mental disorders. Advances in the neurosciences have resulted in the development of new techniques and improvements on old ones that greatly increase our ability to study the brain. Combining such techniques as neuropsychological testing or biochemical analysis with brain imaging techniques extends that ability even further. Current research is increasingly taking multidimensional approaches to the study of mental disorders, integrating data concerning different aspects of brain functioning and behavior into testable hypotheses. That trend is expected to accelerate.

Essential to this effort will be strategies for studying the integrated networks of brain structures that control behaviors. Some mental disorders may be collections of disorder subtypes, indicating that the normal functioning of a network that mediates a behavior can be disrupted at various points. The ultimate goals of research are to understand how brain structures work in concert to produce behavior, how this process is disrupted in mental disorders, and what factors cause it to go awry.

CHAPTER 4 REFERENCES

1. Altshuler, L.L., Conrad, A., Kovelman, J.A., et al., "Hippocampal Pyramidal Cell Orientation in Schizophrenia: A Controlled Neurohistologic Study of the Yakoviev Collection," *Archives of General Psychiatry* 44:1094-1098, 1987.
2. American Psychological Association, *Women and Depression*, E. McGrath, G.P. Keita, B.R. Strickland, and N.F. Russo (eds.) (Washington, DC: American Psychological Association, 1990).
3. Ballenger, J.C., "Toward an Integrated Model of Panic Disorder," *American Journal of Orthopsychiatry* 59:284-293, 1989.
4. Baxter, L.R., "Brain Imaging as a Tool in Establishing a Theory of Brain Pathology in Obsessive Compulsive Disorder," *Journal of Clinical Psychiatry* 51:22-25, 1990.
5. Baxter, L.R., Schwartz, J.M., Guze, B.H., et al., "PET Imaging in Obsessive Compulsive Disorder With and Without Depression," *Journal of Clinical Psychiatry* 51:61-69, 1990.
6. Berger, P.A., and Nemeroff, C.B., "Opioid Peptides in Affective Disorders," *Psychopharmacology: The Third Generation of Progress*, H.Y. Meltzer (ed.) (New York, NY: Raven Press, 1987).
7. Brown, G.M., "Psychoneuroendocrinology of Depression," *Psychiatric Journal of the University of Ottawa* 14:344-348, 1989.
8. Bunney, W.E., and Garland-Bunney, B.L., "Mechanisms of Action of Lithium in Affective Illness: Basic and Clinical Implications," *Psychopharmacology: The Third Generation of Progress*, H.Y. Meltzer (ed.) (New York, NY: Raven Press, 1987).
9. Carpenter, W.T., Buchanan, R.W., Kirkpatrick, B., et al., "Negative Symptoms: A Critique of Current Approaches," *Proceedings of the Workshop on Negative/Positive Schizophrenia, June 29-30, 1990* (Heidelberg: Springer-Verlag, in press).
10. Cleghorn, J.M., Zipursky, R.B., and List, S.J., "Structural and Functional Brain Imaging in Schizophrenia," *Journal of Psychiatric Neuroscience* 16:53-74, 1991.
11. Cornblatt, B., Winters, L., and Erlenmeyer-Kimling, L., "Attentional Markers of Schizophrenia: Evidence From the New York High-Risk Study," *Schizophrenia: Scientific Progress*, S.C. Schulz and C.A.

Tamminga (eds.) (New York, NY: Oxford University Press, 1989).

12. Davis, K.L., Kahn, R.S., Ko, G., et al., "Dopamine in Schizophrenia: A Review and Reconceptualization," *American Journal of Psychiatry* 148:1474-1486, 1991.

13. DeLisi, L.E., "Viral and Immune Hypotheses for Schizophrenia," *Psychopharmacology: The Third Generation of Progress*, H.Y. Meltzer (ed.) (New York, NY: Raven Press, 1987).

14. Dilsaver, S.C., "Generalized Anxiety Disorder," *American Family Physician* 39:137-144, 1989.

15. Dilsaver, S.C., and Coffman, J.A., "Cholinergic Hypothesis of Depression: A Reappraisal," *Journal of Clinical Psychopharmacology* 9:173-179, 1989.

16. Early, T.S., Posner, M.I., Rieman, E.M., et al., "Hyperactivity of the Left Striato-Pallidal Projection. Part I: Lower Level Theory," *Psychiatric Developments* 2:85-108, 1989.

17. Early, T.S., Posner, M.T., Reiman, E.M., et al., "Left Striato-Pallidal Hyperactivity in Schizophrenia. Part II: Phenomenology and Thought Disorder," *Psychiatric Developments* 7:109-121, 1989.

18. Feinberg, I., "Cortical Pruning and the Development of Schizophrenia," *Schizophrenia Bulletin* 15:477-490, 1989.

19. Freudenheim, M., "Seeking Safer Treatments for Schizophrenia," *New York Times*, Jan. 15, 1992, p. 47.

20. Fyer, A.J., Liebowitz, M.R., Gorman, J.M., et al., "Lactate Vulnerability of Remitted Panic Patients," *Psychiatry Research* 14:143-148, 1985.

21. Garza-Trevino, E.S., Volkow, N.D., Cancro, R., et al., "Neurobiology of Schizophrenia Syndromes," *Hospital and Community Psychiatry* 41:971-980, 1990.

22. Glover, V., and Sandler, M., "Tribulin and Stress: Clinical Studies on a New Neurochemical System," *Frontiers of Clinical Neuroscience*, vol. 8, *Neurobiology of Panic Disorder*, J.C. Ballenger (ed.) (New York, NY: Alan R. Liss, 1990).

23. Gold, P.W., and Rubinow, D.R., "Neuropeptide Function in Affective Illness: Corticotropin-Releasing Hormone and Somatostatin as Model Systems," *Psychopharmacology: The Third Generation of Progress*, H.Y. Meltzer (ed.) (New York, NY: Raven Press, 1987).

24. Goodman, W.K., McDougle, C.J., Price, L.H., et al., "Beyond the Serotonin Hypothesis: A Role for Dopamine in Some Forms of Obsessive Compulsive Disorder," *Journal of Clinical Psychiatry* 51:36-43, 1990.

25. Goodwin, F.K., and Jamison, K.R., *Manic-Depressive Illness* (New York, NY: Oxford University Press, 1990).

26. Gorman, J.M., Liebowitz, M.R., Fyer, A.J., et al., "A Neuroanatomical Hypothesis for Panic Disorder," *American Journal of Psychiatry* 146:148-161, 1989.

27. Gorman, J.M., and Papp, L.A., "Respiratory Physiology of Panic," *Frontiers of Clinical Neuroscience*, vol. 8, *Neurobiology of Panic Disorder*, J.C. Ballenger (ed.) (New York, NY: Alan R. Liss, 1990).

28. Hasey, G., and Hanin, I., "The Cholinergic-Adrenergic Hypothesis of Depression Reexamined Using Clonidine, Metoprolol, and Physostigmine in an Animal Model," *Biological Psychiatry* 29:127-138, 1991.

29. Heninger, G.R., and Charney, D.S., "Monoamine Receptor Systems and Anxiety Disorders," *Psychiatric Clinics of North America* 11:309-326, 1988.

30. Janowsky, D.S., and Overstreet, D.H., "Cholinergic Dysfunction in Depression," *Pharmacology and Toxicology* 66(suppl. 3):100-111, 1990.

31. Javitt, D.C., and Zukin, S.R., "Recent Advances in the Phencyclidine Model of Schizophrenia," *American Journal of Psychiatry* 148:1301-1308, 1991.

32. Kaufman, C.A., and Ziegler, R.J., "The Viral Hypothesis of Schizophrenia," *Receptors and Ligands in Psychiatry*, A.K. Sen and T. Lee (eds.) (Cambridge, England: Cambridge University Press, 1987).

33. Kellner, C., and Roy-Byrne, P.P., "Computed Tomography and Magnetic Resonance Imaging in Panic Disorder," *Frontiers of Clinical Neuroscience*, vol. 8, *Neurobiology of Panic Disorder*, J.C. Ballenger (ed.) (New York, NY: Alan R. Liss, 1990).

34. Keshavan, M.S., and Ganguli, R., "Biology of Schizophrenia," *Progress in Basic Clinical Pharmacology*, vol. 3, *The Biological Basis of Psychiatric Treatment*, R. Pohl and S. Gershon (eds.) (Basel: Karger, 1990).

35. Khanna, S., "Obsessive-Compulsive Disorder: Is There a Frontal Lobe Dysfunction?" *Biological Psychiatry* 24:602-613, 1988.

36. Klerman, G., "Future Prospects for Clinical Psychopharmacology," *Psychopharmacology: The Third Generation of Progress*, H.Y. Meltzer (ed.) (New York, NY: Raven Press, 1987).

37. Kovelman, J.A., and Scheibel, A.B., "A Neurohistological Correlate of Schizophrenia," *Biological Psychiatry* 19:1601-1621, 1984.

38. Kupfer, D.J., Frank, E., Jarrett, D.B., et al., "Interrelationship of Electroencephalographic Sleep Chronobiology and Depression," *Biological Rhythms and Mental Disorders*, D.J. Kupfer, T.H. Monk, and J.D. Barchas (eds.) (New York, NY: Guilford Press, 1988).

39. Levin, S., Yurgelun-Todd, D., and Craft, S., "Contributions of Clinical Neuropsychology to the Study of Schizophrenia," *Journal of Abnormal Psychology* 98:341-356, 1989.

40. Lloyd, K.G., Zivkovic, B., Scatton, B., et al., "The GABAergic Hypothesis of Depression," *Progress in Neuropsycho-Pharmacology and Biological Psychiatry* 13:341-351, 1989.

41. Lyon, M., Barr, C.E., Cannon, T.D., et al., "Fetal Neural Development and Schizophrenia," *Schizophrenia Bulletin* 15:149-161, 1989.

42. McNeil, T.F., "Perinatal Influences in the Development of Schizophrenia," *Biological Perspectives of Schizophrenia*, H. Helmchen and T.A. Henn (eds.) (New York, NY: John Wiley & Sons, 1987).

43. Maser, J.D., and Woods, S.W., "The Biological Basis of Panic: Psychological Interactions," *Psychiatric Medicine* 8:121-147, 1990.

44. Mathew, R.J., and Wilson, W.H., "Cerebral Blood Flow in Anxiety and Panic," *Frontiers of Clinical Neuroscience*, vol. 8, *Neurobiology of Panic Disorder*, J.C. Ballenger (ed.) (New York, NY: Alan R. Liss, 1990).

45. Mathew, R.J., and Wilson, W.H., "Anxiety and Cerebral Blood Flow," *American Journal of Psychiatry* 147:838-849, 1990.

46. Meltzer, H., "Serotonergic Dysfunction in Depression," *British Journal of Psychiatry* 155:25-31, 1989.

47. Meltzer, H., "The Mechanism of Action of Novel Antipsychotic Drugs," *Schizophrenia Bulletin* 17:263-287, 1991.

48. Meltzer, H., "Dimensions of Outcome With Clozapine," *British Journal of Psychiatry* 160:46-53, 1992.

49. Murphy, D.L., and Pigott, T.A., "A Comparative Role for Serotonin in Obsessive Compulsive Disorder, Panic Disorder, and Anxiety," *Journal of Clinical Psychiatry* 51(suppl.):53-58, 1990.

50. Murphy, D.L., Zohar, J., Benkelfat, C., et al., "Obsessive-Compulsive Disorder as a 5-HT Subsystem-Related Behavioural Disorder," *British Journal of Psychiatry Supplement* 8:15-24, 1989.

51. Nair, N.P., and Sharma, M., "Neurochemical and Receptor Theories of Depression," *Psychiatric Journal of the University of Ottawa* 14:328-341, 1989.

52. *Newsweek*, "The Promise of Prozac," Mar. 26, 1990, pp. 38-41.

53. Neylan, T.C., and van Kammen, D.P., "Biological Mechanisms of Schizophrenia: An Update," *Psychiatric Medicine* 8:41-52, 1990.

54. North, C.S., "New Concepts of Schizophrenia," *Comprehensive Therapy* 15:8-21, 1989.

55. Nutt, D.J., "The Pharmacology of Human Anxiety," *Pharmacology Therapeutics* 47:233-266, 1990.

56. Pary, R., Tobias, C., and Lippmann, S., "Fluoxetine: Prescribing Guidelines for the Newest Antidepressant," *Southern Medical Journal* 82:1005-1009, 1989.

57. Pasnau, R.O., and Bystritsky, A., "An Overview of Anxiety Disorders," *Bulletin of the Menninger Clinic* 54:157-170, 1990.

58. Pecknold, J.C., "Serotonin Abnormalities in Panic Disorder," *Frontiers of Clinical Neuroscience*, vol. 8, *Neurobiology of Panic Disorder*, J.C. Ballenger (ed.) (New York, NY: Alan R. Liss, 1990).

59. Pickar, D., Breier, A., Hsiao, J.K., et al., "Cerebrospinal Fluid and Plasma Monoamine Metabolites and Their Relation to Psychosis," *Archives of General Psychiatry* 47:641-648, 1990.

60. Pickar, D., Litman, R.E., Konicki, P.E., et al., "Neurochemical and Neural Mechanisms of Positive and Negative Symptoms in Schizophrenia," *Modern Problems in Pharmacopsychiatry* 24:124-125, 1990.

61. Pohl, R., Yeragani, V., Balon, R., et al., "Isoproterenol-Induced Panic: A Beta Adrenergic Model of Panic Anxiety," *Frontiers of Clinical Neuroscience*, vol. 8, *Neurobiology of Panic Disorder*, J.C. Ballenger (ed.) (New York, NY: Alan R. Liss, 1990).

62. Post, R.M., and Weiss, S.R.B., "Non-Homologous Animal Models of Affective Illness: Clinical Relevance of Sensitization and Kindling," *Animal Models of Depression*, G. Koob, C. Ehlers, and D.J. Kupfer (eds.) (Boston, MA: Birkhauser, 1989).

63. Rapoport, J.L., "The Waking Nightmare: An Overview of Obsessive Compulsive Disorder," *Journal of Clinical Psychiatry* 51(suppl.):25-28, 1990.

64. Rapoport, J.L., and Wise, S.P., "Obsessive-Compulsive Disorder: Evidence for Basal Ganglia Dysfunction," *Psychopharmacology Bulletin* 24:380-384, 1988.

65. Redmond, D.E., "Neurochemical Basis for Anxiety and Anxiety Disorders: Evidence From Drugs Which Decrease Human Fear and Anxiety," *Anxiety and the Anxiety Disorders*, A.H. Tuma and J.D. Maser (eds.) (Hillsdale, NJ: Lawrence Erlbaum Associates, 1985).

66. Reifman, A., and Wyatt, R.J., "Lithium: A Brake in the Rising Cost of Mental Illness," *Archives of General Psychiatry* 37:385-388, 1980.

67. Reiman, E.M., "PET, Panic Disorder, and Normal Anticipatory Anxiety," *Frontiers of Clinical Neuroscience*, vol. 8, *Neurobiology of Panic Disorder*, J.C. Ballenger (ed.) (New York, NY: Alan R. Liss, 1990).

68. Reynolds, C.F., Gillin, J.C., and Kupfer, D.J., "Sleep and Affective Disorders," *Psychopharmacology: The Third Generation of Progress*, H.Y. Meltzer (ed.) (New York, NY: Raven Press, 1987).

69. Rickels, K., and Schweizer, E., "Clinical Overview of Serotonin Reuptake Inhibitors," *Journal of Clinical Psychiatry* 51:9-12, 1990.

70. Rothschild, A.J., "Biology of Depression," *Medical Clinics of North America* 72:765-790, 1988.

71. Rubin, R.T., "Pharmacoendocrinology of Major Depression," *European Archives of Psychiatry and Neurological Sciences* 238:259-267, 1989.

72. Sack, D.A., Rosenthal, N.E., Parry, B.L., et al., "Biological Rhythms in Psychiatry," *Psychopharmacology: The Third Generation of Progress*, H.Y. Meltzer (ed.) (New York, NY: Raven Press, 1987).

73. Sandberg, D.P., and Liebowitz, M.R., "Potential Mechanisms for Sodium Lactate's Induction of Panic," *Frontiers of Clinical Neuroscience*, vol. 8, *Neurobiology of Panic Disorder*, J.C. Ballenger (ed.) (New York, NY: Alan R. Liss, 1990).

74. Small, J.G., "Psychiatric Disorders and EEG," *Electroencephalography: Basic Principles, Clinical Applications, & Related Fields*, 2nd ed., E. Niedermeyer and F.H. DaSilva (eds.) (Baltimore, MD: Williams & Wilkins, 1987).

75. Snyder, S.H., "Molecular Strategies in Neuropsychopharmacology: Old and New," *Psychopharmacology: The Third Generation of Progress*, H.Y. Meltzer (ed.) (New York, NY: Raven Press, 1987).

76. Teicher, M.H., "Biology of Anxiety," *Medical Clinics of North America* 72:791-814, 1988.

77. Uhde, T.W., "Caffeine Provocation of Panic: A Focus on Biological Mechanisms," *Frontiers of Clinical Neuroscience*, vol. 8, *Neurobiology of Panic Disorder*, J.C. Ballenger (ed.) (New York, NY: Alan R. Liss, 1990).

78. Uhl, G.R., Jayaraman, A., and Nishimori, S., "Neuropharmacologic Techniques in the Molecular Biology of Schizophrenia," *Advances in Neuropsychiatry and Psychopharmacology*, vol. 1, *Schizophrenia Research*, C.A. Tamminga and S.C. Schultz (eds.) (New York, NY: Raven Press, 1991).

79. U.S. Congress, Office of Technology Assessment, *Biological Rhythms: Implications for the Worker*, OTA-BA-463 (Washington, DC: U.S. Government Printing Office, 1991).

80. van Kammen, D.P., and Gelernter, J.P., "Biochemical Instability in Schizophrenia I: The Norepinephrine System," *Psychopharmacology: The Third Generation of Progress*, H.Y. Meltzer (ed.) (New York, NY: Raven Press, 1987).

81. van Kammen, D.P., and Kelley, M., "Dopamine and Norepinephrine Activity in Schizophrenia: An Integrative Perspective," *Schizophrenia Research* 4:173-191, 1991.

82. van Kammen, D.P., Peters, J., Yao, J., et al., "Norepinephrine in Acute Exacerbations of Chronic Schizophrenia," *Archives of General Psychiatry* 47:161-168, 1990.

83. Waltrip, R.W., Carrigan, D.R., and Carpenter, W.T., "Immunopathology and Viral Reactivation," *Journal of Nervous & Mental Disorders* 178:729-738, 1990.

84. Weinberger, D.R., "Implications of Normal Brain Development for the Pathogenesis of Schizophrenia," *Archives of General Psychiatry* 44:660-669, 1987.

85. Wiesel, F.-A., "Positron Emission Tomography in Psychiatry," *Psychiatric Developments* 1:19-47, 1989.

86. Williamson, P.C., and Kaye, H., "EEG Mapping Applications in Psychiatric Disorders," *Canadian Journal of Psychiatry* 34:680-686, 1989.

87. Winslow, J.T., and Insel, T.R., "Neurobiology of Obsessive Compulsive Disorder: A Possible Role for Serotonin," *Journal of Clinical Psychiatry* 51(suppl.): 27-31, 1990.

88. Wise, R.A., "Neuroleptic-Induced Anhedonia," *Advances in Neuropsychiatry and Psychopharmacology*, vol. 1, C.A. Tamminga and S.C. Schulz (eds.) (New York, NY: Raven Press, 1991).

89. Wyatt, R.J., "Introduction: Side Effects," *Psychopharmacology: The Third Generation of Progress*, H.Y. Meltzer (ed.) (New York, NY: Raven Press, 1987).

90. Wyatt, R.J., Kirch, D.C., and DeLisi, L.E. "Schizophrenia: Biochemical, Endocrine, and Immunological Studies," *Comprehensive Textbook of Psychiatry*, vol. 1, 5th ed., H.I. Kaplan and B.J. Sadock (eds.) (Baltimore, MD: Williams & Wilkins, 1989).

91. Zohar, J., Insel, T., and Rasmussen, S. (eds.), *The Psychobiology of Obsessive-Compulsive Disorder* (New York, NY: Springer Publishing, 1991).

92. Zuckerman, M., *Psychobiology of Personality* (Cambridge, England: Cambridge University Press, 1991).

Chapter 5

The Genetics of
Mental Disorders

CONTENTS OF CHAPTER 5

The Genetics of Mental Disorders

Few theories in biology provoke as heated a debate as the notion that human behavior in general, and mental disorders in particular, have a genetic basis. While there could be no more potent evidence of a biological basis than the identification of causative genes, none has yet been found. On the other hand, opponents of this theory characterize it as deterministic, casting behavioral genetics as the enemy of free will. Furthermore, discriminatory social policies, linked to genetic theories of behavior and mental disorders in the past, are an ever present specter in this field.

On this stage of invective and praise, the search for genes linked to mental disorders continues, propelled by one of the all-time largest research projects in the history of biology—the Human Genome Project—and supported by the primary funding agency for research into mental disorders, the National Institute of Mental Health (NIMH) (table 5-1). This gene hunt has resulted in claims of success in finding genes for bipolar disorder and schizophrenia, only to be followed by contradictory data and withdrawal of claims.

Despite the polemics and clashing research findings, there remains powerful evidence from multiple sources that many mental disorders, including the ones considered in this report, have a genetic component. The only evidence to date that mental disorders are *caused*, at least in part, by biological factors comes from genetic studies. However, the inheritance of mental disorders is far from simple, and nongenetic factors also play a role. This chapter summarizes what is known about the inheritance of schizophrenia, major mood disorders, and anxiety disorders. A technical section explains why specific genes are so difficult to find. Finally, the chapter considers some of the implications of what is known about the inheritance of these conditions. First, the basis of inheritance is reviewed.

BASIC GENETIC CONCEPTS

In nearly every cell of the body, instructions for making proteins—the chemicals required for the function and structure of cells—are encoded in genes, the fundamental units of heredity. Humans have 50,000 to 100,000 genes, as many as half of which function primarily in the brain. The existence of these now famous substrates of inheritance was predicted long before modern chemistry or microscopy could resolve the minute structure of the cell. By crossbreeding pea plants and meticulously observing the resulting colors and shapes, the Augustinian monk Gregor Mendel (1822-1884) hypothesized that offspring receive discrete elements of inheritance from their parents.

Genes are made up of deoxyribonucleic acid (DNA), a double-stranded molecule that twists into a helix (figure 5-1). Complementary chemical subunits, called base pairs, tether the two strands of the helix: guanine with cytosine and adenine with thymine. The linear sequence of bases in each strand of DNA forms the genetic code. It is this sequence of bases in genes that determines the structure of proteins and regulates cell activity. In all, an estimated 3.3 billion base pairs constitute the human genome, of which only a small fraction—1 to 3 percent—is believed to code for proteins.

Genes, along with intervening regions of DNA that do not appear to code for proteins, are folded into rod-shaped bodies, or chromosomes. Each human cell except gametes (eggs and sperm) contains 23 pairs of chromosomes: 22 pairs of autosomes and 1 pair of sex chromosomes, either two

Table 5-1—NIMH Genetic Research Investment, Fiscal Year 1991[a]

	Total costs of genetic research	Number of grants	Genetics as a percent of budget
Division of Clinical Research	$25,629,833[b]	88	15%
Division of Basic Brain and Behavioral Sciences ..	$13,351,201	55	10.9%
NIMH total	$38,981,043	143	8.7%

[a]These figures represent funding for research where the primary focus is human genetics of mental disorders.
[b]$2,090,812, or 8.14 percent, of the Division of Clinical Research's genetics budget, is devoted to Diagnostic Centers Cooperative Agreement.

SOURCE: National Institute of Mental Health, 1992.

Figure 5-1—Substrates of Inheritance

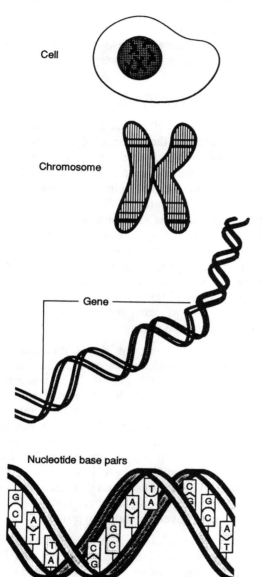

Series of thousands to millions of base pairs form genes, the substrates of inheritance. Genes, which are strewn along chromosomes in the cell nucleus, code for specific proteins.

SOURCE: Office of Technology Assessment, 1992.

X chromosomes, in women, or an X and a Y chromosome, in men. Each gene has a specific address, or locus, on the chromosomes, with two versions, or alleles, of each gene inherited from each parent. If the two alleles at a particular locus are identical, the individual is said to be homozygous; when the two alleles differ, heterozygous. Some alleles are dominant, requiring only one copy to cause expression of a trait, or phenotype (figure 5-2). In such cases, an individual expresses the dominant phenotype regardless of whether the hereditary information for a trait, or genotype, is homozygous or heterozygous. Other alleles are recessive and require two copies of the allele for expression of the trait. In other words, the individual must be homozygous for the gene, with two recessive alleles, in order to express the recessive phenotype. Of course, the inheritance of traits can be much more complex. Many traits reflect the action of several genes as well as the environment. Or a gene may not be expressed, even when present. These complexities have important implications for the study of mental disorders.

Eggs and sperm have only 23 chromosomes (22 autosomes and one sex chromosome), and these form the genetic contribution from our parents—that is, we receive one set of chromosomes from each. During the production of gametes, the 23 pairs of chromosomes are duplicated in the parent cell, endowing it with four copies of each chromosome (figure 5-3). The parent cell divides twice, producing

Figure 5-2—A Simple Pattern of Inheritance

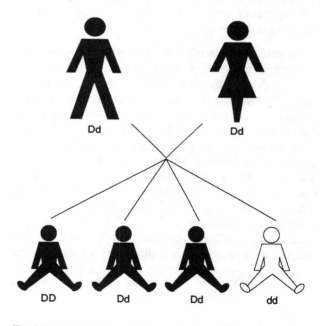

The father and mother both have a dominant version, or allele, of a gene (D) and a recessive version (d). Both express the dominant trait, indicated by shading. Each offspring has a 75 percent chance of receiving either one or two copies of the dominant allele and therefore expressing the dominant trait. One out of four times an offspring will receive two recessive versions of the gene and exhibit the recessive trait, shown in white.

SOURCE: Office of Technology Assessment, 1992.

four gametes, each with a single copy of the 23 chromosomes. However, the production of gametes does not simply involve the separation of chromosome pairs—considerable genetic reshuffling also occurs. The pairs of chromosomes line up near each other before their final departure to separate gametes. As the pairs of chromosomes draw near one another, they actually exchange segments. This segment exchange—or recombination—has important implications for linkage analysis, a technique used to map genes.

STUDYING THE INHERITANCE OF MENTAL DISORDERS

Observers have long noticed that behavioral traits, such as mental disorders, tend to run in families, suggesting the involvement of genetic factors. However, the genetics of human behavioral traits is more difficult to study than other phenotypes. Aside from the ethical impossibility of human breeding experiments and the relatively long time between generations, the phenotype itself is complex.

> Behavior ... is not just another phenotype. Because behavior involves the functioning of the whole organism rather than the action of a single molecule, a single cell, or a single organ, behavior is the most complex phenomenon that can be studied genetically ... (83).

Despite these difficulties, methods have been developed to take advantage of "natural" breeding studies. Observing the prevalence and pattern of behavioral traits among related individuals helps illuminate their genetic basis. Charles Darwin's cousin, Francis Galton (1822-1911), launched this approach to the study of the genetics of human behavior. The prodigious Galton explored the inheritance of intelligence, developed new statistical methods for analyzing such traits, and introduced the study of twins (85). Unfortunately, his work also ushered in the ugly era of eugenics in this century (box 5-A).

Classic investigations into human inheritance include adoption, twin, and family studies. These approaches seek to answer the following questions: Are these traits inherited? What is the relative contribution of genetic versus nongenetic factors?[1] What is the pattern of inheritance? Is the trait

Figure 5-3—The Chromosome Swap in Meiosis

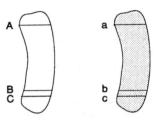

Chromosomes, with alleles of genes A, B, and C, come together in pairs before gametes are formed in meiosis.

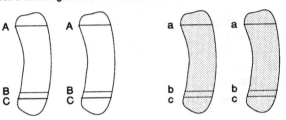

Each chromosome in the pair duplicates itself.

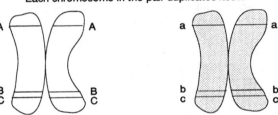

Chromosomes attach to each other.

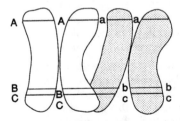

Crossing over upon breaking and rejoining of chromosomes.

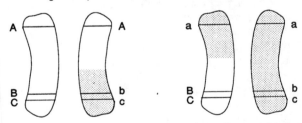

Chromosomes with new gene combinations after crossing over. Alleles that are far apart—e.g., A and B—may be separated during meiosis. Alleles that are close together—e.g., B and C—are less likely to be separated.

SOURCE: Office of Technology Assessment, 1992.

---

[1] Nongenetic, or so-called environmental, factors may include biological, psychological, or social components. Thus, the now passé nature versus nurture debate does not necessarily boil down to biological versus psychosocial factors.

Box 5-A—Eugenics and Mental Disorders

In Nazi Germany and the United States during the earlier part of this century, people with mental disorders were among the initial targets of eugenic policies. People with mental disorders were subjected to immigration restrictions, involuntary sterilization, and extermination. While moderns deny that such practices could be repeated, the record of eugenics and its historical link to mental disorders raise uncomfortable questions: Is the new age of genetics a harbinger of a new age of eugenics? Are people with mental disorders especially vulnerable?

Eugenics enjoys a long, well-bred intellectual pedigree, with the cousin of Charles Darwin, Sir Francis Galton, as its modern forefather. Galton coined the term "eugenics" in 1883, christening the scientific pursuit of improved inborn human qualities through judicious matings: positive eugenics. Prior to Galton, eugenic notions can be traced back as far as Plato's *Republic*, wherein the philosopher also proposes positive eugenic practices. Of course, the human genetic pool can be distilled by other means. Negative eugenics refers to the systematic attempt to minimize the passing of deleterious genes by reducing or preventing the reproduction of individuals carrying such genes.

A number of scientific discoveries planted the seeds of eugenic policies in the 19th and 20th centuries. Galton himself observed that many accomplished men of his day were linked by blood lines, which led to his belief that proper matings could produce a race with enhanced intellectual, behavioral, and physical characteristics. In addition, Galton, as well as others, developed statistical techniques that permitted the quantitative analysis of inherited traits.

While these and other scientific advances were the seeds of eugenics, they were not solely responsible for such policies in the United States. Social, political, and economic factors of the late 19th and early 20th centuries fertilized the growth of the eugenics movement. National attention was increasingly focused on social issues of unemployment, criminality, prostitution, and chronic alcoholism. Also, concerns arose that increased immigration from southern and eastern Europe was drawing the United States away from its "Anglo-Saxon superiority."

At the Federal level, eugenic policies took the form of increasingly restrictive immigration laws. Eugenicists, asserting the simple inheritance of such traits as lunacy, epilepsy, alcoholism, pauperism, criminality, and feeblemindedness, proffered scientific rationales for excluding individuals from entry to the United States. It is important to note that while authentic advances in genetics seeded the eugenics movement, they provided no evidence for the simple inheritance of the traits mentioned above.

Eugenic considerations also prompted States to enact laws regarding compulsory sterilization. In 1907, Indiana passed the first law legalizing the compulsory sterilization of inmates at the State reformatory; by 1931, 30 States had passed compulsory sterilization laws applying to individuals categorized as feebleminded, alcoholic, epileptic, sexually deviant, or mentally ill. Individuals with mental disorders made up half of the 64,000 persons in this country sterilized for eugenic reasons between 1907 and 1964. When eugenic sterilization laws were challenged in 1927, the Supreme Court ruled the practice was constitutional.

What is the current status of eugenic policies in the United States? While immigration laws still restrict the entry of people with mental disorders, denial of entry is not based on eugenic principles, but rather on concerns about whether behavior associated with a disorder poses a threat. State sterilization laws still stand, as does the 1927 Supreme Court ruling upholding them. As of 1987, compulsory sterilization laws remained on the books in 22 States; however, these laws are rarely invoked.

The current application of immigration and compulsory sterilization laws suggests that eugenics is not a major concern at this time. Furthermore, the understanding that mental disorders do not have a simple genetic basis and that nongenetic factors play an important role would seem to limit the potential of eugenic policies. Perhaps most important, American repulsion by the Nazi legacy and the emphasis in this country on individual reproductive rights also make State-determined eugenic policies unlikely. But indirect pressure not to have children may well come to bear on individuals seen to have a greater genetic risk of mental disorders; society may brand them irresponsible or immoral for transmitting disorders to their children. Given the financial strain posed by mental disorders today and the stigma attached to them, in conjunction with scientific advances, it is possible that these factors could unlock what some call a backdoor to eugenics.

SOURCES: T. Duster, *Backdoor to Eugenics* (New York, NY: Routledge, 1990); K.L. Garver and B. Garver, "Eugenics: Past, Present, and Future," *American Journal of Human Genetics* 49:1109-1118, 1991; I.I. Gottesman, *Schizophrenia Genesis: The Origins of Madness* (New York, NY: W.H. Freeman, 1991); D.J. Kevles, *In the Name of Eugenics* (New York, NY: Knopf, 1985); D. Suzuki and P. Knudtson, *Genethics: The Clash Between the New Genetics and Human Values* (Cambridge, MA: Harvard University Press, 1989); N.A. Holtzman, *Proceed with Caution: Predicting Genetic Risks in the Recombinant DNA Era* (Baltimore, MD: The Johns Hopkins University Press, 1989).

dominant? Recessive? Determined by more than one gene?

Adoption studies, though variable in design, compare the presence of a trait among biological versus adoptive family members or other control groups. They attempt to disentangle the influence of genes from that of the environment and can provide powerful evidence of a genetic effect. Generally, they do not rule out the effect of nongenetic factors that preceded adoption, such as possible prenatal influences. While few adoption studies have evaluated the genetics of anxiety disorders, they provide evidence about the inheritance of mood disorders and schizophrenia.

Twin studies compare how often identical twins, who are genetically identical, and fraternal twins, who have the genetic similarity of nontwin siblings, are similar, or concordant, for a trait. A high concordance rate for a trait among identical twins versus fraternal twins usually demonstrates a genetic basis for the trait. The absence of 100 percent concordance among identical twins shows that nongenetic factors also play a role in producing the trait.

Twin studies raise several issues, including the certainty with which identical twins versus fraternal twins are identified; the way in which twins are sampled; the assumption that identical and fraternal twins experience the environment identically; the definition of concordance; and the statistical methods for measuring concordance (39,85). All of these factors must be weighed when evaluating data from twin studies.

Of all the traditional approaches to studying genetics, family studies have been used most frequently to evaluate mental disorders. Such studies consider whether a trait runs in families. The familial nature of a trait is essential for proving it is inherited; however, such data do not conclusively demonstrate the genetic basis of a trait, since family members share not only genes but also their environment.

Showing that a trait is more prevalent within a family than in a control population suggests the importance of genetic factors. The observation that a trait is more common among first-degree relatives— parents, siblings, and offspring—than more distant ones strengthens the genetic hypothesis. The way in which a trait is distributed among family members may also elucidate the mode of inheritance. For example, if a trait is never passed from father to son, an X-linked gene is implicated. More complicated quantitative techniques may reveal other aspects of the mode of inheritance. While family studies provide part of the foundation for the genetic theory of mental disorders, they have not resolved how these disorders are inherited.

Classic genetic studies are quite useful. And data from these studies form the sole existing support for the genetic basis of mental disorders. This research produces the bottom line of genetic influence, that is, distinguishing the relative influence of heredity from that of the environment (84). But there is a limit to what classic genetic studies can reveal. They cannot identify a specific gene defect. Because of this limitation, researchers have been eager to apply the new, powerful tools of modern genetics to the study of mental disorders.

The search for the molecular genetic underpinnings of mental disorders in the last several years has involved mostly the technique of linkage analysis. Linkage analysis can determine whether a single gene makes a major contribution to a trait and where that gene is located. A positive finding of linkage shows that a nearby gene plays an important role in the inheritance of the investigated trait. It maps the gene to a location on the chromosomes; it does not isolate the specific gene or reveal its function.

Linkage analysis takes advantage of the fact that although alleles for genes of most traits are inherited independently—since they lie on different chromosomes or are so far apart on a single chromosome that they are separated during the chromosome segment exchange that occurs during meiosis— those lying close together on the same chromosome are usually inherited together. Their loci, or chromosomal positions, are linked (see figure 5-3). The actual distance between two loci can be estimated by determining how frequently the alleles at those sites are inherited together. If the alleles for two traits are passed on together 90 percent of the time (and 10 percent of the time they are not), they are said to have a 10 percent recombination fraction, which corresponds to roughly 1 million base pairs. A recombination fraction of 50 percent indicates that the alleles for two genes are not linked; they are far removed from each other on a single chromosome or on separate chromosomes.

Linkage analysis uses genetic markers—traits or DNA sequences—with known chromosomal addresses. In the past, traits such as color blindness or blood type served as markers; however, they were quite limited in their usefulness. There were not very many of them, and they lacked variability, an important feature in a genetic marker. The surge in popularity of linkage analysis in the last decade reflects the discovery of new breeds of genetic markers, including restriction fragment length polymorphisms, or RFLPs (pronounced rif' lips), and, more recently, microsatellite repeat markers (7,11). These markers derive from variation in the very DNA sequence, revealed by the techniques of molecular genetics. And because these markers span the entire genome, they enable investigators to search for linked genes, regardless of their location.

Linkage analysis is used to distinguish two questions: Given the way a trait is distributed within a family under investigation, does the responsible gene lie within a short and specified distance from the genetic marker? Or is it so far away from the marker that the gene was inherited independently? That is to say, are the two loci (for the gene of interest and the genetic marker) likely to be linked or not in this family? The probability that either of the questions is true is expressed in the form of an odds ratio. Traditionally, an odds ratio of 1,000 to 1 has been taken as proof of linkage (75): It is 1,000 times more likely that the gene loci are linked than not. An odds ratio of less than 1 to 100 has been regarded as proof against linkage. Odds ratios are typically transformed into LOD scores, their base 10 logarithm. Therefore a LOD score of 3 ($\log_{10} 1,000/1$) or greater is considered evidence of linkage; linkage is rejected with a LOD score of -2 ($\log_{10} 1/100$) or less.

Upon finding a LOD score of nearly 7—placing the likelihood of linkage at 10 million to 1—a researcher would seem to have near absolute proof of linkage. In fact, such a finding has been reported for schizophrenia (96). But, as with all statistical tests, certain assumptions must hold true if the results are to be meaningful. And there is always a chance that a positive finding is spurious, a random occurrence. For example, with a LOD score of 3, there is a 1 in 20 chance that the finding of linkage is spurious. The confusion and controversy that surround the gene search in mental disorders stem from the fact that these conditions violate the rules and assumptions of linkage analysis. The problems associated with this method are considered in a subsequent section, but first, the available evidence

that these conditions have a genetic basis is summarized.

GENETICS OF SCHIZOPHRENIA

Classic genetic studies show that schizophrenia has a genetic component (for review, see 38,39,49,54, 102). Data from family studies lead to estimates that first-degree relatives of an individual with schizophrenia have approximately 10 times the general risk of developing the disorder. Twin and adoption studies also implicate genetic factors. Although estimates vary, data consistently show that a person whose identical twin has schizophrenia is at higher risk for schizophrenia than a person whose fraternal twin has the disorder (table 5-2). Adoption studies indicate that schizophrenia runs in biological but not adoptive families (53). These data also point to a genetic relationship between schizophrenia and other disorders, such as schizotypal personality disorder (50).

Clearly, schizophrenia has a genetic component. But genetics is not the whole picture. Twin studies indicate that genetic factors do not entirely account for the development of schizophrenia; an identical twin of someone with schizophrenia exhibits the disorder approximately 30 to 50 percent of the time. Thus, nongenetic factors must also be important. Furthermore, important questions about genetics persist. Even though having a family member with schizophrenia increases the likelihood of developing the disorder, many family members do not develop schizophrenia, and 80 to 90 percent of individuals with schizophrenia have no first-degree relative with the disorder (38). The distribution of schizophrenia within families is not consistent with any simple pattern of inheritance. Studies generally rule out the

Table 5-2—Relatives' Risk of Schizophrenia

Relationship	Risk (%)
First degree	
Parents	5.6
Siblings	10.1
Children	12.8
Children of two parents with schizophrenia ...	46.3
Second degree	
Half siblings	4.2
Uncles/aunts	2.4
Nephews/nieces	3.0
Grandchildren	3.7

SOURCE: Adapted from I.I. Gottesman, *Schizophrenia and Genetic Risks* (Arlington, VA: National Alliance for the Mentally Ill, 1984).

Chapter 5—The Genetics of Mental Disorders • *107*

action of a single gene without determining whether a couple of genes, or many genes, are important in producing schizophrenia.

A report that an uncle and nephew with schizophrenia shared a chromosome defect—an extra copy of part of chromosome 5—impelled the search for a schizophrenia gene on this chromosome (8,31,51, 62,95). Linkage to chromosome 5 was asserted soon thereafter in a study of seven British and Icelandic families (96). A simultaneously reported study in a separate kindred in Sweden ruled this linkage out (52). Subsequent studies have since rejected a link between chromosome 5 and schizophrenia (2,26,41, 47,63,77,93).

Studies have evaluated the linkage of schizophrenia to the classic genetic marker, the HLA (human-leukocyte-associated) antigen system on chromosome 6. The HLA antigen system is a collection of genes important for immune function. An early study provided only weak evidence of linkage to the HLA system (106), and four subsequent studies ruled out linkage to the HLA system and a wide variety of other classical markers (1,14,36,60). While schizophrenia has not been linked to a region of the X chromosome thought to play a role in bipolar disorder (23; see later discussion), preliminary data support linkage to a region that lies at the ends of the X and Y chromosomes (18).

GENETICS OF MOOD DISORDERS

What do classic genetic studies indicate about the inheritance of mood disorders? Identical twins share mood disorders more frequently than do fraternal twins (for review, see 32,61,74,103,105). For example, data show that the identical twin of an individual with bipolar disorder would exhibit that disorder three times more often than would a fraternal twin (32) (figure 5-4). Parents, siblings, and children of individuals with bipolar disorder or major depression more commonly develop these disorders, although the estimated incidence among family members varies among studies. Only a few adoption studies have evaluated the inheritance of mood disorders. Data from these studies generally support the role of inheritance in mood disorders (for review, see 32,74).

The heritability of mood disorders appears to be correlated with the severity of the condition. Bipolar disorder has the largest genetic component of all mood disorders, and recurring bouts of depression

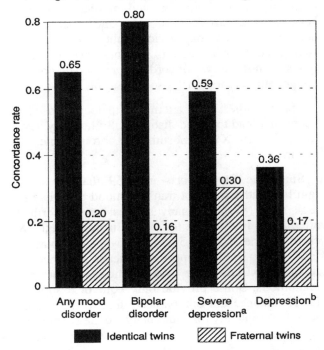

Figure 5-4—Mood Disorders Among Twins

Graphically depicted data were derived from evaluation of 110 pairs of twins. Identical twins shared mood disorders, especially bipolar disorder, more frequently than fraternal twins.

[a]Three or more episodes of depression.
[b]Less than three episodes of depression.

SOURCE: Adapted from A. Bertelsen, B. Harvald, and M. Hauge, "A Danish Twin Study of Manic-Depressive Disorders," *British Journal of Psychiatry* 130:330-351, 1977.

appear to be more directly heritable than a single episode. Also, major depression that has an earlier age of onset may be more heritable. Family and twin studies suggest a genetic link between depression and bipolar disorder. For example, identical twins, who often share the same mood disorder, not infrequently have different forms (10). Similarly, first-degree relatives of a person with bipolar disorder are at greater risk of developing *any* mood disorder than the general population (32). But the genetic overlap between major depression and bipolar disorder is not complete (110). For example, while rates of major depression are greatly increased among the relatives of an individual with bipolar disorder, the opposite is not true: The relatives of an individual with major depression are not at a much higher risk for developing bipolar disorder.

Family and twin studies demonstrate the importance of genetic factors in both bipolar disorder and major depression. However, studies do not reveal a simple pattern of inheritance, nor do they implicate the action of a single gene. The genetic relationships between major depression and bipolar disorders, between schizoaffective disorder and mood disorders, as well as among various subtypes of depression are not clear (see ch. 3). And since identical twins are not always concordant for mood disorders, nongenetic factors must also play a role.

Many studies have attempted to locate specific genes that lead to mood disorders. So far, they have focused on the X chromosome and chromosomes 11 and 6.

Since the first reports in 1969 that, in some families, fathers do not transmit mood disorders to their sons (87,117), many studies have described attempts to find a gene for mood disorders on the X chromosome (6,24,30,34,35,57,66-71). Although a few of the studies report significant evidence of linkage—a LOD score over 3—the results are not unanimous. Some provide only equivocal support for X linkage, and others, according to their LOD scores, completely rule out linkage to the X chromosome.

What explains these conflicting data? The use of a specific marker, the Xg blood group, accounts for some of the inconsistencies. Studies using the Xg blood group, which is located far from the other markers used to date, have never shown linkage. The remaining discrepancies may result from genetic heterogeneity: Genetic factors leading to mood disorders may vary among families.

The finding of X linkage in more than one study supports the hypothesis that a gene on that chromosome leads to mood disorders in some families. Nonetheless, doubts about the X linkage of mood disorders persist. The report of linkage to one marker, the F9 marker, does not easily square with positive findings for other, somewhat distant markers. Another study of 10 families without male-to-male transmission failed to map mood disorders to the X chromosome, despite the prediction that many such families would display this linkage (9,92). And while there has been disagreement about the pedigrees used in this study refuting X linkage (3,29,42,116), the results question how frequently a gene on the X chromosome accounts for inherited cases of mood disorders, even in families without father-to-son transmission.

The scientific and popular press heralded a report linking mood disorders to chromosome 11 among a group of Amish families in Pennsylvania (27). The Amish are an ideal population for studying the genetics of all kinds of disorders, especially mental disorders. They are the progeny of a small group of people who emigrated from Europe in the early 18th century (27). Since they seldom marry outside their own community, they have preserved a relatively homogeneous genetic heritage. Also, due to their religious convictions, they forswear the use of drugs and alcohol, abuse of which may confound the diagnosis of mood disorders.

The results of the Amish study conflicted with two reports on non-Amish families published about the same time (25,43). These studies ruled out linkage of mood disorders to chromosome 11 in nine families. Furthermore, results from a followup study of the same Amish families 2 years later disputed the original findings (48). The reanalysis, which included new family members and a change of diagnosis in two individuals due to the subsequent onset of mood disorders, also excluded the possibility that mood disorders are linked to a gene on chromosome 11.

Several studies have evaluated the possible linkage of mood disorders to the HLA system on chromosome 6 (12,36,46,55,56,97-101,108,109,114, 115). Four produced evidence of linkage, with one reporting odds of approximately 10^8 to 1 (109). However, there are questions concerning the methods used in some of these studies. Gershon (33), for example, points out that the remaining studies produced no evidence of linkage. Therefore, no strong evidence fixes a gene for mood disorders on chromosome 6. Other studies, not described here, provide equivocal evidence, at best, for linkage of mood disorders to other chromosome markers (105).

GENETICS OF ANXIETY DISORDERS

Panic disorder and obsessive-compulsive disorder (OCD) appear to have a genetic component, although inheritance of these disorders has undergone less experimental scrutiny than that of schizophrenia and mood disorders. While several family studies have been conducted, only a few twin studies and no adoption studies have analyzed the inheritance of these anxiety disorders. Further studies are necessary to discern the role of genetics in these disorders.

Several family studies have found higher rates of panic disorder among first-degree relatives of a person with panic disorder than among control populations (79,112). Also, there appears to be a greater frequency of agoraphobia—the fear of being in public places—with panic disorder among family members (21). These family studies have also distinguished between panic disorder and other disorders. For example, data indicate that panic disorder is distinct from generalized anxiety disorder (112) but that families of individuals with both panic disorder and depression are at increased risk of depression, panic disorder, and other conditions (20). Thus, the data indicate that panic disorder does run in families. Information from the few twin studies performed to date suggests that panic attacks, if not panic disorders, have a heritable component (21,104). No adoption studies of panic disorder have been conducted (104).

Based on the observed pattern of panic disorder in families, researchers have begun the search for genetic linkage. A recent linkage study provides preliminary evidence that a gene found on chromosome 16 might influence panic disorder (20-22); other linkage studies are underway (111).

Investigators of the genetics of OCD have used both family and twin studies; there are no adoptive studies (107). Data from family studies suggest that OCD has a genetic component (13,81,86,107), as do data from twin studies (13,81). They also suggest a link between OCD and Tourette's syndrome (80,82). No data from linkage studies of OCD have been reported to date.

THE CHALLENGE OF MAPPING GENES FOR MENTAL DISORDERS

Although evidence from multiples sources indicates that schizophrenia, bipolar disorder, and major depression, as well as panic disorder and OCD, have a genetic component, linkage studies have not succeeded in locating specific genes for these disorders. Attempts to pin mental disorders to specific chromosomes have produced acclaimed reports of linkage and subsequent contradiction of findings (89). These conflicting results have been analyzed in a series of papers (5,33,59,72,89,91). Two basic, unanswered questions confound linkage analysis of mental disorders: What accounts for the complex genetics of mental disorders? And what is inherited?

What Accounts for Complex Genetics?

Linkage analysis has achieved spectacular success in mapping diseases with a simple genetic basis, such as Huntington's disease and cystic fibrosis. Such diseases are rare in the general population, and a single gene can easily account for their occurrence. Mental disorders, like many cancers, Alzheimer's disease, and diabetes mellitus, present a much more complicated picture of inheritance. Although they also tend to run in families, they are common in the general population and no single gene can account for all cases.

Several factors may contribute to the complex pattern of inheritance of mental disorders, thus confounding linkage analysis:

- Distinct factors, genetic or nongenetic, may lead independently to a disorder.
- A gene that sometimes produces a particular disorder may not always do so.
- Several genes acting in concert may be necessary to produce a disorder.
- Nongenetic factors contribute to the development of a disorder.

The most optimistic explanation for inconsistent linkage results is genetic heterogeneity—that is, one gene leads to a disorder in some families, while a different gene operates in others. With this explanation, reports mapping a mental disorder to a specific chromosome in some families but refuting linkage in others can both be correct.

Several types of evidence may implicate genetic heterogeneity. Reports of linkage to different chromosomes may support this hypothesis. Distinct clinical profiles, symptoms, patterns of inheritance, and other biological measures among families may also indicate the action of separate genes (89). Given the complex characteristics of schizophrenia and mood disorders, it would be surprising if they did not have a heterogeneous basis. Some data suggest subtypes of these disorders; e.g., major depression seems to be more concentrated in families when it has an early age of onset (113). In general, however, clinical subsets of these disorders are not firmly established, and linkage studies (as well as diagnostic classification systems) have not incorporated them. On the contrary, many linkage studies have included a wide spectrum of mental disorders.

Experts caution against interpreting conflicting linkage results alone as proof of genetic heterogeneity. Only replication of a finding of linkage provides strong evidence that a nearby gene leads to the disorder (5,32,89). Furthermore, evidence of linkage to more than one gene is required to prove that a disorder is genetically heterogeneous.

Separate genes operating among and even within families make the search for linkage more difficult. One strategy is to study large families with many members who are afflicted with mental disorders (5). A single, large family, especially one that is relatively isolated, is more likely to be genetically homogeneous. The presence of a disorder in many family members also predicts, but does not prove, that a single gene is the culprit.

This approach has some disadvantages. Large families with many members showing a mental disorder are relatively rare. Also, a single gene that produces schizophrenia or mood disorders in certain families may only rarely do so in the general population. In this event, the finding of linkage will not lead to a genetic test that is generally useful. Of course, mapping a mental disorder to a specific gene, even in a few families, may lead to improved understanding of the disorder.

So far, this discussion has focused on the possible genetic heterogeneity of mental disorders. Various nongenetic factors may also be responsible. That is, a disorder may be produced by genetic or nongenetic factors. In fact, nongenetic factors can produce a phenocopy of a disorder—that is, symptoms that mirror the genetically derived disorder. For example, depression produced by genetic factors may be symptomatically indistinguishable from depression provoked by external factors. While diagnostic criteria ferret out conditions obviously caused by a known and distinct factor, such as chemically induced symptoms, it is currently impossible to identify some phenocopies.

Sometimes a trait is not expressed even though the gene coding for it is present. In other words, only a fraction of persons carrying a particular gene actually display the trait. This is called incomplete penetrance. The causes of incomplete penetrance are unknown, although it is believed that modifying genes or other factors may thwart gene expression. Akin to incomplete penetrance is variable expressivity, where expression of a disorder varies in individuals with the gene from very severe symptoms to

nearly none at all. The complex pattern of inheritance of mental disorders is commonly attributed, at least in part, to this phenomenon.

There are other unexplained aspects of the genetics of mental disorders. For example, if a single gene causes a disorder, is it dominant or recessive? How many alleles are there? While incomplete penetrance and these other unknown factors complicate linkage analysis, they need not preclude it (16,19,37). Linkage studies commonly consider a range of estimates for these variables and factor in such considerations as age of onset, cohort effect, and nonrandom mating, which often occurs in mental disorders (see ch. 3) (5). Accounting for all of these variables and unknowns does, however, require statistical adjustments, since they violate the assumptions of LOD score analysis (15,90).

Given the unknown parameters of inheritance, the sib-pair method of analysis offers some advantages in the search for genes linked to mental disorders (89). This method is based on the fact that, if a marker and a trait are linked, pairs of siblings who share a trait will be more likely to have the same genetic marker than could be expected by chance. The sib-pair method does not require prior knowledge of the mode of inheritance, as does the LOD score method. Furthermore, this approach does not require extended pedigrees, which may be difficult to find.

Although the problems discussed thus far complicate linkage analysis, they do not rule it out as a reasonable research approach. However, successful linkage analysis relies on a single gene making a major contribution to a disorder. While research has not resolved the number of genes involved in producing mood disorders or schizophrenia, data do suggest that a single gene is unlikely to make a major contribution in most cases of schizophrenia or mood disorders (89,105).

Why, then, does linkage analysis remain a serious research endeavor? First, a major-gene effect, at least in some families, has not been ruled out in major mood disorders and schizophrenia. A large, systematic linkage study, though expensive, is the only available method likely to answer the question, Is a single gene linked to these mental disorders? Such an approach could then locate a major gene if it exists in the families studied or rule out the presence of such a gene. Also, new techniques and methods of analysis are being advanced all the time, possibly resulting in new ways of searching for genes. Another rationale for continued linkage analysis is that a gene may contribute in a large way to these mental disorders in a few families. Single genes have been linked to a fraction of cases of other complex disorders, such as Alzheimer's disease (94). Unfortunately, studies have not identified families where prior evidence suggests that a single gene produces a mental disorder (89).

What if, as suspected by some observers, many genes, each with a very small effect, underlie these disorders? There is little likelihood that linkage analysis could locate one of many minor genes. Other techniques would be required (e.g., see 58).

The absence of 100 percent concordance for schizophrenia and mood disorders between identical twins implicates the importance of nongenetic factors in the genesis of these disorders (4). Other types of studies also point out that genetic factors and the environment, nature *and* nurture so to speak, produce mental disorders (95). Nongenetic factors may range from exposure to a chemical or virus to social interactions. Research has not identified these factors precisely (58,88); however, mapping a major gene that leads to increased susceptibility to a mental disorder may facilitate research into nongenetic factors (4,28,78,95).

What Is Inherited?

In order to map a gene, it is crucial to identify correctly the inherited trait, or phenotype. While the problems mentioned above are common to all complex disorders, uncertainty about what is inherited plagues mental disorders especially.

How well does the current classification of mental disorders define the inherited phenotype? Researchers disagree. Some are confident that rigorous use of the available diagnostic classifications will serve genetic research well. Others are uncomfortable that these diagnostic classes have not been validated and have no biological marker. It is perhaps ironic that while psychiatry looks hopefully to genetic research for help in refining systems of disorder classification (95), questions in the current classification system may impede genetic research.

When performing a linkage study, this question emerges: Are some disorders genetically related? For example, should a study attempting to map the gene for schizophrenia include only individuals with

schizophrenia? Or should it include individuals with other forms of psychosis too? Individuals with any mental disorder?

Family studies provide some clues about the genetic relationship among disorders. For example, data suggest that bipolar disorder is genetically related to depression (32). Schizophrenia appears to run in families with schizotypal personality disorder and possibly other types of psychotic disorders (17,49). Agoraphobia and panic disorder appear to be genetically related (76), as do OCD and Tourette's syndrome (80,82). Further studies are needed to establish which disorders appear together in families and thus may be genetically related.

In practice, linkage studies have generally taken the approach of doing multiple analyses of different sets of mental disorders, ranging from core diagnoses to a broad spectrum of disorders. Two points warrant consideration. First, statistical accommodation is necessary for multiple analyses. Second, decisions concerning which diagnoses to include in each analysis must precede the study.

Instead of using an entire diagnostic class for linkage analysis, such as depression, some subset of the class may more accurately reflect the inherited trait, for example, recurrent bouts of depression or depression with an early age of onset. Although the identification of such "phenotype markers" is in its infancy, there are several potentially useful biological and psychological markers for specific subsets of disorders. Response to drug treatment is one such possibility, and it forms the basis of pharmacogenetics (64). Similar responsiveness to the same drugs may identify individuals with genetically related disorders. Tsuang and Faraone (105) review data supporting the conclusion that individuals who respond well to certain antidepressant agents tend to have relatives who respond well to these agents. In general, linkage analysis has not yet incorporated such markers.

Another possible answer to the question, What is inherited? is illustrated by research into abnormal eye movements and schizophrenia (44,45). Individuals with schizophrenia sometimes have a problem with smooth-pursuit eye movements (SPEM); that is, they may have difficulty maintaining a focus on moving objects. Approximately 65 percent of individuals with schizophrenia, versus 8 percent of the general population, have problems with SPEM. Furthermore, data suggest a genetic link between schizophrenia and these eye-movement abnormalities. Forty-five percent of the parents and siblings of individuals with schizophrenia exhibit SPEM abnormalities. Both identical twins exhibit schizophrenia or problems with SPEM, or both, 80 percent of the time. On this basis, researchers are looking for a gene that accounts for either schizophrenia or abnormal eye movement (51,65).

Ultimately, clues about what is inherited may suggest specific genes that underlie mental disorders. Identifying such candidate genes will enable researchers to target their search for linkage. One candidate gene was the gene that codes for the D_2 receptor. This receptor binds the brain chemical dopamine. Antipsychotic agents, which are used to treat schizophrenia, also bind to the D_2 receptor (see ch. 4). However, studies aimed at mapping schizophrenia to the gene for the D_2 receptor failed to establish linkage (51,73). One of several other candidate gene approaches sought to link bipolar disorder to a receptor for another brain chemical, serotonin (41); it also failed to establish linkage. The absence of a known etiology for mental disorders has thwarted the candidate gene approach to linkage analysis so far. However, continued advances in molecular biology and neuroscience will undoubtedly provide information on new possible targets for candidate gene searches.

IMPACT OF GENETIC RESEARCH

Optimism generally surrounds today's genetic research into mental disorders. The modern-day sleuth—the molecular genetics researcher—is on the trail of perhaps the most enigmatic of all human afflictions. High hopes for an improved understanding of mental disorders and better, more rational treatments are pinned to this research.

This typically American enthusiasm for scientific progress may benefit from some temperance. Undoubtedly, genetic research will advance our understanding of at least some mental disorders, but rapid achievement of this goal is not likely. Researchers caution that identifying the location of relevant genes may require several years. And mapping a gene is only the first step in understanding the etiology of a mental disorder. The next step involves identifying the specific gene, which can take years. For example, the location of the gene for Huntington's disease was found in 1983 (40), but the gene has yet to be identified. Understanding how a gene's

action is translated into something as complex as a mental disorder will probably demand a great deal of further research.

But genetic research has already had some important effects. One has been on the general perception of mental disorders (see ch. 7). Our overwhelming acceptance of the hereditary basis for mental disorders is astonishing. Only two decades ago, the idea that psychosocial factors produced schizophrenia dominated scientific thought, leading, for example, to the pervasive and brutally stigmatizing stereotype of the "schizophrenogenic" mother (see ch. 7).

Family, adoption, and twin studies in the 1960s and 1970s established a solid theoretical basis for the role of genetics in mental disorders. These data, coupled with the revolution in genetics, fueled the emphasis on genetic research and focused the public spotlight on it. The frequent newspaper headlines and increasing number of books for the layperson evidence the spreading perception that mental disorders are inherited.

What is the impact of this perception that mental disorders are inherited? Perhaps more than any other type of research, genetics identifies mental disorders as biological. Thus, proponents of the biological-medical model of mental disorders generally support and commend this research. In a review article on genetics and mental disorders, leaders in the psychiatric community state that "wider recognition of the biological basis for mental illnesses (derived from genetic research) may allow these illnesses, finally, to be seen as similar to other medical problems" (78).

Spurious interpretation of the fact that genetic factors contribute to mental disorders can result in the belief that genes are destiny. This interpretation is founded on the false assumptions that human behavior is simply programmed by genes and that no useful intervention—barring a eugenic approach—can be developed. In fact, an environmental intervention can be successful in treating a genetic condition, as exemplified by phenylketonuria, or PKU. PKU is a single-gene defect that, if untreated, leads to mental retardation. This result can be prevented if a diet low in a particular amino acid (phenylalanine) is provided during the early years of life.

A few voices caution against the overemphasis on genetic factors in mental disorders, noting that genetics does not completely account for these disorders and that a single-gene cause is unlikely to be found (58,83). What danger is there in overemphasizing the role of genetics? Although considered unlikely today, past enthusiasm for genetics led to atrocious abuses, such as the sterilization of individuals with mental disorders (see box 5-A). In this era of tight competition for research support, funding for genetic research may supplant support for other types of research. Some fear that unfulfilled expectations of quickly finding a particular gene or a new treatment may lead to impatience, disappointment, perhaps even a backlash against genetic research.

Since there is an increasing appreciation of the genetic component of mental disorders, it is not surprising that patients and family members would seek advice on the inheritance of these disorders. What information can genetic counseling provide on mental disorders (box 5-B)? At this point, one cannot unequivocally predict whether an individual will or will not develop a disorder (table 5-3). Genetic counseling can only provide a general estimate of risk for a disorder. While relatives are at increased risk of a mental disorder, estimates of risk are not easily adapted to individuals. They vary among studies (105) and are not specific—an individual's risk may exceed or fall short of average estimates. One important message of genetic counseling is that family members do not usually face a large threat of developing a disorder. For example, on average only 10 to 15 percent of individuals with schizophrenia or mood disorders, on average, will have a child with the disorder. Given that family members face a relatively low risk of developing a mental disorder, genetic counseling is often in the position of putting patients and family members—who may have overestimated their risk of a severe disorder—at ease (95).

Individuals could receive much more specific information during genetic counseling once genetic tests for mental disorders have been developed.

Genetic tests are typically the first spin-off from the successful mapping of a gene for a disorder, preceding treatment advances by many years. While no such tests are available now, and it may be somewhat premature to raise concerns about genetic testing for mental disorders, data point to the importance of genetic factors. Therefore, tests for a genetic predisposition to some mental disorders may be technically feasible in the future. Our current understanding of the genetics of mental disorders makes a single, highly predictive genetic test that is useful across the general population unlikely. Data from genetic studies predict that such genetic tests could possibly take the following forms:

- A major gene found in a subset of families with a disorder could lead to the development of a genetic test. It would be highly predictive of mental disorders within a few families but not useful in other families.

- Discovery of a gene that contributes to the development of a disorder, but alone cannot produce the disorder, may lead to a genetic test for increased susceptibility. This scenario is commonly envisioned for many disorders that are produced by genetic and nongenetic factors, such as diabetes, some cancers, coronary heart disease, and hypertension. Not everyone testing positive for the gene will develop the disorder. On a far more positive note, such individuals may be able to control their destiny by avoiding known risk factors.

SUMMARY AND CONCLUSIONS

Advances in genetics have bequeathed an increasing understanding of how simple traits are inherited, what the cellular and molecular substrates of inheritance are, and, more recently, the identity of genes in human disease. Interest in probing the inheritance of human behavior has paralleled our increasing knowledge of genetics. However, the study of human

Table 5-3—Risk of Mental Disorders (In percent)

	Schizophrenia	Bipolar disorder	Major depression	Obsessive-compulsive disorder	Panic disorder
To general population	1.0	0.8	4.9	2.6	1.6
To first-degree relative (parent, child, or sibling)	9.0-13.0[a]	4.0-9.0	5.9-18.4	25.0	15.0-24.7

[a]46 percent when both parents affected.

SOURCE: K. Berg and D.G. Kirch, National Institute of Mental Health, 1992.

Box 5-B—Genetic Counseling for Mental Disorders

According to researchers and other experts, individuals with mental disorders and their families have become increasingly interested in knowing the risk of inheriting these conditions. Such information is relayed in the context of genetic counseling, a clinical service that provides an individual and sometimes his or her family with information about heritable conditions. Unfortunately, empirical data on mental disorders and genetic counseling are sorely lacking.

Genetic counseling for mental disorders apparently occurs quite rarely. Who does seek it? Some individuals in the early stages of their disorder seek genetic counseling on the impact the disorder is likely to have on a potential spouse or children. The majority of genetic counseling requests come from relatives of affected individuals concerned about incipient or potential mental disorders in another family member or reproductive issues. Prospective spouses may also request information regarding both their partner and their potential offspring.

The accepted aim of genetic counseling is to provide information. It is generally held that genetic counseling should be nondirective and show the highest respect for the requester's autonomy. While it is no simple task to relay complicated concepts of risk, it is perhaps even more difficult to do so in a nondirective manner. Furthermore, individuals request genetic information for a reason: to make reproductive decisions, to seek comfort or assuage fears. Genetic counseling in general is concerned with the psychological effects of receiving frightening information; given the psychopathology in mental disorders, this concern will most likely be amplified. For this reason, some people believe that psychiatrists should provide genetic counseling. However, many physicians have less-than-adequate knowledge of genetics. And no professional organization (e.g., American Psychiatric Association) or government institution (e.g., the National Institute of Mental Health) has put forth guidelines on the practice of genetic counseling for mental disorders.

A common concern of individuals seeking genetic counseling for mental disorders is reproductive decisions: Should we have children? Various factors may come to bear on such a decision, including the perceived risks and burdens of a mental disorder among offspring. Current risk estimates are not specific and generally are not very high. Thus, as stated by one genetic researcher, "Avoiding childbearing is not necessary, even from the most hardheaded primary prevention viewpoint."

One measure of the burden of a disorder arises from its clinical profile: age of onset, associated morbidity, available treatment, and cost of treatment. From this standpoint, mental disorders pose a considerable burden. They usually emerge in early adulthood and are often chronic. Although there is no cure, treatments that control the symptoms of mental disorders are available. Genetic counseling should deliver information regarding possible treatment, course, and community resources. This becomes crucial for the decisionmaking process insofar as awareness, early diagnosis, and provision of the correct treatment can limit the burden of the disorder.

There is also a subjective component to estimating the burden of a disorder in offspring. First, the desire for children can be strong. Furthermore, patients and their families assess the burden quite differently. In one study of schizophrenia, 92 percent of well family members versus 25 percent of affected individuals viewed schizophrenia

behavior and mental disorders has always proved difficult.

Methods traditionally used to examine the genetics of mental disorders include adoption, twin, and family studies. Data from these approaches indicate that mental disorders are at least in part inherited. Adoption, twin, and family studies reveal that schizophrenia has a genetic component. Twin and family studies, in particular, point to the importance of genetic factors in bipolar disorder and major depression. The heritability of these mood disorders seems to correlate with severity; bipolar disorder appears to have the clearest genetic component, followed by recurring bouts of major depression.

The inheritance of panic disorder and of OCD has undergone less scrutiny; however, based on data largely from family studies, it appears that genetic factors are involved. Data also indicate that nongenetic factors play a role in all of the mental disorders examined in this report. Questions concerning the inheritance of these disorders remain: specifically, the precise definition of what is inherited and the number of genes involved.

Spectacular advances in molecular genetics have enabled researchers to locate specific genes for diseases caused by a major gene. However, despite early claims of success and evidence from multiple sources that schizophrenia, bipolar disorder, and as a severe, debilitating disorder entailing extreme burden. With regard to childbearing decisions, 29 percent of parents versus 66 percent of affected individuals reported that they would have children (either in hindsight or in the future), given their present understanding of schizophrenia.

Another concern sometimes voiced when considering the burden of a mental disorder, especially bipolar disorder, relates to its possible link with creativity. Historical analysis and some systematic studies increasingly support this link. The concern is whether the creative output balances the burden of a severe mental disorder. The link between mental disorders and creativity raises the question, What is the value of a human being with a mental disorder? Does it lie in his or her creative output or contribution to society? Or does it emerge from the simple fact that he or she is a human being? While the creative output of individuals with mental disorders can be a source of pride, this consideration may pit the interests of society against those of the individual.

Prominent psychiatric geneticists generally reject directive counseling on reproductive decisions, emphasizing the benefit of genetic information for the individual, the rather low risk of inheriting these disorders, and their treatability. Exceptions to the prohibition against directive counseling are generally supported when severely affected individuals are involved or both spouses are afflicted. Risk to offspring greatly increases when both parents are affected. Also, pregnancy may severely exacerbate the symptoms of a mental disorder. Research concerning pregnancy, childbirth, and childrearing in persons with mental disorders, while limited, reveals possible complicating factors for both mother and offspring, including birth complications, potential teratogenic and other negative effects of psychotropic drugs on offspring, and the effect of pregnancy and the postpartum period on the mother's mental disorder, such as increased symptoms or heightened severity of symptoms.

Given the reluctance to counsel against childbearing, the question arises, How is information about the genetics of mental disorders useful to affected individuals and their families? As previously mentioned, it may relieve excessive fears of passing on the disorder to offspring. It also enhances the likelihood of early intervention. Being alert to early symptoms of a disorder will permit early treatment, perhaps forestalling the most debilitating symptoms. Unfortunately, knowledge about genetic risk does not open the door to prevention. No known interventions can prevent the development of severe mood disorders or schizophrenia. This potential scenario underscores the need for research into the prevention of mental disorders.

SOURCES: E.S. Gershon, "Genetics," *Manic-Depressive Illness*, F.K. Goodwin and K.R. Jamison (eds.) (New York, NY: Oxford University Press, 1990); E.S. Gershon, National Institute of Mental Health, personal communication, 1991; I.I. Gottesman, *Schizophrenia Genesis: The Origins of Madness* (New York, NY: W.H. Freeman, 1991); K.K. Kidd, Yale University, personal communication, 1991; M. Lappe and J.A. Brody, "Genetic Counseling: A Psychotherapeutic Approach to Autonomy in Decision Making," M.A. Sperber and L.F. Jarvik (eds.), *Psychiatry and Genetics: Psychological, Ethical, and Legal Considerations* (New York, NY: Basic Books, 1976); J. Marks, Sarah Lawrence College, personal communication, 1991; P.M. Schulz, "Patient and Family Attitudes About Schizophrenia: Implications for Genetic Counseling," *Schizophrenia Bulletin* 8:504-513, 1982; S.D. Targum and E.S. Gershon, "Pregnancy, Genetic Counseling, and the Major Psychiatric Disorders," *Genetic Diseases in Psychiatry, Maternal Effects and Fetal Outcome* J.D. Schuluan and J.L. Simpson (eds.) (New York, NY: Academic Press, 1981); M.T. Tsuang, "Genetic Counseling for Psychiatric Patients and Their Families," *American Journal of Psychiatry* 135:1465-1475, 1978; U.S. Congress, Office of Technology Assessment, *Genetic Monitoring and Screening in the Workplace*, OTA-BA-455 (Washington, DC: U.S. Government Printing Office, 1990).

major depression have a genetic component, linkage studies have failed so far to find specific genes for these disorders. Gene searches are difficult because these mental disorders probably are caused by more than one gene, both genetic and nongenetic factors contribute to them in an unknown way, and identification of the phenotype is difficult.

The complexity of the genetics of mental disorders and past failures to locate specific genes should not promote a pessimistic view of this research. Rather, our knowledge to date points out the need for various types of studies and can serve as a guide for future research endeavors. Furthermore, we can look to continued advances in molecular genetics and analytical techniques to help discern the specifics about the genetics of mental disorders. A wise investment of research dollars would support a broad effort, including continued family, twin, and adoption studies, the development of analytical methods for complex genetics, the search for major and minor genes using various approaches, and the investigation of nongenetic factors.

What is the impact of all this excitement in the field of genetics? Commentators have noted that the public increasingly views mental disorders as inherited, in sharp contrast to only a couple of decades ago. There is also an air of expectation that genetics will improve our understanding and treatment of these disorders. It is important that such hopes be tempered with realism. A long-term investment in this research is necessary, given the complexity of these disorders. At this point, the clinical implications of these data are limited; therefore, only limited information about the risk of inheritance can be provided to persons with mental disorders and their families. Finally, past abuses of genetic knowledge and the potential for a genetic test for mental disorders remind us of the necessity for great care in the use of genetic information and underscore the need to consider the social, ethical, and legal implications of this research.

CHAPTER 5 REFERENCES

1. Andrew, B., Watt, D.C., Gillespie, C., et al., "A Study of Genetic Linkage in Schizophrenia," *Psychological Medicine* 17:363-375, 1987.

2. Aschauer, H.N., Aschauer-Treiber, G., Isenberg, K.E., et al., "No Evidence for Linkage Between Chromosome 5 Markers and Schizophrenia," *Human Heredity* 40:109-115, 1990.

3. Baron, M., "Bipolar Pedigrees" (letter), *Archives of General Psychiatry* 48:671-672, 1991.

4. Baron, M., "Genes, Environment and Psychopathology," *Biological Psychiatry* 29:1055-1057, 1991.

5. Baron, M., Endicott, J., and Ott, J., "Genetic Linkage in Mental Illness: Limitations and Prospects," *British Journal of Psychiatry* 157:645-655, 1990.

6. Baron, M., Risch, N., Hamburger, R., et al., "Genetic Linkage Between X-Chromosome Markers and Bipolar Affective Illness," *Nature* 326:289-292, 1987.

7. Barr, C.L., and Kidd, K.K., "New Molecular Techniques for Genetic Linkage Studies," *Biological Psychiatry*, vol. 2, G. Racagni, N. Brunello, and T. Fukuda (eds.) (Amsterdam: Excerpta Medica, 1991).

8. Bassett, A.S., Jones, B.D., McGillivray, B.C., et al., "Partial Trisomy Chromosome 5 Cosegregating With Schizophrenia," *Lancet* 1:799-801, 1988.

9. Berrettini, W.H., Goldin, L.R., Gelernter, J., et al., "X-Chromosome Markers and Manic-Depressive Illness," *Archives of General Psychiatry* 47:366-373, 1990.

10. Bertelsen, A., Harvald, B., and Hauge, M., "A Danish Twin Study of Manic-Depressive Disorders," *British Journal of Psychiatry* 130:330-351, 1977.

11. Botstein, D., White, R.L., Skolnick, M., et al., "Construction of a Genetic Linkage Map in Man Using Restriction Fragment Length Polymorphisms," *American Journal of Human Genetics* 32:314-331, 1980.

12. Campbell, J., Crowe, R.R., Goeken, N., et al., "Affective Disorder Not Linked to HLA in a Large Bipolar Kindred," *Journal of Affective Disorders* 7:45-51, 1984.

13. Carey, G., and Gottesman, I.I., "Twin and Family Studies of Anxiety, Phobic and Obsessive Disorders," *Anxiety: New Research and Changing Concepts* (New York, NY: Raven Press, 1981).

14. Chadda, R., Kulhara, P., Singh, T., et al., "HLA Antigens in Schizophrenia: A Family Study," *British Journal of Psychiatry* 149:612-615, 1986.

15. Clerget-Darpoux, F., Babron, M.-C., and Bonaiti-Pellie, C., "Assessing the Effect of Multiple Linkage Tests in Complex Diseases," *Genetic Epidemiology* 7:245-253, 1990.

16. Clerget-Darpoux, F., Bonaiti-Pellie, C., and Hochez, J., "Effects of Misspecifying Genetic Parameters in LOD Score Analysis," *Biometrics* 42:393-399, 1986.

17. Cloninger, C.R., von Knorring, L., Sigvardsson, S., et al., "Clinical Predictors of Familial Psychopathology: Principles, Methods, and Findings," *Relatives at Risk for Mental Disorder*, D.L. Dunner, E.S. Gershon, and J.E. Barrett (eds.) (New York, NY: Raven Press, 1988).

18. Collinge, J., Delisi, L.E., Boccio, A., et al., "Evidence for a Pseudo-Autosomal Locus for Schizophrenia Using the Method of Affected Sibling Pairs," *British Journal of Psychiatry* 158:624-629, 1991.

19. Cox, D.J., Hodge, S.E., Marazita, M.L., et al., "Some Effects of Selection Strategies on Linkage Analysis," *Genetic Epidemiology* 5:289-297, 1988.

20. Crowe, R.R., "Panic Disorder: Genetic Considerations," *Journal of Psychiatric Research* 24(suppl. 2):129-134, 1990.

21. Crowe, R.R., Noyes, R., Persico, T., et al., "Genetic Studies of Panic Disorder and Related Conditions," *Relatives at Risk for Mental Disorders*, D.L. Dunner, E.S. Gershon, and J.E. Barrett (eds.) (New York, NY: Raven Press, 1988).

22. Crowe, R.R., Noyes, R., Wilson, A.F., et al., "A Linkage Study of Panic Disorder," *Archives of General Psychiatry*, 44:933-937, 1988.

23. Delisi, L.E., Crow, T.J., Davies, K.E., et al., "No Genetic Linkage Detected for Schizophrenia to Xq27-q28," *British Journal of Psychiatry* 158:630-634, 1991.

24. Del Zompo, M., Bocchetta, A., Goldin, L.R., et al., "Linkage Between X-Chromosome Markers and

Manic-Depressive Illness," *Acta Psychiatrica Scandinavia* 70:282-287, 1984.

25. Detera-Wadleigh, S.D., Berrettini, W.H., Goldin, L.R., et al., "Close Linkage of c-Harvey-*ras*-1 and the Insulin Gene to Affective Disorder Is Ruled Out in Three North American Pedigrees," *Nature* 325:806-808, 1987.

26. Detera-Wadleigh, S.D., Goldin, L.R., Sherrington, R., et al., "Exclusion of Linkage to 5q11-13 in Families With Schizophrenia and Other Psychiatric Disorders," *Nature* 340:391-393, 1989.

27. Egeland, J., Gerhard, D.S., Pauls, D.L., et al., "Bipolar Affective Disorders Linked to DNA Markers on Chromosome 11," *Nature* 325:783-786, 1987.

28. Erlenmeyer-Kimling, L., Cornblatt, B., and Fleiss, J., "High-risk Research in Schizophrenia," *Psychiatric Annals* 9:38-51, 1979.

29. Feldman, E., "Bipolar Pedigrees" (letter), *Archives of General Psychiatry* 48:673, 1991.

30. Fieve, R.R., Mendlewicz, J., and Fleiss, J.L., "Manic-Depressive Illness: Linkage With the Xg Blood Group," *American Journal of Psychiatry* 130:1355-1359, 1973.

31. Gelernter, J., and Kidd, K.K., "The Current Status of Linkage Studies in Schizophrenia," *Genes, Brain, and Behavior*, P.R. McHugh and V.A. McKusick (eds.) (New York, NY: Raven Press, 1991).

32. Gershon, E.S., "Genetics," *Manic-Depressive Illness*, F.K. Goodwin and K.R. Jamison (eds.) (New York, NY: Oxford University Press, 1990).

33. Gershon, E.S., Martinez, M., Goldin, L.R., et al., "Genetic Mapping of Common Diseases: The Challenges of Manic-Depressive Illness and Schizophrenia," *Trends in Genetics* 6:282-287, 1990.

34. Gershon, E.S., Mendlewicz, J., Gastpar, M., et al., "A Collaborative Study of Genetic Linkage of Bipolar Manic-Depressive Illness and Red/Green Colorblindness," *Acta Psychiatrica Scandinavia* 61:319-338, 1980.

35. Gershon, E.S., Targum, S.D., Matthyssee, S., et al., "Color Blindness Not Closely Linked to Bipolar Illness: Report of a New Pedigree Series," *Archives of General Psychiatry* 36:1423-1430, 1979.

36. Goldin, L.R., Clerget-Darpoux, F., and Gershon, E.S., "Relationship of HLA to Major Affective Disorder Not Supported," *Psychiatry Research* 7:29-45, 1982.

37. Goldin, L.R., Martinez, M.M., and Gershon, E.S., "Sampling Strategies for Linkage Studies," *European Archives of Psychiatry and Clinical Neuroscience* 240:182-187, 1991.

38. Gottesman, I.I., *Schizophrenia Genesis: The Origins of Madness* (New York, NY: W.H. Freeman, 1991).

39. Gottesman, I.I., and Shields, J., *Schizophrenia: The Epigenetic Puzzle* (Cambridge: Cambridge University Press, 1982).

40. Gusella, J.F., Wexler, N.S., Conneally, P.M., et al., "A Polymorphic Marker Genetically Linked to Huntington's Disease," *Nature* 306:234-238, 1983.

41. Hallmayer, J., Maier, W., Ackenheil, M., et al., "Evidence Against Linkage of Schizophrenia to Chromosome 5q11-q13 Markers in Systematically Ascertained Families," *Biological Psychiatry* 31:83-94, 1992.

42. Hebebrand, J., "A Critical Appraisal of X-Linked Bipolar Illness," *British Journal of Psychiatry* 160:7-11, 1992.

43. Hodgkinson, S., Sherrington, R., and Gurling, H., "Molecular Genetic Evidence for Heterogeneity in Manic Depression," *Nature* 325:805-806, 1987.

44. Holzman, P.S., "Eye Movement Dysfunctions and Psychosis," *International Review of Neurobiology* 27:179-205, 1985.

45. Holzman, P.S., and Matthysse, S., "The Genetics of Schizophrenia: A Review," *Psychological Science* 1:279-286, 1990.

46. Johnson, G.F.S., Hunt, G.E., Robertson, S., et al., "A Linkage Study of Manic-Depressive Disorders With HLA Antigens, Blood Groups, Serum Proteins, and Red Cell Enzymes," *Journal of Affective Disorders* 3:43-58, 1981.

47. Kaufman, C.A., DeLisi, L.E., Lehner, T., et al., "Physical Mapping, Linkage Analysis of a Putative Schizophrenia Locus on Chromosome 5Q," *Schizophrenia Bulletin* 15:441-452, 1989.

48. Kelsoe, J.R., Ginns, E.I., Egeland, J.A., et al., "Reevaluation of the Linkage Relationship Between Chromosome 11p Loci and the Gene for Bipolar Affective Disorder in the Old Order Amish," *Nature* 342:238-243, 1989.

49. Kendler, K.S., "The Genetics of Schizophrenia and Related Disorders," *Relatives at Risk for Mental Disorder*, D.L. Dunner, E.S. Gershon, and J.E. Barrett (eds.) (New York, NY: Raven Press, 1988).

50. Kendler, K.S., Gruenberg, A.M., and Strauss, J.S., "An Independent Analysis of the Copenhagen Sample of the Danish Adoption Study of Schizophrenia, II: The Relationship Between Schizotypal Personality Disorder and Schizophrenia," *Archives of General Psychiatry* 38:982-984, 1981.

51. Kennedy, J.L., and Giuffra, LA., "Recent Developments in Genetic Linkage Studies of Schizophrenia," *Advances in Neuropsychiatry and Psychopharmacology*, vol. 1, *Schizophrenia Research*, C.A. Tamminga and S.C. Schulz (eds.) (New York, NY: Raven Press, 1991).

52. Kennedy, J.L., Giuffra, LA., Moises, H.W., et al., "Evidence Against Linkage of Schizophrenia to

Markers on Chromosome 5 in a Northern Swedish Pedigree,'' *Nature* 336:167-170, 1988.

53. Kety, S.S., "Mental Illness in the Biological and Adoptive Relatives of Schizophrenic Adoptees: Findings Relevant to Genetic and Environmental Factors in Etiology,'' *American Journal of Psychiatry* 140:720-727, 1983.

54. Kety, S.S., Rosenthal, D., Wender, P.H., et al., "Mental Illness in the Biological and Adoptive Families of Adopted Schizophrenics,'' *American Journal of Psychiatry* 128:302-308, 1971.

55. Kidd, K.K., Egeland, J.A., Molthan, L., et al., "Amish Study: IV. Genetic Linkage Study of Pedigrees of Bipolar Probands,'' *American Journal of Psychiatry* 141:1042-1048, 1984.

56. Kruger, S.D., Turner, W.J., and Kidd, K.K., "The Effects of Requisite Assumptions on Linkage Analyses of Manic-Depressive Illness With HLA,'' *Biological Psychiatry* 17:1081-1099, 1982.

57. Leckman, J.F., Gershon, E.S., and McGinniss, M.H., "New Data Do Not Suggest Linkage Between the Xg Blood Group and Bipolar Illness,'' *Archives of General Psychiatry* 36:1435-1441, 1979.

58. McClearn, G.E., Promin, R., Gora-Maslak, G., et al., "The Gene Chase in Behavioral Science,'' *Psychological Science* 2:222-228, 1991.

59. McGue, M., and Gottesman, I.I., "The Genetic Epidemiology of Schizophrenia and the Design of Linkage Studies,'' *European Archives of Psychiatry and Clinical Neuroscience*, 240:174-181, 1991.

60. McGuffin, P., Festenstein, H., and Murray, R.M., "A Family Study of HLA Antigens and Other Genetic Markers in Schizophrenia,'' *Psychological Medicine* 13:31-43, 1983.

61. McGuffin, P., and Katz, R., "The Genetics of Depression and Manic-Depressive Disorder,'' *British Journal of Psychiatry* 155:294-304, 1989.

62. McGuffin, P., and Owen, M., "The Molecular Genetics of Schizophrenia: An Overview and Forward View,'' *European Archives of Psychiatry and Clinical Neuroscience* 240:169-173, 1991.

63. McGuffin, P., Sargeant, M., Hetti, G., et al., "Exclusion of a Schizophrenia Susceptibility Gene From the Chromosome 5Q11-q13 Region: New Data and a Reanalysis of Previous Reports,'' *American Journal of Human Genetics* 47:524-535, 1990.

64. McGuffin, P., and Sargeant, M.P., "Genetic Markers and Affective Disorder,'' *The New Genetics of Mental Illness*, P. McGuffin and R. Murray (eds.) (Oxford, Great Britain: Butterworth-Heinemann Ltd., 1991).

65. Matthysse, S., Holzman, P.S., and Lange, K., "The Genetic Transmission of Schizophrenia: Application of Mendelian Latent Structure Analysis to Eye Tracking Dysfunction in Schizophrenia and Affective Disorder,'' *Journal of Psychiatric Research* 20:57-67, 1986.

66. Mendlewicz, J., and Fleiss, J.L., "Linkage Studies With X-Chromosome Markers in Bipolar (Manic-Depressive) and Unipolar (Depressive) Illness,'' *Biological Psychiatry* 9:261-294, 1974.

67. Mendlewicz, J., Fleiss, J.L., and Fieve, R.R., "Evidence for X-Linkage in the Transmission of Manic-Depressive Illness,'' *Journal of the American Medical Association* 222:1624-1627, 1972.

68. Mendlewicz, J., Fleiss, J.L., and Fieve, R.R., "Linkage Studies in Affective Disorders: The Xg Blood Group and Manic-Depressive Illness,'' *Genetic Research in Psychiatry*, R.R. Fieve, K. Rosenthal, and H. Brill (eds.) (Baltimore, MD: Johns Hopkins University Press, 1975).

69. Mendlewicz, J., Linkowski, P., Guroff, J.J., et al., "Color Blindness Linkage to Bipolar Manic-Depressive Illness: New Evidence,'' *Archives of General Psychiatry* 36:1442-1447, 1979.

70. Mendlewicz, J., Linkowski, P., and Wilmotte, J., "Linkage Between Glucose-6-Phosphate Dehydrogenase Deficiency and Manic-Depressive Psychosis,'' *British Journal of Psychiatry* 137:337-342, 1980.

71. Mendlewicz, J., Simon, P., Sevy, S., et al., "Polymorphic DNA Marker on X Chromosome and Manic Depression,'' *Lancet* 1:1230-1231, 1987.

72. Merikangas, K.R., Spence, M.A., and Kupfer, D.J., "Linkage Studies of Bipolar Disorder: Methodologic and Analytic Issues,'' *Archives of General Psychiatry* 46:1137-1141, 1989.

73. Moises, H.W., Gelernter, J., Grandy, D.K., et al., "Exclusion of the D2-dopamine Receptor Gene as Candidate Gene for Schizophrenia in a Large Pedigree From Sweden,'' abstract, First World Congress on Psychiatric Genetics, Cambridge, England, 1989.

74. Moldin, S.O., Reich, T., and Rice, J.P., "Current Perspectives on the Genetics of Unipolar Depression,'' *Behavior Genetics* 21:211-242, 1991.

75. Morton, N.E., "Sequential Tests for the Detection of Linkage,'' *American Journal of Human Genetics* 7:277-318, 1955.

76. Noyes, R., Crowe, R.R., Harris, E.L., et al., "Relationship Between Panic Disorder and Agoraphobia: A Family Study,'' *Archives of General Psychiatry* 43:227-232, 1986.

77. Owen, M., Crawford, D., and St. Claire, D., "Localisation of a Susceptibility Locus for Schizophrenia on Chromosome 5,'' *British Journal of Psychiatry* 157:123-127, 1990.

78. Pardes, H., Kaufmann, C.A., Pincus, H.A., et al., "Genetics and Psychiatry: Past Discoveries, Cur-

rent Dilemmas, and Future Directions,'' *American Journal of Psychiatry* 146:435-443, 1989.

79. Pauls, D.L., Bucher, K.D., Crowe, R.R., et al., "A Genetic Study of Panic Disorder Pedigrees," *American Journal of Human Genetics* 32:639-644, 1980.

80. Pauls, D.L., and Leckman, J.F., "The Inheritance of Gilles de la Tourette's Syndrome and Associated Behaviors: Evidence for Autosomal Dominant Transmission," *New England Journal of Medicine* 315:993-997, 1986.

81. Pauls, D.L., Raymond, C.L., Robertson, M., "The Genetics of Obsessive-Compulsive Disorder: A Review," *Psychobiology of Obsessive-Compulsive Disorder*, 1991.

82. Pauls, D.L., Towbin, K.E., Leckman, J.F., et al., "Gilles de la Tourette Syndrome and Obsessive Compulsive Disorder: Evidence Supporting an Etiological Relationship," *Archives of General Psychiatry* 43:1180-1182, 1986.

83. Plomin, R., "Behavioral Genetics," *Genes, Brain, and Behavior*, P.R. McHugh and V.A. McKusick (eds.) (New York, NY: Raven Press, 1991).

84. Plomin, R., personal communication, 1992.

85. Plomin, R., DeFries, J.C., and McClearn, G.E., *Behavioral Genetics: A Primer* 2nd ed. (New York, NY: W.H. Freeman, 1990).

86. Rasmussen, S.A., and Tsuang, M.T., "Clinical Characteristics and Family History in DSM-III Obsessive-Compulsive Disorder," *American Journal of Psychiatry* 143:317-322, 1986.

87. Reich, T., Clayton, P.J., and Winokur, G., "Family History Studies: V. The Genetics of Mania," *American Journal of Psychiatry* 125:64-75, 1969.

88. Reiss, D., Plomin, R., and Hetherington, E.M., "Genetics and Psychiatry: An Unheralded Window on the Environment," *American Journal of Psychiatry* 148:283-291, 1991.

89. Risch, N., "Genetic Linkage and Complex Diseases, With Special Reference to Psychiatric Disorders," *Genetic Epidemiology* 7:3-16, 1990.

90. Risch, N., "A Note on Multiple Testing Procedures in Linkage Analysis," *American Journal of Human Genetics* 48:1058-1064, 1991.

91. Risch, N., "Genetic Linkage: Interpreting Lod Scores," *Science* 255:803-804, 1992.

92. Risch, N., and Baron, M., "X-Linkage and Genetic Heterogeneity in Bipolar Related Major Affective Illness: Re-analysis of Linkage Data," *Annals of Human Genetics* 46:153-166, 1982.

93. St. Clair, D., Blackwood, D., Muir, W., et al., "No Linkage of Chromosome 5q11-q13 Markers to Schizophrenia in Scottish Families," *Nature* 339:305-309, 1989.

94. St. George-Hyslop, P.H., Tanzi, R.E., Polinshy, R.J., et al., "The Genetic Defect Causing Familial

Alzheimer's Disease Maps on Chromosome 21," *Science* 235:885-890, 1987.

95. Schulz, S.C., "Genetics of Schizophrenia: A Status Report," *Review of Psychiatry*, vol. 10, A. Tasman and S.M. Goldfinger (eds.) (Washington, DC: American Psychiatric Press, 1991).

96. Sherrington, R., Brynjolfsson, J., Petursson, H., et al., "Localization of a Susceptibility Locus for Schizophrenia on Chromosome 5," *Nature* 336:164-169, 1988.

97. Smeraldi, E., and Bellodi, L., "Possible Linkage between Primary Affective Disorder Susceptibility Locus and HLA Halotypes," *American Journal of Psychiatry* 139:1232-1234, 1981.

98. Smeraldi, E., Negri, F., Melica, A.M., et al., "HLA System and Affective Disorders: A Sibship Genetic Study," *Tissue Antigens* 12:270-274, 1978.

99. Suarez, B.K., and Croughan, J., "Is the Major Histocompatibility Complex Linked to Genes that Increase Susceptibility to Affective Disorder? A Critical Appraisal," *Psychiatry Research* 7:19-27, 1982.

100. Suarez, B.K., and Reich, T., "HLA and Major Affective Disorder," *Archives of General Psychiatry* 41:22-27, 1984.

101. Targum, S.D., Gershon, E.S., Van Eerdewegh, M., et al., "Human Leukocyte Antigen System Not Closely Linked to or Associated With Bipolar Manic-Depressive Illness," *Biological Psychiatry* 14:615-636, 1979.

102. Tienari, P., Sorri, A., Lahti, I., et al., "Interaction of Genetic and Psychosocial Factors in Schizophrenia," *Acta Psychiatrica Scandinavia* 71:19-30, 1985.

103. Torgersen, S., "Genetic Factors in Moderately Severe and Mild Affective Disorders," *Archives of General Psychiatry* 43:222-226, 1986.

104. Torgersen, S., "Twin Studies in Panic Disorder," *Neurobiology of Panic Disorder*, J.C. Ballenger (ed.) (New York, NY: Alan R. Liss, 1990).

105. Tsuang, M.T., and Faraone, S.V., *The Genetics of Mood Disorders* (Baltimore, MD: Johns Hopkins University Press, 1990).

106. Turner, W.J., "Genetic Markers for Schizotaxia," *Biological Psychiatry* 14:177-205, 1979.

107. Turner, W.J., Beidel, D.C., and Nathan, R.S., "Biological Factors in Obsessive-Compulsive Disorders," *Psychological Bulletin* 97:430-450, 1985.

108. Turner, W.J., and King, S., "Two Genetically Distinct Forms of Bipolar Affective Disorder," *Biological Psychiatry* 16:417, 1981.

109. Turner, W.J., and King, S., "BPD2 An Autosomal Dominant Form of Bipolar Affective Disorder," *Biological Psychiatry* 18:63-87, 1983.

110. Weissman, M.M., "The Affective Disorders: Bipolar Disorder and Major Depression," *Concepts of*

Mental Disorders, McClelland and Kerr (eds.) (London: England, 1991).

111. Weissman, M.M., personal communication, 1992.

112. Weissman, M.M., "Panic Disorder: Epidemiology and Genetics," *Proceedings of the Consensus Development Conference on Treatment of Panic Disorder*, Sept. 25-27, 1991 (Bethesda, MD: National Institutes of Health, in press).

113. Weissman, M.M., Wickramaratne, P., Merikangas, K.R., et al., "Onset of Major Depression in Early Adulthood. Increased Familial Loading and Specificity," *Archives of General Psychiatry* 41:1136-1143, 1984.

114. Weitkamp, L.R., Pardue, L.H., and Huntzinger, R.S., "Genetic Marker Studies in a Family With Unipolar Depression," *Archives of General Psychiatry* 37:1187-1192, 1980.

115. Weitkamp, L.R., Stancer, H.C., Persad, E., et al., "Depressive Disorders and HLA: A Gene on Chromosome 6 That Can Affect Behavior," *New England Journal of Medicine* 305:1301-1306, 1981.

116. Winokur, G., "Bipolar Pedigrees" (letter), *Archives of General Psychiatry* 48:671, 1991.

117. Winokur, G., Clayton, P.J., and Reich, T., *Manic Depressive Illness* (St. Louis, MO: C.V. Mosby, 1969).

Chapter 6
Research Effort and Issues

CONTENTS OF CHAPTER 6

Box

Figures

Tables

This chapter describes the funding of research into the biology of mental disorders and discusses issues surrounding the conduct of that research. The conduct of this research is shaped by many forces, including scientific developments, the availability of resources, and public support for it. Advances in the neurosciences have especially increased interest in the biology of mental disorders and have fostered the expansion of research in this field. These developments have influenced the decisions of policymakers regarding funding levels and priorities for research.

Beyond funding decisions, a number of issues affect scientists' ability to carry out this research. Some of these issues are unique to the study of the biology of mental disorders. They involve specific methodological and technical considerations associated with experiments. Other issues are related to the willingness of individuals to participate in research and their awareness of the need for this research and what is required to carry it out. Impediments associated with these issues can slow the rate of progress in this field.

This chapter provides an analysis of the funding decisions that have been made regarding research into the biology of mental disorders. It also examines the issues associated with this research and describes some actions that have been, and can be, taken to lessen their retarding influence.

RESEARCH EFFORT

Improving the understanding of mental disorders—both their causes and treatments—requires financial support for research, including (but not limited to) basic neuroscience research and research devoted specifically to the biology of mental disorders.

Federal sources of funding are the most important delimiting factor in this research.

Decisions about the amount and distribution of research dollars reveal the priority society places on addressing mental disorders and the thinking about where the greatest advances are likely to occur. In this section, the Office of Technology Assessment (OTA) examines both the financial support for mental health research in general and the investment in research on the biological factors that contribute to mental disorders. The major source of this funding is the National Institute of Mental Health (NIMH), the oldest and largest institute of the Alcohol, Drug Abuse, and Mental Health Administration (ADAMHA), within the U.S. Department of Health and Human Services.

National Institute of Mental Health

Figure 6-1 presents the funding of NIMH from 1970 until the present, adjusted for inflation.[1] Total funding and funding for research and services are presented. This breakdown represents the dual role of NIMH: conducting and supporting research and research training on the biological, behavioral, public health, and social science aspects of mental disorders; and conducting research on the development and improvement of mental health services and supporting such services. Research funding[2] includes extramural research, intramural research, and research training, while service funding includes service programs,[3] services research, and clinical training.[4] From 1970 until the early 1980s, NIMH experienced a decrease in its budget. Since the early 1980s, this trend has been reversed (see later discussion), although the total NIMH budget for 1992 is less than for 1970.

---

[1] To eliminate the effect of inflation, the NIMH budget was converted into constant 1987 dollars using the gross domestic product deflator as the price index (12).

[2] Research funding is defined, in this chapter, as that extramural research supported by the Division of Basic Brain and Behavioral Sciences and the Division of Clinical Research and intramural research; it excludes the extramural budget of the Division of Applied and Services Research, which supports services research and the portion of the intramural budget devoted to services research. It also excludes funds for AIDS research.

[3] Figures for 1970-81 do not include funding of services programs which were continued under block grants to the States starting in 1982 (see later text). Service activities that continued to be funded by NIMH are service planning and demonstration projects, programs related to the legal protection and advocacy for individuals with mental disorders, and programs for the homeless.

[4] While clinical training also includes aspects of research training, the major focus of the clinical training programs is to prepare professionals to enhance the effectiveness of services to persons with mental disorders.

Figure 6-1—NIMH Budget, Fiscal Years 1970-92

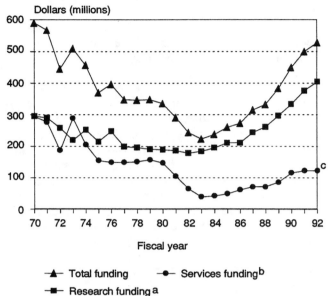

The research, services, and total budgets of NIMH from 1970 until the present.

NOTE: Figures converted to constant 1987 dollars using the 1992 gross domestic product deflator.

[a] Research includes funding for research training and all extramural and intramural research, excluding funding for services research (see text).

[b] Services include services programs, services research, and clinical training. Figures for 1970-1981 do not include funding of services programs that were continued under block grants to the states starting in 1982.

[c] 1991 and 1992 figures are estimates. 1992 figures are based on the assumption that the price index is going to stay constant at its 1991 level.

SOURCE: Office of Technology Assessment from figures supplied by National Institute of Mental Health, 1992.

The history of NIMH funding is an indication of the priority that has been placed on research into mental disorders. In the past, others have noted an underfunding of mental disorders research by examining such factors as the costs of mental disorders to society and the number of people affected (17). Another indication of relative support can be derived by comparing the research funding and social costs of mental disorders to those of cancer and heart disease (table 6-1). The latter were chosen for comparison to mental disorders because they exact comparable costs from society (1,44). The costs of

all these disorders were derived in a similar manner.[5] If the total cost to society of mental disorders, including dementia (42), is compared with the total 1985 budget of NIMH and the portion of the budget of the National Institute on Aging devoted to dementia research, one finds that for every $100 of social costs, $.30 was spent on research. In comparison, for every $100 of social costs of cancer (41), $1.63 was spent on research, and for every $100 of social costs of heart disease (44), $.73 was spent on research.

A similar underfunding of research into mental disorders is apparent when the average annual rates of increase in the NIMH and National Cancer Institute (NCI) budgets are compared. When adjusted for inflation using the gross domestic product (GDP) deflator as the price index, the purchasing power of the total NIMH budget dropped an average of 1 percent per year between 1970 and 1991. During the same period, NCI's purchasing power increased an average of 5 percent per year. If the same comparisons are made for just the 1980s, however, this trend is reversed: Not only does the purchasing power of the NIMH budget increase, it increases faster than the purchasing power of the NCI budget (an average of 3.0 percent per year compared to 0.7 percent).[6] Thus, while research into mental disorders receives less support than research into cancer and heart disease, relative to their respective costs to society, it has increased somewhat in the last 10 years.

Figure 6-2 shows the research and services budgets of NIMH between 1980 and 1992 (29). The average annual real rate of increase in research funding between 1980 and 1992 was 6.7 percent. After 1986, the rate of increase accelerated to 11.5 percent. The increase in NIMH's research budget in 1987 constant dollars between 1991 and 1992 is 7.7 percent, which is less than the 11.5 percent average annual real rate of increase between 1986 and 1992. Nonetheless, if the trend between 1986 and 1992 continues through the 1990s, it would compensate for the years when research on mental disorders did not keep up with inflation or with the advances in

---

[5] Costs of mental disorders, cancer, and heart disease include direct health-related costs (treatment, support) and indirect health-related costs (morbidity costs, the value of goods and services that were not produced, and mortality costs, the value of future output lost due to premature death). Costs of mental disorders also include nonhealth-related costs, such as losses in productivity due to time spent to care for a family member with a mental disorder (see box 2-A).

[6] To compare NIMH budgets between 1970 and 1991 and between 1980 and 1991, the share of categorical Federal support for service programs was subtracted from total NIMH budgets between 1970 and 1981. After 1981, categorical Federal support for service programs is no longer part of the NIMH budget.

Table 6-1—Comparison of Costs and Research Funding, Fiscal Year 1985

Illness	Costs[a] ($ millions)	Total budget of principal Federal institution[b] ($ millions)	Dollars spent on research per $100 of cost to society
Mental disorders	103,691[c]	310[d]	0.30
Cancer (malignant neoplasms only) ..	72,494	1,184	1.63
Heart disease	69,000	501	0.73

[a]D.P. Rice, S. Kelman, L.S. Miller, et al., *The Economic Costs of Alcohol and Drug Abuse and Mental Illness: 1985*, report submitted to the Office of Financing and Coverage Policy, Alcohol, Drug Abuse, and Mental Health Administration, U.S. Department of Health and Human Services (San Francisco, CA: Institute for Health and Aging, University of California, 1990); D.P. Rice, T.A. Hodgson, and F. Capell, "The Economic Burden of Cancer, 1985: United States and California," *Cancer Care and Cost: DRGs and Beyond*, R.M. Scheffler and N.C. Andrews (eds.) (Ann Arbor, MI: Health Administration Press Perspectives, 1989); T. Thom, Health Statistician, Division of Epidemiology and Clinical Applications, National Heart, Lung, and Blood Institute, National Institutes of Health, personal communication, 1991.
[b]National Institute of Mental Health, National Cancer Institute, and National Heart, Lung, and Blood Institute budgets.
[c]Costs of mental disorders include costs of dementia.
[d]Figure includes $29 million for funding of dementia research by the National Institute on Aging.

SOURCE: Office of Technology Assessment, 1992.

Figure 6-2—NIMH Budget, Fiscal Years 1980-92

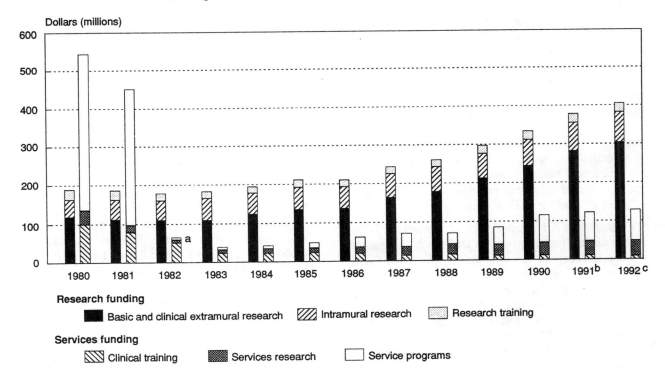

Funding of the components of the research and services budgets of NIMH.

NOTE: Figures converted to constant 1987 dollars using the 1992 gross domestic product deflator.
[a]Decrease reflects initiation of State block grants.
[b]1991 and 1992 figures are estimates.
[c]1992 figures based on assumption of constant price index.

SOURCE: Office of Technology Assessment from figures supplied by National Institute of Mental Health, 1992.

Table 6-2—Funding of Extramural and Intramural NIMH Research, Fiscal Year 1991[a]

NIMH research	Funding ($ millions)	Percent of research budget
Extramural		
Division of Basic Brain and Behavioral Sciences	124.2	25.7
Division of Clinical Research	169.6	35.1
Division of Applied Sciences and Services Research	42.0	8.7
AIDS	62.3	12.8
Total	398.1	82.3
Intramural	85.7	17.7
Total	483.8	100.0

[a]Funding for research training is included in budgets for extramural and intramural research.
SOURCE: National Institute of Mental Health, 1991.

funding for other diseases. In 1991, research funding made up 75 percent of the total funding for research and services.

Before 1982, the single most important aspect of services funding was the service programs—the categorical Federal support of community mental health and social services programs (figure 6-2).[7] The drastic decline in NIMH funding for services in 1982 reflects the end of an era of categorical Federal support. Almost all of these service programs were later continued under five block grants, administered by ADAMHA, to the States (36). When the categorical support is subtracted from services funding in 1980 and 1981, NIMH's purchasing power in this area dropped an average of 1.1 percent per year between 1980 and 1992. Since 1986, however, NIMH's purchasing power in this area has increased an average of 13.4 percent per year, reflecting the overall increase in NIMH funding.

Funding of all extramural and intramural NIMH research in 1991 is given in table 6-2.[8] Extramural research received 82 percent of the total NIMH research budget. To analyze the recent research emphasis at NIMH, the two divisions of extramural research—the Division of Basic Brain and Behavioral Sciences and the Division of Clinical Research—are examined. These two divisions account for 74 percent of the extramural budget and 61 percent of NIMH's total research budget.

The Division of Basic Brain and Behavioral Sciences

The Division of Basic Brain and Behavioral Sciences (DBBBS) consists of seven branches that

support brain and behavioral research aimed at furthering the understanding of mental disorders (figure 6-3). DBBBS was formed in 1989, when the Division of Basic Science was reorganized to reflect the diversity of research areas being supported by the division and to allow more efficient administration of the large number of research grants being funded (58). The three branches of the Division of Basic Science (i.e., Neuroscience Research, Health and Behavior Research, and Behavioral Research) were restructured into the current seven branches. The restructuring and renaming of the division also reflected an increased emphasis at NIMH on the role of behavioral research in understanding mental disorders (27).

Budget figures provided by NIMH divide the funding of DBBBS into two components—behavioral research (Basic Behavioral and Cognitive Sciences Research Branch, Personality and Social Processes Research Branch, and Basic Prevention and Behavioral Medicine Research Branch) and biological research (Molecular and Cellular Neuroscience Research Branch, Cognitive and Behavioral Neuroscience Research Branch, Neuroimaging and Applied Neurosciences Research Branch, and Psychopharmacology Research Branch) (29). Since the latter four branches directly concentrate on brain mechanisms related to mental disorders, an analysis of their funding provide a rough estimate of DBBBS support for research into the biological factors that contribute to mental disorders. However, because of the interaction of biology and behavior in mental disorders, research projects often overlap. Thus, a project funded by one of the biological branches may include behavioral aspects in its design; conversely,

[7] Funding for these service programs is included in the budget figures for 1980 and 1981 in figure 6-2.

[8] In this table, budget figures for extramural and intramural research include support of research training.

Figure 6-3—Structure of the Division of Basic Brain and Behavioral Sciences

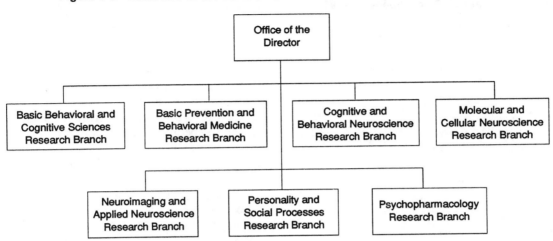

The NIMH Division of Basic Brain and Behavioral Sciences is made up of seven research branches.

SOURCE: Office of Technology Assessment, 1992.

Table 6-3—Distribution of Research Funds by the Division of Basic Brain and Behavioral Sciences (DBBBS), Fiscal Year 1991

Research branch	Funding ($ millions)	Percent of research budget
Basic Behavioral and Cognitive Sciences	13.5	11.5
Personality and Social Processes	18.4	15.6
Basic Prevention and Behavioral Medicine	12.4	10.5
Molecular and Cellular Neuroscience	22.3	19.0
Cognitive and Behavioral Neuroscience	22.0	18.7
Neuroimaging and Applied Neuroscience	14.2	12.1
Psychopharmacology	14.8	12.6
Total	$117.6[a]	100.0

[a]This total does not include $6.6 million of the DBBBS budget allocated to the Contracts and Interagency Agreements and the Small Business Innovation Research Program.

SOURCE: National Institute of Mental Health, 1991.

a study that is funded through one of the behavioral branches may have a biological component to it.

Table 6-3 shows the distribution of funds among the research branches of DBBBS for 1991. Of the $117.6 million research budget of the DBBBS,[9] 38 percent is allocated to the three behavioral branches and 62 percent to the four biological branches (29). Figure 6-4 presents the funding of biological and behavioral research, adjusted for inflation, for 1988 through 1992. Both areas show a steady increase—biological by 70 percent, with an average annual real rate of increase of 14.5 percent, and behavioral research by 38 percent, with an average annual rise of 8.5 percent—indicating consistent and strong

support. The portion of the total DBBBS budget devoted to biological research, adjusted for inflation, increased from 60 percent in 1988 to 65 percent in 1992. Taken as an indicator of funding for the study of biological factors associated with mental disorders, these figures reveal vigorous support. The average 14.5 percent annual rate of increase is above the 11.5 percent rate for the total NIMH research budget between 1986 and 1992 (see previous discussion).

Division of Clinical Research

The Division of Clinical Research (DCR) consists of six research-oriented branches and one that supports programs in mental health education (see

[9] The $6.6 million of the DBBBS budget allocated to the Contracts and Interagency Agreements and Small Business Innovation Research Program is not included in this analysis.

Figure 6-4—Funding of the Division of Basic Brain and Behavioral Sciences, Fiscal Years 1988-92

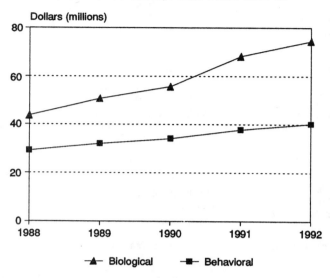

The funding of the Division of Basic Brain and Behavioral Sciences broken down into biological and behavioral research (see text).

NOTE: Figures converted to constant 1987 dollars using the 1992 gross domestic product deflator.

SOURCE: Office of Technology Assessment from figures supplied by National Institute of Mental Health, 1992.

ch. 7) (figure 6-5) (26). Table 6-4 shows the distribution of funding among the six research branches in 1991 (29). Two of these branches support studies of specific mental disorders considered in this report—the Schizophrenia Research Branch and the Mood, Anxiety, and Personality Disorders Research Branch. These two branches account for the largest share—50.4 percent—of the $169.6 million total research budget of the DCR for 1991.

Trends in support for specific areas of mental disorders research can be discerned by examining the funding of the DCR branches. Figure 6-6 illustrates that funding, adjusted for inflation, for 1980 through 1992 (29). One notable trend is the increase in funding of research related to schizophrenia. From 1986 until the present, the Schizophrenia Research Branch experienced a 156 percent increase in funding, with an annual average real rate of increase of 17.4 percent. The other branches saw an annual average increase of 10.7 percent over the same period. The Mood, Anxiety, and Personality Disorders Research Branch also experienced consistently higher-than-average funding during this

period. The Prevention Research Branch is the only branch to have experienced a net decline in funding (-20.5 percent) between 1980 and 1992.

NIMH Centers

NIMH also supports research on mental disorders through specialized centers administered by DBBBS and DCR. These centers foster collaborative research in specific areas, bringing together teams of researchers who contribute various skills to the research projects. Funding for these centers is included in the overall budgets for these divisions. DBBBS administers three types of centers, all of whose major research emphasis is the biology of mental disorders (table 6-5). Of the $9.0 million total support for DBBBS centers in 1991, $5.4 million (60 percent) funded the five Centers for the Neuroscience of Mental Disorders. All five focus specifically on schizophrenia. Their purpose is to integrate research on schizophrenia with neuroscience approaches to brain function and dysfunction. The second group—the Centers for Neuroscience Research—consists of three centers funded with $3.2 million. The goal of these centers is to pursue novel and innovative research on specialized areas of neuroscience related to mental disorders. Currently, there is only one center in the third group— Functional Brain Imaging Center for the Study of Mental Disorders. NIMH plans to add new centers to this group in the next several years in order to expand multidisciplinary research on brain imaging technologies.

DCR provided $22.4 million for 23 research centers in 1991 (table 6-6) (28). These centers focus on four areas of mental disorders research— schizophrenia, mood disorders, child, and aging. The research of 19 of these centers can be characterized as biological (28), accounting for 82 percent ($18.4 million) of the total DCR research center budget. The remaining four centers, one in each of the four areas, conduct research related to psychosocial factors. Sixteen of the centers are involved in research related to either schizophrenia or mood disorders. These 16 receive $14.4 million, or 64 percent of the DCR research center budget.

In addition to these research centers, NIMH also funds 10 gene-bank diagnostic centers that collect blood samples and diagnostic data from patients and their families for use in genetic studies of mental disorders (see ch. 5).

Figure 6-5—Structure of the Division of Clinical Research

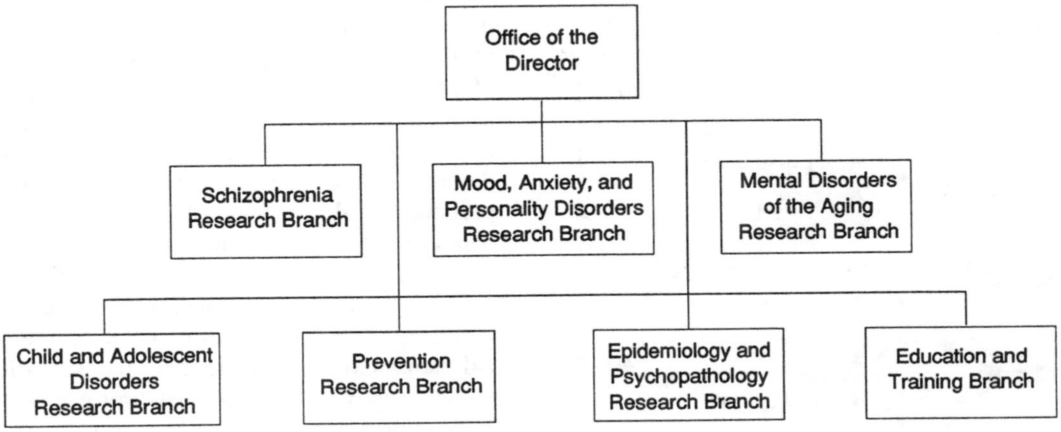

The NIMH Division of Clinical Research is made up of six research branches and an education and training branch.

SOURCE: Office of Technology Assessment, 1992.

Table 6-4—Distribution of Research Funds by the Division of Clinical Research, Fiscal Year 1991

Research branch	Funding ($ millions)	Percent of research budget
Schizophrenia Research	42.3	24.9
Mood, Anxiety, and Personality Disorders Research	43.0	25.4
Mental Disorders of the Aging Research	24.6	14.5
Child and Adolescent Disorders Research	27.0	15.9
Prevention Research	12.7	7.5
Epidemiology and Psychopathology Research	20.0	11.8
Total	169.6	100.0

SOURCE: National Institute of Mental Health, 1991.

Summary of NIMH Funding

Since NIMH is the principal Federal institution that plans and supports research on mental disorders, its funding and the research emphasis within it provide a fairly accurate illustration of the overall research emphasis in the United States. Over the past decade, total support of NIMH has increased, reversing a previous trend of undersupport. This is particularly evident in the increases in funding that have occurred since 1986. OTA's analysis indicates that NIMH is a multifaceted organization, responsible for many things, including research on biological, behavioral, public health, and sociological aspects of mental disorders, with an emphasis on biological research.

The extramural research funding of DBBBS and DCR supports studies on a variety of biological, behavioral, and social science aspects of mental disorders. Analysis of the distribution of this funding reveals two areas of emphasis. First is the emphasis on basic research related to biological factors associated with mental disorders, an emphasis that overlaps with the recommendations of the National Advisory Mental Health Council (51). Over half the total budget of DBBBS is devoted to funding those branches that emphasize biology; with four exceptions, all of the research centers funded by DCR and DBBBS emphasize biological research. The second emphasis is research on the severe mental disorders included in this report: schizophrenia and mood and anxiety disorders. In 1991, the two branches of DCR devoted to research on these disorders received 50.3 percent of the total DCR budget, and since 1986 the Schizophrenia Research Branch has experienced the highest rate of growth of any DCR branch. Also, the majority of research centers (16 out of 23) funded by DCR focus

Figure 6-6—Funding of the Division of Clinical Research, Fiscal Years 1980-92

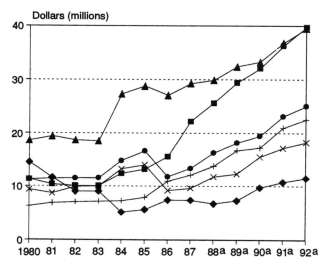

Dollars (millions)

- ■— Schizophrenia
- +— Mental disorders of the aging
- ●— Child and adolescent disorders
- ▲— Mood, anxiety, and personality disorders
- ✕— Epidemiology and psychopathology
- ◆— Prevention

Funding of the six research branches of the Division of Clinical Research.

NOTE: Figures converted to constant 1987 dollars using the 1992 gross domestic product deflator.
aFigures include research training.
SOURCE: Office of Technology Assessment from figures supplied by National Institute of Mental Health, 1992.

specifically on these disorders. The emphasis on schizophrenia research again coincides with recommendations of the National Advisory Mental Health Council (52).

Other Federal Agencies

Although NIMH is the principal Federal institution that funds research related to mental disorders, others contribute. One such Federal agency, the Department of Veterans Affairs (VA), specifically funds research on mental disorders. In fiscal year 1991, the VA spent approximately $15 million on some 230 research projects related to mental disorders (31). Of this $15 million, approximately $700,000 supports various projects at three centers devoted to the study of the neurobiology of schizophrenia (i.e., Denver VA Hospital, Bronx VA Hospital, West

Haven VA Hospital) (7). The remaining funds support research into various aspects of mental disorders, including biological factors (31). The total VA medical research budget for fiscal year 1991 was $216 million (4). It has been noted that there is a disparity between VA medical research expenditures and VA clinical costs regarding mental disorders (4). Mental disorders account for 40 percent of all VA bed days, while 7 percent of research monies are allocated to mental disorders research. A report recently completed by the VA Advisory Committee for Health Research Policy recommended the creation of a Health Research Advisory Council to identify and set priorities for those areas with the greatest promise of enhancing VA health care (4). This council would be a mechanism for addressing issues such as the disparity related to mental disorders. Table 6-7 shows VA funding of research projects related to mental disorders for fiscal years 1986 through 1991.

The remainder of Federal funding in this area is devoted to support of neuroscience research. As previously discussed (see ch. 2), neuroscience is an interdisciplinary field encompassing many different areas. Research in the neurosciences fuels the study of the biological factors that contribute to mental disorders. While not all neuroscience projects are directly applicable to mental disorders, research in many areas (e.g., cellular and molecular neuroscience, neurochemistry, neuropharmacology) all contribute to the foundation that supports the study of biological mechanisms associated with mental disorders.

Many Federal institutions have programs devoted to various aspects of neuroscience research (figure 6-7). In fact, Federal funding for this broadly defined area of research was more than $1 billion in 1990 (48). Federal funding institutions include NIMH (see earlier discussion) as well as the National Institute on Drug Abuse and the National Institute on Alcohol Abuse and Alcoholism and a number of institutes within the National Institutes of Health (NIH). The National Institute of Neurological Disorders and Stroke (NINDS) is the major source of such funding at NIH, with an expenditure of almost $500 million in fiscal year 1990 (figure 6-7). Other institutes at NIH that fund neuroscience research are the National Institute on Aging, National Eye Institute, National Institute on Deafness and Other Communication Disorders, National Institute on Child Health and Human Development, National

Table 6-5—Research Centers Funded by the Division of Basic Brain and Behavioral Sciences

Center	Number	Funding ($ millions)
Neuroscience of Mental Disorders	5	5.4
Neuroscience Research	3	3.2
Functional Brain Imaging for the Study of Mental Disorders	1	0.4
Total	9	9.0

SOURCE: National Institute of Mental Health, 1991.

Table 6-6—Clinical Research Centers Funded by the Division of Clinical Research

Area of research	All centers Number	Funding ($ millions)	Centers doing biological research Number	Funding ($ millions)
Aging	5	3.9	4	3.1
Schizophrenia	8	7.8	7	6.5
Mood disorders	8	8.8	7	7.9
Child	2	1.9	1	0.9
Total	23	22.4	19	18.4

SOURCE: National Institute of Mental Health, 1991.

Table-6-7—Department of Veterans Affairs Funding of Mental Disorders Research, Fiscal Years 1986-91

Fiscal year	Funding ($ millions)	Projects (no.)
1986	8.8	119
1987	8.6	198
1988	11.0	204
1989	12.6	221
1990	14.6	214
1991[a]	15.0	230

[a]Estimated.
SOURCE: U.S. Department of Veterans Affairs, 1992.

Institute of Environmental Health Sciences, and the National Institute of Dental Research. Other Federal agencies funding neuroscience research include the Department of Veterans Affairs, the National Science Foundation,[10] the Department of Energy, the Department of Defense, the National Institute on Disability and Rehabilitation Research, the National Aeronautics and Space Administration, the Environmental Protection Agency, the Department of Agriculture, the Centers for Disease Control, and the Food and Drug Administration.

The diversity of Federal organizations that fund this research necessitates interagency communication. An official channel for such communication has been set up through the Office of Science and Technology Policy's Federal Coordinating Council for Science, Engineering, and Technology (FCCSET —pronounced ''fix-it''). FCCSET provides a forum for coordinating executive research and development activities; it has received special attention from the President's Science Adviser and has proven itself a workable mechanism in coordinating research in such areas as high-performance computing (48). Among the leadership for FCCSET's neuroscience subcommittee (Subcommittee on Brain and Behavioral Sciences) are senior agency personnel from the chief Federal agencies funding neuroscience research, namely, NIMH and NINDS.

Nonfederal Support

State and private sources also support research on mental disorders, but these sources have generally been very limited (21,43). This funding is not limited to research on the biology of mental disorders, but rather supports all types of mental health research. A survey conducted in 1987 found that of the 45 States that provided figures, 26 funded some aspect of mental health research (i.e., services research and research into understanding mental disorders) (table 6-8) (43). Funding for this research, approximately $17 million in 1985, represented no more than 0.3 percent of the total State expenditures for mental health. Factors that affected a State's likelihood of funding research were its population,

[10] Recently, the National Science Foundation reorganized its research structure for neuroscience and behavioral research. Box 6-A describes this reorganization.

Figure 6-7—Distribution of Federal Support of Neuroscience Research, Fiscal Year 1990

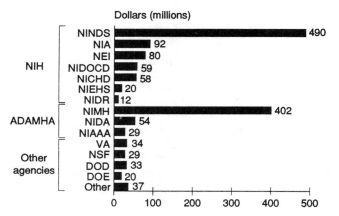

Dollars (millions)

Funding of neuroscience research by various Federal agencies.

NOTE: NIH = National Institutes of Health; ADAMHA = Alcohol, Drug Abuse, and Mental Health Administration; NINDS = National Institute of Neurological Disorders and Stroke; NIA = National Institute on Aging; NEI = National Eye Institute; NIDOCD = National Institute on Deafness and Other Communication Disorders; NICHD = National Institute on Child Health and Human Development; NIEHS = National Institute on Environmental Health Sciences; NIDR = National Institute of Dental Research; NIMH = National Institute of Mental Health; NIDA = National Institute on Drug Abuse; NIAAA = National Institute on Alcohol Abuse and Alcoholism; VA = U.S. Department of Veterans Affairs; NSF = National Science Foundation; DOD = U.S. Department of Defense; DOE = U.S. Department of Energy; Other = National Institute on Disability and Rehabilitation Research, National Aeronautics and Space Administration, Environmental Protection Agency, U.S. Department of Agriculture, Centers for Disease Control, and U.S. Food and Drug Administration.

SOURCE: Office of Technology Assessment, adapted from E. Pennisi and D. Morgan, "Brain Decade Scientists Court Support," *The Scientist* 4:8, 1990.

Table 6-8—States Funding Mental Health Research, Fiscal Year 1985

Arizona	New York
California	North Carolina
Colorado	Ohio
Connecticut	Oklahoma
Florida	Oregon
Georgia	Pennsylvania
Hawaii	Rhode Island
Illinois	South Carolina
Indiana	Tennessee
Iowa	Texas
Maryland	Utah
Massachusetts	Virginia
Michigan	Washington

SOURCE: B.A. Ridge, H.A. Pincus, R. Blalock, et al., "Factors That Influence State Funding for Mental Health Research," *Hospital and Community Psychiatry* 40:377-382, 1989.

which affects levels of available funds, and the existence of other research support and research facilities. The survey also noted that the political environment and the individual characteristics of State leaders, both of which are susceptible to the influence of lobbying and advocacy activity, play a role in determining whether State funds will be allocated for mental health research.

Foundations are another nonfederal source of funding for research. Since foundations possess uncommitted funds that can be used to support new projects relatively quickly, they represent a more flexible source of funds than government entities (21). An analysis of foundation funding for mental health research during the period from 1983 to 1985[11] revealed that of the 4,402 foundations reviewed, 63 had an interest in mental health and 15 of these 63 had made grants for mental health research (21). In addition, 29 foundations that did not list mental health as an interest had given grants for mental health research. These grants encompassed all aspects of mental health research. Of the 44 foundations that had made grants to mental health research—only 1 percent of the foundations reviewed—almost half had a national orientation and over half held assets of $50 million or more.

The National Alliance for Research on Schizophrenia and Depression (NARSAD) is a source of foundation funding for research into the biology of mental disorders. NARSAD is the largest private sector, noncorporate funder of mental disorders research (30). It was founded in 1986 by the major citizen's organizations in mental illness advocacy and services—National Alliance for the Mentally Ill, National Mental Health Association, National Depressive and Manic Depressive Association—to be their research arm. All of NARSAD's funds for research are raised through gifts from the public. Since 1987, the alliance has funded 424 research grants with $16 million. The Stanley Foundation also supports research into the biology of mental disorders, focusing on severe mental disorders, including schizophrenia and mood disorders, with approximately $1.5 million a year. Finally, the Scottish Rite Foundation, which was founded in 1935, has long funded mental disorders research, focusing explicitly on understanding the nature and causation of schizophrenia. It funds approximately 25 grants a year with $750,000.

---

[11] The period of time for which information from all foundations was available.

Box 6-A—Neuroscience at the National Science Foundation

In January 1992, two new directorates were established at the National Science Foundation (NSF). The Directorate for Social, Behavioral, and Economic Sciences (SBE) and the Directorate for Biological Sciences (BIO) replaced the Directorate for Biological, Behavioral, and Social Sciences. This reorganization was spurred by congressional pressures to increase the emphasis on the behavioral and social sciences at NSF. The result was the formation of SBE to fund such research.

This reorganization also had a direct effect on neuroscience research at NSF. Previously, neuroscience projects were funded primarily through the Division of Behavioral and Neural Sciences within the Directorate for Biological, Behavioral, and Social Sciences. Under the reorganization, the behavioral component is now included in SBE, while the neural component is part of BIO. Neuroscience research is now housed in the Division of Integrative Biology and Neuroscience within BIO. The Neuroscience Program/Cluster is the major program funding neuroscience research, with a budget of $30.6 million in fiscal year 1992. It is divided by topic into seven program elements. These include neural mechanisms of behavior, neuroendocrinology, sensory systems, synaptic mechanisms, neuronal and glial mechanisms, developmental neuroscience, and computational, cognitive, and theoretical neurobiology.

The establishment of a directorate devoted to behavioral and social sciences was greeted with enthusiasm within those scientific communities. However, the initial announcement of this reorganization resulted in some trepidation within the neuroscience community. There were fears that neuroscience research was going to be dispersed among different disciplines: for example, that cellular neuroscience was to be part of a general program on cell biology and that developmental neuroscience was to be part of a developmental biology program. There were concerns that this would represent a dismantling of neuroscience research support at NSF, concerns that were allayed by the establishment of the current organizational structure.

The fact that neuroscience research will no longer share a common directorate with psychology and cognitive sciences suggests a separation of brain and behavioral research; however, under the new organization there are plans to maintain linkages of these disciplines through initiatives that cut across directorates. An example is an initiative in cognitive science that will involve a total of five NSF directorates. More recently, a Decade of the Brain working group was established that cuts across four directorates. While language, cognitive, and social behavior are now housed in the SBE directorate, the Division of Integrative Biology and Neurosciences has a program cluster in physiology and behavior that includes support for animal behavior in both field and laboratory settings.

SOURCES: M. Baringa, "Neuroscience at Risk at NSF," *Science* 254:643, 1991; M. Clutter, "Neuroscience at NSF: Opportunities From Change," *Neuroscience Newsletter* 23(1):8, 1992; "Neuro Nerves Calmed," *Science* 255:680-681, 1992; "NSF Directorate: Yes!" *APS Observer* 4(6):1,28-31, 1992; K. Olsen, Leader, Neuroscience Program, National Science Foundation, personal communication, February/May 1992.

RESEARCH ISSUES

Other factors besides financial support influence the environment in which research into the biology of mental disorders takes place. OTA has identified several issues in this research that, if not addressed, can hamper progress. These issues relate to the development of animal models of mental disorders, the study of clinical populations, and the training of individuals to conduct this research. Some of these issues are unique to the study of the biology of mental disorders; others, while not confined to this area of research, are particularly pertinent to it. The unique nature of attempting to understand complex human behavior and how it sometimes goes awry, as well as public and professional attitudes toward mental disorders, can present impediments to research. The stigma of mental disorders and the lack

of awareness among the public, patients and their families, and medical personnel as to the requirements of this research present difficulties. These factors affect many aspects of research, ranging from basic scientific concerns to ethical implications.

Addressing these issues will result in a more supportive environment for research. This section discusses the problems associated with using animals as models of mental disorders and examines the impact of the debate over the use of animals in biomedical research. A number of general issues associated with the use of patients in research on mental disorders are described. Two specific issues—the collection and banking of brain tissue for study and the conduct of clinical trials with medication-free subjects—are discussed. Finally, concerns about the number of clinician-researchers available to conduct research are also discussed. Initiatives that have been undertaken to address these issues are described, and areas for additional action are presented.

Animal Models of Mental Disorders

As in other areas of biomedical research, animal models play an important role in advancing the understanding of mental disorders. In designing animal models for the study of human diseases, scientists seek to develop in animals disorders that resemble aspects of human pathology. Ideally, an animal model of a disorder is identical to the human disorder in cause, symptoms, underlying mechanisms, and responsiveness to treatment. In reality, this ideal is rarely achieved. Disruption of the processes that control thoughts and emotions is particularly difficult to replicate in nonhumans. The delusional thinking of schizophrenia, the despair of depression, and the fear and dread of anxiety disorders are all complex cognitive-emotional states. As a result, a model encompassing all attributes of a mental disorder is probably impossible to achieve; certainly, no such model exists now (16).

Even though human mental disorders cannot be modeled exactly in animals, useful animal models exist. At the most basic level, fundamental information about the anatomy, molecular biology, chemistry, and other functions of the brain can be gained from animal studies. Also, animal models have been designed to study and evaluate specific aspects of a mental disorder (table 6-9), including the basic biological mechanisms that may contribute to its symptoms, the hypothesized causes, and the drugs used for treatment.

One important issue to consider in animal research is the choice of species. The decision as to which species is most appropriate is made by considering the purpose of the model, the design of the experiment, and what kind of information is sought. In studying basic neurobiological mechanisms, which are often the same across species, any species can be used. For example, information about how a drug interacts with a receptor can be gathered in any species that has that receptor. For models of more complex behaviors, mammals are the most appropriate species (table 6-9). The use of primates is particularly important in the study of mental

disorders since they most closely resemble humans in their behavior and brain structure.

As more is learned about a disorder, new areas of interest are identified for study. For example, positron emission tomography (PET) imaging studies have shown that decreased activity in the frontal cortex is a common characteristic of persons with schizophrenia (ch. 4). Scientists have used this information to investigate the frontal cortex in animals, particularly primates, using various experimental techniques on these animals that could not be used on patients (13) (table 6-9). Thus, recent progress in the neurosciences has ushered in a new phase in the use of animals for the study of mental disorders.

Some aspects of human mental disorders are particularly difficult to replicate in animals, such as the social withdrawal and blunted emotional responsiveness seen in schizophrenia (15,51,57). The development of models encompassing these characteristics would yield valuable information and represents an area for future research.

As in other areas of biomedical research, the controversy surrounding the use of experimental animals has had an impact on research into mental disorders (34). The debate encompasses a range of positions, from animal welfare to animal rights (50). Animal welfare generally concerns proper treatment, shelter, and care of animals used in studies; animal rights is the concept that animals have intrinsic rights equal to human rights (50). As a result, some advocates of animal rights argue that animals should not be used for any human purpose, including biomedical research (50).

Federal laws, State laws, and guidelines written by executive branch agencies all regulate the use of animals (46). The Animal Welfare Act, which was enacted in 1966, is the primary Federal law setting requirements for the care and use of animals in research. As a result of increased concern about the care and use of animals, the Animal Welfare Act was amended in 1985 to enhance the requirements for animal care. To enforce the amended act, the U.S. Department of Agriculture (USDA) has issued a series of new regulations and standards for the use of animals in a variety of settings, including biomedical research (54 F.R. 36112; 54 F.R. 36123; 55 F.R. 28879; 56 F.R. 6426). At the same time, new regulations were also enacted under the Public Health Service's (PHS) Guidelines for Animal Care

Table 6-9—Animal Models of Mental Disorders

Disorder	Features	Species typically used
Schizophrenia		
Amphetamine-induced psychosis	Administration of amphetamine produces schizophrenia-like symptoms.	Rats, mice, primates
Primate prefrontal cortex	Surgical damage to prefrontal cortex produces schizophrenia-like deficits in visual tracking	Primates
Depression		
Learned helplessness	Animals exposed to unpredictable stimuli, with no control over occurrence, exhibit stress and some of the same behaviors seen in depression.	Rats
Maternal separation	Infants separated from their mothers exhibit some behaviors roughly analogous to depression.	Primates, rats, hamsters
Mania		
Drug- and surgically induced hyperactivity	Various drugs and destruction of certain areas of the brain produce a persistent hyperactivity that shares some features of mania.	Rats
Bipolar Disorder		
Sensitization and kindling	Using either repeated administration of stimulant drugs or low-level electrical brain stimulation, patterns of behavior are produced that mimic the progressive, increased frequency of cycling between mania and depression that occurs in bipolar disorder.	Rats
Anxiety		
Conflict model	Animals both rewarded and punished for performing a task exhibit anxious behavior.	Various species
Social interaction	Placing two males in an unfamiliar setting and bright light produces less social interaction, which is overcome with antianxiety drugs.	Rats
Drug-induced or brain-stimulated anxiety	Various drugs and electrical stimulation of certain brain regions produce anxiety-like behavior.	Rats
Open-field paradigm	Rodents exposed to large, open, novel, well-lit areas exhibit high rates of activity that are decreased by antianxiety drugs.	Rodents
Genetic models	A strain of rats and a line of pointer dogs exhibit increased reactivity and "nervousness".	Rats, dogs
Obsessive-compulsive disorder		
Spontaneous paw licking	Some species of dogs lick their paws to the point of causing physical damage, a behavior thought to share features of OCD.	Dogs
Displacement behaviors	Normally fixed patterns of activity (e.g., pecking, grooming, digging, head turning) that can become excessive under stress (e.g., captivity) are thought to be related to the ritualistic behaviors seen in OCD.	Various species

SOURCE: Office of Technology Assessment, 1992.

and Use. These guidelines oversee the use of animals in all settings funded by the PHS and are generally used in most animal facilities throughout the public and private sectors. Both the new USDA and PHS regulations impose more stringent standards for the care, handling, housing, and use of animals in biomedical research than had previously been in place. The PHS regulations cover all animals used in research, while the USDA regulations exclude rodents and birds. In January 1992, a Federal judge ruled that the USDA regulations should be expanded to include rodents and birds (8).

Implementation of these regulations has increased the costs of conducting research. The USDA estimated that capital expenditures (e.g., renovation of animal housing, construction of aseptic surgical facilities, new equipment) for all establishments and persons affected by the new USDA regulations would be $876 million over the first 2 to 3 years (54 F.R. 10831). The USDA also estimated that the regulations would increase annual operating costs by $207 million (54 F.R. 10831). These figures do not take into account the costs of including rodents and birds under the regulations.

The actions of animal rights groups have compelled many institutions to initiate more rigorous security precautions to safeguard their facilities and personnel, thereby incurring additional costs (34). Concern about such actions prompted Congress to pass a bill (S. 544, Animal Research Facilities Protection Act of 1991) that makes it a Federal crime to vandalize facilities used for research or to remove animals from such facilities.

It is feared that the controversy over the use of animals in research will impede research in other ways (34). Apprehension regarding possible adverse actions by animal activists can affect decisions about types of research protocols to be used and the species selected for study. As previously mentioned, primates are crucial to research on the biological factors in mental disorders. It has been noted that the combined effects of increased financial costs of new regulations and activities of animal activists have particularly constrained the use of primates in biomedical research (23).

Clinical Research

Clinical research involves two broad areas—the development and testing of potential new treatments and the conduct of studies aimed at unveiling the underlying pathology and causes of a disorder. Thus, it includes studies that use human subjects in various types of experiments, the collection of tissue samples (e.g., blood, cerebrospinal fluid) for analysis, and the examination of donated brains from people who have died. Regardless of the type of clinical research being conducted, several general issues emerge. These relate to the recruitment and selection of subjects, the inclusion of representative populations in clinical studies, and the costs of conducting this research. This section discusses these general issues and describes the issues associated with two specific research situations—the banking and use of postmortem brain tissue and clinical studies with medication-free subjects.

Whatever the research, subjects must be recruited to participate in studies. The willingness of individuals to participate in such studies is often linked to their awareness of the need for subjects. Also, the stigma and negative attitudes associated with mental disorders (see ch. 7) can lessen the willingness of individuals to participate in studies. A variety of approaches are used to recruit subjects. Sometimes volunteers are recruited through an advertisement or public service announcement describing, for example, the symptoms of a disorder and announcing the need for subjects in a study. Patient support and advocacy groups often inform their members of the need for subjects. Usually, such individuals are screened over the telephone and then in person to determine their eligibility for a particular research project. Most often, however, subjects are recruited from patients receiving treatment, on an inpatient or outpatient basis, at a clinic or medical center.

Regardless of the source of subjects, participants in a research protocol in any area of biomedical research must provide their informed consent to participate (6). Informed consent is a large and complex topic that has been addressed extensively elsewhere (47). Briefly, U.S. Department of Health and Human Services (DHHS) regulations guide informed consent in all research funded by DHHS; in addition, these regulations are widely used as guidelines in institutions that do not receive Federal funding (47). The regulations specify that informed consent for participation in a study is governed by each institution's Institutional Review Board (IRB).[12]

Obtaining informed consent from patients with mental disorders raises some unique problems (6). In order to provide informed consent, the possible benefits and risks associated with an experimental procedure must be explained to the individual. He or she must understand these factors, rationally weigh them, and then make a decision as to whether or not to participate. The nature of some mental disorders may make an individual incompetent to render such a decision and thus to provide informed consent. In some cases, if the disability associated with a disorder is permanent, the individual can be declared legally incompetent and a guardian appointed to make decisions for him or her. In that case, the guardian can provide consent for participation in research. However, most individuals with mental disorders are not declared legally incompetent, since they are capable of making decisions related to their welfare when their disorder is under control (6). Thus, the ability of individuals with a mental disorder to understand what they are being asked to consent to can vary, depending on their condition. As a result, the question of whether a person is providing a valid informed consent must be care-

---

[12] IRBs review the medical, legal, and ethical aspects of all proposed research projects using human subjects.

fully determined based on his or her competency at the time. It is the role of the IRBs and researchers to ensure that the decision truly represents informed consent.

Once subjects are recruited, their appropriateness for inclusion in an experimental protocol must be determined. The validity of a study's results is dependent on the selection of a homogeneous experimental group made up of individuals who have all been accurately diagnosed as having the same disorder. A number of factors can complicate this selection process. As discussed in chapters 3 and 5, some mental disorders that are classified as a single disorder, such as schizophrenia, may actually consist of subtypes. Also, patients frequently have multiple disorders. Depression is frequent, for example, among patients with obsessive-compulsive disorder. Finally, the familiarity of investigators with diagnostic issues surrounding a disorder, such as the existence of subtypes, may vary. These factors can result in lack of homogeneity among subjects within a study or across different studies. Heterogeneity within and across samples can confound the results of studies or make it difficult to compare results of different studies. One of the problems that has beset research into the biological factors associated with mental disorders is the difficulty of replicating findings, even though the same methods are used and the same disorders are being studied. Some of this difficulty is due to the selection of experimental subjects (52).

NIMH has suggested that some of these problems can be partially alleviated by ensuring that research teams include a clinical investigator who is aware of the diagnostic and clinical issues related to the disorder being studied (52). To make it easier to find individuals with such expertise, NIMH has suggested establishing diagnostic centers that could provide consultation and intensive short-term training in diagnostic and other clinical issues (52). Such centers could result in a more integrated and coherent approach to clinical diagnosis.

It is difficult to estimate how many clinical studies of mental disorders are conducted each year, but there are clearly hundreds. Study populations may vary in size from 15 or 20 patients to several hundred patients at various facilities. Sample size is determined by the goal of the study. If it involves new drug development, several hundred patients are required to discern the safety and effectiveness of the experimental drug.

In general, adults between the ages of 18 and 55 to 60 are included in these studies. Adolescents and children pose special problems in clinical research, both in terms of consent and because in some cases there is no clear-cut diagnosis during the very early stages of a disorder. Persons over the age of 55 or 60 are frequently excluded from clinical research because they are likely to have other illnesses that require medications, which would complicate the investigation. As a result, adolescents, children, and the elderly are understudied populations in whom significant mental disorders can occur and for whom a variety of important questions related to cause and treatment frequently go unanswered. Clearly, research does focus on some disorders that are relatively specific to childhood (e.g., attention deficit disorder with hyperactivity) or later life (e.g., senile dementia of the Alzheimer type), but these age groups are infrequently studied for disorders such as depression and schizophrenia.

Women of childbearing age are often excluded from experimental drug trials because of the potentially damaging effects of such drugs on conception and fetal development. To some extent this concern is driven by fear of litigation. Sponsors and investigators fear that if a woman conceives while taking an experimental drug, despite their warnings against such action, they will be found liable for any damage to the fetus. This policy results in a situation where efficacy is more clearly established in men than it is in women. Some have argued that the policy of denying women of childbearing age the opportunity to participate in clinical trials is demeaning to women.

The prevalence and expression of some mental disorders vary by sex. For example, depression is twice as prevalent among women as men (see ch. 3), and schizophrenia often has an earlier onset and more difficult course in men than women (see ch. 3). Thus, understanding mental disorders requires that women be included in clinical trials and that gender differences be studied specifically. Concern about the lack of such studies, and other issues related to women's health, resulted in congressional calls for a greater emphasis in this area (11). Accordingly, the PHS initiated an Action Plan for Women's Health (56) that outlines the goals established by PHS agencies in regard to these issues (33). The Office of

Women's Health, within PHS, will be in charge of monitoring its progress.

ADAMHA has set a number of goals related to mental disorders research as part of this plan. These goals augment the NIH/ADAMHA policy on the inclusion of women in research first established in 1986 and updated in 1990 (54). These include increasing research initiatives concerned with sex-related differences in mental disorders and promoting and enforcing a policy regarding the inclusion of women in clinical research. Steps to achieve these goals include identifying specific areas for future study and requiring that all applications and proposals for clinical research funding include women in their research protocol, where appropriate. When women are to be excluded, there must be justification for doing so. In addition, ongoing research studies will be monitored to ensure that they comply with the policy.

The finding that ethnic groups may differ in their sensitivities to drugs indicates the need to consider ethnic differences when studying the biology of mental disorders (14). Such ethnic differences and other public health concerns regarding minorities led ADAMHA and NIH to establish a policy in 1987 (updated in 1990) regarding the inclusion of minorities in research (55). This policy requires that applicants for research funding give appropriate attention to inclusion of minorities in study populations, unless compelling scientific or other justification for not including minorities is provided. While the purpose of the policy is the inclusion of minorities in studies, it also encourages attention to gaps in knowledge about specific U.S. racial and ethnic minorities and health problems that significantly affect them. As with the policy regarding the inclusion of women in research, this policy is intended to ensure that every effort is made to include minorities in applications for clinical research funds. Failure to comply with the policy is sufficient grounds for not receiving a research award.

A final factor that affects clinical research, including research into mental disorders, is the changing landscape of health-care financing in the United States. While a discussion of the effects of cost-containment efforts on clinical research is beyond the scope of this report, it is important to note that costs associated with mental disorders research have traditionally been enfolded in the costs of clinical care (39). That is, diagnostic and treatment procedures that are normally administered to a patient as part of their care may also be used in research. Implementation of measures to control health-care costs may disrupt this traditional piggy-backing of clinical research studies onto standard clinical care (39). As a result, other mechanisms for covering these costs will need to be developed. These could include efforts by academic health centers to manage existing budgets in a way that will allow them to continue to participate in clinical research, private funding of research, and additional research funding from Federal sources (39).

Brain Banks

Federal agencies and researchers have emphasized the importance of postmortem brain tissue samples for the study of mental disorders (38,51,52). Brains from deceased patients can be examined for anatomical and morphological abnormalities, and samples of brain tissue can be assayed to discern any changes in pharmacological and chemical activity (see ch. 4). Without doubt, the most crucial issue in regard to the study of brains after death is lack of availability (24,25,52): There is agreement in the scientific community that the demand for tissue— which has increased in parallel with the emphasis on research into the biological factors of mental disorders—far exceeds the available supply. There is also a great need for control tissue, from unaffected individuals, for comparison with the pathological samples. Factors related to the handling and distribution of tissue and issues associated with the donation of brains by patients and their families hamper the collection of brains (25).

Currently, two centers in the United States, which have been in operation for about 25 years, are funded to serve specifically as brain banks (24,51). One is located at Harvard University and one at the VA's Wadsworth Medical Center in West Los Angeles. The operations of both banks are cofunded by NIMH and NINDS. In addition, both receive some support from private institutions. The Harvard University brain bank was federally supported at a level of $350,000 in fiscal year 1990, $374,000 in fiscal 1991, and a projected $400,000 in fiscal 1992 (58). Federal support for the VA facility in fiscal 1990 was approximately $330,000 (58).

These centers supply tissue samples to researchers upon request. Their inventories consist of brains from patients with a variety of neurological and psychiatric disorders, as well as from normal individuals. Samples from neurological patients comprise the bulk of these collections. Figures from the Harvard brain bank indicate that of their current inventory of 944 brains, 94 are from individuals who had some form of mental disorder, 116 are from controls, and the remainder are from patients with neurological conditions (45). The VA bank has a current inventory of 1,149 brains, of which 121 are from patients with mental disorders and 202 from controls (45). It must be kept in mind, however, that when a request for tissue is received, it is usually for a specific region of the brain, depending on the disorder being studied. For example, studies of schizophrenia often examine areas of the frontal cortex. As a result, although the brain bank may have a brain from a patient with schizophrenia on hand, there may be no more tissue remaining from the frontal cortex. In 1991 the Harvard brain bank received written requests for samples from 233 cases of patients with mental disorders (22). This number is an underestimate of the actual demand, since many initial inquiries are made by telephone, and if they cannot be met, a written request is never made.

These banks have established standardized procedures for storing tissue—namely, freezing one half of a donated brain and placing the other half in formaldehyde (24). This allows tissue from the same individual to be studied using either chemical or anatomical techniques. However, many new methodologies cannot use tissue that has been stored in either fashion and require different handling procedures. In order for tissue samples to be useful, therefore, it is necessary to coordinate handling procedures with experimental needs (25). These methodological problems, and the fact that the demand for tissue has grown rapidly over the past few years, have led to the establishment of 15 to 20 additional brain collections at various institutions in the United States. In general, these collections have been established by individual research groups conducting studies on brain tissue. The expenses of maintaining the collections are met by funding sources that support the ongoing research. Often, the researchers who maintain the collections enter into collaborations with other scientists to share samples. As a result, an informal network has developed among neuroscientists regarding where brain samples might be obtained.

It is crucial to have complete medical records and histories of persons whose brains are being studied

in order to correctly diagnose the clinical disorder and provide information about treatment history and the presence of other medical conditions. Samples from medical examiners are frequently from suicide victims or homeless individuals whose medical records are inaccessible or nonexistent. Absence of proper categorization and information about other factors that might affect the outcome of experiments severely limits the usefulness of collected tissue. This is especially important regarding control samples, where it is critical that the individual not suffer from a mental disorder. From the patient's and survivors' perspective, it is essential that mechanisms be in place to ensure confidentiality. The comprehensiveness of such safeguards could affect the decision by patients and their families to donate tissue. It has been proposed that some of these impediments can be lessened by the creation of a national registry of voluntarily preregistered, prediagnosed tissue donors (51). This would ensure that tissue would be available from patients with a recorded, comprehensive medical history.

In an effort to improve the acquisition process and to better disseminate information about the availability of sources of brain tissue from various centers, NIMH has created a task force to make recommendations on how to coordinate these efforts (24). A number of suggestions are under consideration, including using a private institution under contract to NIMH as a clearinghouse for the collection and distribution of brain tissue. An example of the type of organization that could serve such a function is the National Disease Research Interchange, a private, nonprofit foundation funded by NIH that is involved with the procurement and distribution of other organs and tissues for research purposes. The NIMH task force is also identifying other needs related to the collection of brains for research. These include designing systems to address the problem of the limited samples of tissue available from persons with specific disorders, especially bipolar disorder, and the pressing need for tissue from normal individuals that can be used as experimental controls (24).

Beyond the concerns raised by the handling and distribution of tissue, other issues related to brain donation play a significant role in availability. While the specifics for donation may vary by locale, in general, arrangements for donation of brain tissue, as for all organs and tissues for transplantation and research purposes, are made according to the guidelines provided by the Uniform Anatomical Gift Act of 1987.[13] That act prohibits compensation for such donation. If a patient desires to donate tissue, he or she can sign a document of gift, a legally valid donation that is carried out upon his or her death. Also, once an individual has died, the family has authority to consent to donation. In some cases, patients with mental disorders are not capable of providing consent for donation (see earlier discussion of informed consent), and unlike the donation of other organs, the stigma and negative attitudes associated with mental disorders (see ch. 7) may inhibit the willingness of individuals to donate. Also, the severely mentally ill are often estranged from their families, making it difficult to find family members quickly to give permission for a brain donation. Finally, there is a lack of awareness among patients, their families, and the general public of the acute need for brain tissue. The result is that patients and their families often do not make arrangements for donation of tissue that could be useful to researchers. It has been proposed that increased education of patients, their families, and the public regarding the research community's need for brain tissue to study could enhance efforts to acquire brain samples (24,25,52).

Even in cases where a donation has been arranged by patient and family alike, retrieval of the tissue can be difficult (25). Often it is difficult to make arrangements to deliver the body to an appropriate facility with a pathologist to collect the sample. The increased costs and declining number of autopsies present another obstacle. Even when an individual dies in a setting that allows an autopsy, fewer of these procedures are performed, and brain tissue is rarely examined and collected for study. Another factor contributing to this problem is the lack of awareness among medical examiners of the need for tissue samples for research into mental disorders.

In summary, a variety of factors contribute to the shortage of brain tissue available for study. The NIMH task force has been instituted to recommend ways of enhancing the system for collecting and distributing tissue and coordinating tissue handling with the needs of researchers. The establishment of a clearinghouse and a national registry for brain donation are possible means of reaching these goals.

Institution of such a system will require that special attention be paid to concerns about the privacy of patients and families that participate. Other measures needed to increase tissue donation involve educating the public and relevant medical personnel to the acute need for such tissue. These education efforts could be implemented by the Federal Government, patient advocacy groups, or professional organizations. Finally, any efforts to decrease the stigma and negative attitudes associated with mental disorders could affect the willingness of patients and their families to donate tissue.

Clinical Studies With Medication-Free Subjects

Studies using subjects who have mental disorders and who are not taking medications are critical in investigating the underlying biology of a disorder, in establishing the effectiveness of new treatments, and in addressing biological and psychosocial factors leading to relapse. The medications used to treat mental disorders have a variety of effects on biological characteristics, particularly neurotransmitter systems in the brain. In order to study the biological factors contributing to a disorder, it is necessary to eliminate the potentially confounding effects of drug treatment. Drug effects can last for varying periods, depending upon the specific measure of interest; they may persist for weeks, months, or years following discontinuation of use (10,20). As a result, there may be a need to study not only medication-free patients, but in some situations patients who have never been treated with drugs.

There are several obstacles to identifying and recruiting patients who have never received any prior treatment. Persons experiencing the onset of the more severe mental disorders, such as schizophrenia or bipolar disorder, are frequently hospitalized during a crisis and may be admitted first through an emergency room or taken to a municipal hospital. In most cases, some treatment will be administered immediately, and it may be 24 to 48 hours before the patient is admitted to a ward where clinical research might be taking place. If a system is in place to do so, such individuals can be identified by the first treatment contact and referred immediately to the research team. There are relatively few municipal hospitals where such systems are in place. Often patients, particularly those with private insur-

---

[13] The Uniform Anatomical Gift Act (UAGA) was first drafted in 1968 by the National Conference of Commissioners on Uniform State Laws. It addresses the donation and receipt of human cadavers or parts of cadavers for research, education, therapy, or transplantation. The UAGA was updated in 1987 (47).

ance, are admitted to a private hospital or a psychiatric unit in a general hospital. Like municipal hospitals, few of these hospitals have clinical research programs in place.

In those settings where there is an ongoing research program, a patient will be referred to a research team before treatment is administered, although it can still be difficult to recruit patients into clinical research during the initial stages of the illness. Withholding treatment or using an experimental treatment cannot be done without the informed consent of the patient (see earlier discussion). It is especially important that the patient understand the possible risks associated with these experimental protocols. A potential personal sacrifice is often involved, even for those patients who are willing and able to give informed consent. A drug-free interval may mean the prolongation or reappearance of a psychotic episode, depression, or anxiety state. Also, depending on the experiment, participating in a research protocol may mean taking an experimental drug or placebo when a known effective treatment is available. This would require either altruism or dissatisfaction with prior treatment on the part of the patient. In most trials involving new drug development, the investigator makes a commitment to provide alternative standard treatment if the patient does not improve during the course of the trial as a result of being on the placebo or an experimental compound. As with other types of research, the IRB must review experimental protocols to ensure that prospective subjects are informed of all contingencies and that informed consent is obtained.

If investigators wish to study patients who have been previously treated, the patients may need a lengthy drug washout. This can be a considerable challenge. Managing patients without medication for many days or weeks can be difficult, often requiring hospitalization and close monitoring by hospital personnel. Moreover, it is difficult to justify inpatient care for insurance reimbursement purposes if it is not standard treatment. Further complicating many cases, it is often unclear how long a washout is necessary to eliminate the undesirable drug effect, because the research needed to establish this has not been conducted.

As a result of these factors, the cost of care during a drug washout or clinical study can be an important obstacle to the conduct of research. The cost of each

hospital day can range from $300 to over $1,000; thus a 2-week washout or a 6-week experimental drug trial can result in a significant number of unreimbursed bed days. Assuming a daily bed cost of $400, supporting one such bed for an entire year would require $146,000. In regard to Federal support for these expenses, bed costs can be included in the funding available to the Clinical Research Centers supported by NIMH. Few center directors choose to use funds in this fashion, however, since this would divert an enormous proportion of their total funding from other priorities (28). This contrasts with NIH's General Clinical Research Centers Program, which includes specific provisions for bed costs (39). In the recent past, the pharmaceutical industry has recognized the obstacle created by bed costs and some companies have provided support. It is difficult at present to document either the extent of such support or the overall impact that it is having on research.

There are several other reasons why patients may need to be hospitalized. In many cases it may be important to monitor or control diet, use of alcohol, nicotine, activity levels, and use of over-the-counter medication to eliminate variables that might influence measures of interest. In addition, to study biological factors in one disorder, it is frequently necessary to have a control group of either normal subjects or individuals with a different condition. Recruiting and assessing such reference groups under similarly controlled conditions is facilitated in an inpatient setting.

Thus, a number of obstacles hamper clinical studies of medication-free patients or patients who have never been on medication. However, the importance of such studies for understanding the biology of mental disorders and developing treatments for them requires that these obstacles be overcome. High inpatient costs and the costs and other problems associated with drug washout periods are substantial obstacles to these studies. Reevaluation of the funding mechanisms to support these studies is an important initiative to address these obstacles. Developing systems to promote the identification and recruitment of appropriate patients is another action that could facilitate these studies.

Training of Clinician-Researchers

As previously discussed, research into the biology of mental disorders relies heavily on clinical research. Carrying out this research requires the skills of many different professionals, including neuroscientists (usually individuals with a Ph.D. in neuroscience or other disciplines such as physiology, anatomy, psychology, biochemistry), physicians (M.D.s), and clinical psychologists (persons with a Ph.D. in clinical psychology). Often, in order to bring these diverse skills to a research project, studies are conducted as collaborations among teams of researchers. Given the importance of experimental protocols that use patients, it is not surprising that there is a significant role for individuals who are trained as both clinicians and researchers. However, while the number of neuroscientists has increased in the last 20 years (see ch. 2), many experts and organizations have expressed concern about the shortage of clinician-researchers in the United States engaged in mental disorders research (2,3,5,9,19,35,52, 53). The training to be a clinician is different from that needed to be a researcher, and often the two are separated in the fields of psychology and psychiatry. The result is that clinically trained professionals (e.g., psychiatrists, clinical psychologists) may not be trained to do research (52).

Concerns within the medical community about the lack of clinical researchers are not confined to the field of psychiatry. A 1990 report from the Institute of Medicine noted an apparent decline in the overall number of clinician-researchers, as indicated by a 15 percent decrease in the number of physicians applying for grants for the first time to NIH between 1965 and 1985 and a slight decrease in the number of physicians reporting research activity between 1983 and 1986 (18). The added burden of conducting research, coupled with the reduced financial incentives associated with many research positions compared to private practice, lead some young physicians to opt for a career of clinical practice. In the field of psychiatry, there are additional factors that contribute to this situation.

Traditionally, there has not been a strong emphasis on research in psychiatry (9). This can be seen in the results of recent surveys examining research activities in departments of psychiatry across the United States (32,37). For example, in one survey, only 26 percent of psychiatry faculty members with an M.D. degree spent at least 20 percent of their time in research-related activities (37). The authors of that survey compared their results to those of a survey of internal medicine departments, which found that 42 percent of M.D. faculty members had

a similar level of involvement in research. Another measure of the low level of research activity in psychiatry departments is the percentage of departments with ongoing research. This same survey of psychiatry departments indicated that 50 percent of the faculty conducting research are located at 13 percent of the schools (37). This concentration of researchers within a few departments of psychiatry coincides with earlier data showing that in 1983, 77 percent of all grants awarded by NIMH went to 10 percent of psychiatry departments (9).

An important factor associated with research activity is exposure to research and research training during clinical training (32,35,37). One survey found that 67 percent of researchers, compared to 36 percent of nonresearchers, had a medical school background that included research experience (37). Similar results were obtained in another survey, which found that among faculty members who were not exposed to research training in medical school, 26 percent did not go on to conduct research, whereas only 9 percent of those who had medical school research training never engaged in research (32). The association of postdoctoral research training with current research activity is even more striking, with 63 percent of active researchers having had such training, compared to 11 percent of nonresearchers (37). These results indicate the importance of research experience and training in determining future research activities. The lack of research activity in psychiatry departments results in an environment in which students have little or no opportunity to observe and experience ongoing research.

Some suggestions, such as developing and expanding opportunities for medical students to be involved in an intensive research experience, have been made to enhance recruitment of clinician-researchers (2,35). Other suggestions include requiring all resident physicians to receive some experience in planning or conducting empirical research and establishing a formal research track for psychiatry residents who are interested in research careers. The willingness of medical specialties to accommodate students doing research during their residencies varies. The National Advisory Mental Health Council has observed that psychiatry is a specialty in which more can be done to encourage exposure to research during residency (52). Also, the importance of established researchers as mentors to students has been noted (2,9,19,32,35,52). Reinforcing this is the observation that many of the skills required of a clinician-researcher are not easily taught through a standard curriculum (9). The presence of an experienced individual who can serve as a teacher and role model to a young person early in his or her professional education has been cited as a significant factor in the development of many research careers (2,9,19,32,35,52,).

Within psychology, there is a distinction between clinical and nonclinical psychologists. Nonclinical psychologists have research training in fields that can contribute to the study of the biology of mental disorders. These individuals have skills that are distinct from those of clinical psychologists and for which clinical researchers' skills cannot substitute. Thus, the concern about research training for clinical psychologists includes the need for individuals who can complement them in nonclinical areas of investigation.

It has been estimated that over half of all clinical psychology students do not pursue research careers (40). There are several factors that contribute to this (27). In general, the accreditation requirements for programs that award a Ph.D. in clinical psychology, while including research requirements, emphasize clinical practice. Also, the trend among students in recent years has been toward clinical practice instead of research. As with M.D.s, part of the reason for this is the disparity between the financial incentives available to practicing clinicians and research clinicians. Evidence of this trend is seen in the increasing popularity of programs and specific professional schools that award a doctor of psychology degree (Psy.D.) rather than a doctor of philosophy. These programs are practitioner-oriented and involve little, if any, research training. Another factor that inhibits the role of clinical psychologists in research is that departments of psychology at universities are usually located within a college of liberal arts and do not have ready access to patients with severe mental disorders. As a result, many clinical psychologists who are involved in research do not study biological factors related to mental disorders (28).

Recently, NIMH convened a task force to make specific recommendations about the recruitment of investigators into clinical research careers (53). According to the task force:

> Many of these recommendations will not require major new investments of funds, but reflect a focusing and targeting of available resources. Others

require new funding approaches and mechanisms, but these are achievable within the authorities of the NIMH.

Several of the task force's recommendations relate to expanding research opportunities for students, residents, and junior faculty. These include:

- Establishing research clerkships for medical students in laboratories;
- Using summer workshops at research facilities to expose residents and fellows to various topics in the field;
- Promoting and funding the development of research curriculums as part of residency programs in psychiatry; and
- Developing supplemental grants, to be awarded to established principal investigators, to support a variety of student activities related to the development of a research career.

The task force also recommended that research career development information be organized and distributed to predoctoral and postdoctoral students, psychiatry residents, and junior faculty members. It was suggested that this information could best be disseminated through professional societies that have large student memberships, such as the American Psychological Association, the American Psychological Society, and the American Psychiatric Association.

The principal source of Federal funding for clinician-researcher training related to psychology and psychiatry is NIMH. Funding for clinician-researcher training comes from two sources within NIMH that support research training in general. National Research Service Awards (NRSA) are training awards funded by the research training budget of NIMH (see earlier discussion). Since 1986, the research training budget of NIMH has experienced an average annual real rate of increase of 5 percent (figure 6-1). However, when adjusted for inflation, the 1991 budget of $26.9 million is $23.6 million—$2 million less than the 1980 budget. Thus, the recent period of growth in funding has not compensated for an earlier period of decline. In addition to the NRSA training awards, non-NRSA awards, which are funded through NIMH research funds, also support research training.

There are a number of NRSA and non-NRSA training mechanisms (49). Three programs specifically support the training of clinician-researchers

(28), two of which are non-NRSA awards. The Academic Award program is for clinicians (i.e., clinical psychologists, physicians, nurses, social workers) who would like to conduct research as well as maintain a clinical practice. This support is awarded to an individual for 5 years. In fiscal year 1991 the program supported 21 persons, half of them psychiatrists and half clinical psychologists, with $2.2 million. The Scientist Development Award for Clinicians is for clinicians who want to become full-time researchers. Funding for this program was $2.0 million in fiscal 1991, supporting 20 individuals. Finally, the NRSA M.D.-Ph.D. Predoctoral Fellowship program provides tuition and a stipend for persons to complete all the requirements for obtaining both degrees. NIMH funded 15 such students in fiscal 1991 with total funding of $349,000.

In addition to these specific awards, there are other general research training programs. These include other non-NRSA awards such as the Scientist Development Award, the Level 2 Research Scientist Development Award, the First Independent Research Scientist Trainee (FIRST) Awards, and the other grants that make up the NRSAs. Other NRSA grants include awards to institutions to support training (e.g., Institutional Research Training Grants) and awards to individuals (e.g., individual fellowships and Minority Access to Research Career Awards). Any of these programs can fund the training of clinician-researchers. For example, of the 137 FIRST awards made in 1990 by NIMH, 40 (29 percent) supported physician-investigators (28), while of the 996 NRSA awards given in 1985, 70 (7 percent) went to physicians (37).

A dearth of psychiatric clinician-researchers is also evident in the VA system (4). As with NIMH, the VA maintains a career development program to provide training for researchers. In the period from 1987 to 1990, 11 out of 297 awards went to psychiatrists. As in other settings, a major obstacle to recruiting and retaining clinician-researchers in the VA system is the inability to compete with salaries offered in private practice. In an effort to resolve this problem to some extent, Congress passed legislation in April 1991 authorizing ''special pay'' increases for VA physicians based on length of service, whether they work in medical specialties facing extraordinary difficulties or in geographic areas with special needs (4).

In summary, there is concern about the lack of emphasis placed on the training of clinician-researchers in the field of mental disorders research. As a result, there is a need for strategies to increase the recruitment of qualified individuals into research training programs. Integral to this effort will be enhancing the incentives to pursue a research career, increasing financial support for training programs, and modifying attitudes within the psychiatric and psychological communities regarding clinical and research training. While there is clearly a role for Federal institutions in this endeavor, the NIMH task force highlighted the crucial role that academic institutions, particularly departments of psychiatry, must play in fostering a supportive environment for research training.

SUMMARY AND CONCLUSIONS

The pace of research into understanding the biological factors that contribute to mental disorders is determined by the level of financial support it receives and the environment in which it is conducted. In the past, underfunding and lack of a supportive environment have impeded progress in this research. Actions to counter some of these trends have been taken in recent years, although impediments do still exist.

Analysis of the funding of NIMH reveals that a trend toward underfunding has been reversed over the past decade. In particular, the last 5 years have seen a steady increase in allocations to NIMH. The distribution of these funds indicates that research into understanding biological factors related to mental disorders is a high priority. Another priority is research furthering the understanding of the severe disorders considered in this report. These areas of research emphasis, coupled with the support of basic neuroscience research at a number of Federal institutions, hold out the promise that during the next decade there will be a significant increase in the understanding of the role biological factors play in severe mental disorders.

While some of the financial constraints that have hampered this research in the past have eased, there are still issues which need to be addressed to ensure that the promise of increased funding can be realized. OTA identified a number of issues that can impede progress in this field, including the ability to use animals to study mental disorders, issues related to the study of clinical populations, and the training of clinician-researchers. Some of these overlap with other areas of research, but all are especially relevant to the study of the biology of mental disorders. The unique nature of trying to understand the human mind, coupled with the traditional character of public attitudes toward mental disorders, makes these issues particularly pertinent to this area of research.

Overcoming the impediments posed by these issues will create a more supportive environment for research. Doing so will require action by professional and consumer organizations, changes in policy of Federal agencies, and initiatives spurred by congressional action. On the one hand, the issue of using animals to model mental disorders is a scientific one and is best addressed by continued support of research. On the other hand, policy decisions regarding the broader controversy surrounding the use of animals in biomedical research will also have an impact on this research. The issues associated with the study of clinical populations, such as increasing tissue resources and facilitating the conduct of these studies, are related to individuals' attitudes and awareness about what is required to conduct this research. Impediments can be lessened by educating the public, patients and families, and medical personnel to the needs of the research community and by decreasing the stigmatizing attitudes that can hamper the willingness of individuals to participate in research. Impediments associated with the banking of tissues and the conduct of studies with medication-free patients can be lessened by enhancing the resources for, and support of, these enterprises. Increasing the number of clinician-researchers will require an adjustment in the emphasis placed on research training within professional and academic institutions, as well as the support of programs to carry out this training.

Actions have been taken to address some of these issues. As a result of congressional initiatives, policies have been instituted within PHS regarding the inclusion of special populations in clinical research. Also, NIMH has convened task forces on increasing the collection and banking of brain tissue and the training of clinician-researchers. While these initial steps will enhance the research environment, additional efforts are needed. For example, education programs for increasing public and patient awareness need to be enhanced, and specific concerns, such as the costs of clinical research and stimulating interest among clinicians in conducting

research, still need to be addressed. These will require the implementation of additional programs and policies by NIMH. The role of Congress in this effort is to specify issues that could be better addressed by these agencies and to facilitate their ability to respond to them.

CHAPTER 6 REFERENCES

1. American Cancer Society, *Cancer Facts & Figures— 1985* (New York, NY: American Cancer Society, 1985).
2. American Psychiatric Association, "Research Training: Scientific Inquiry and the 'Next Generation,' " *Psychiatric Research Report* 1(3):1,7, 1986.
3. American Psychiatric Association, "Research Training: NIMH and the 'Next Generation,' " *Psychiatric Research Report* 1(4):1,9, 1986.
4. American Psychiatric Association, "An Update on Psychiatric Research in the Department of Veterans Affairs," *Psychiatric Research Report* 6(2):1,6-7,11-14, 1991.
5. American Psychiatric Association, *Psychiatric Research: Profiles for the Future; Mental Illness, Drug Abuse & Alcoholism Research FY 1991* (Washington, DC: American Psychiatric Press, 1991).
6. Brakel, J.B., Parry, J., and Weiner, B.A., *The Mentally Disabled and the Law* (Chicago, IL: American Bar Foundation, 1985).
7. Broadwell, R.D., Medical Research Service, Veterans Health Administration, Department of Veterans Affairs, Washington, DC, personal communication, March 1992.
8. Burd, S., "Federal Judge Says Scope of Animal-Welfare Laws Must Not Exclude Protection of Rats, Mice, Birds," *Chronicle of Higher Education*, Jan. 22, 1992, p. A27.
9. Burke, J.D., Pincus, H.A., and Pardes, H., "The Clinician-Researcher in Psychiatry," *American Journal of Psychiatry* 143:968-975, 1986.
10. Campbell, A., and Baldessarini, R.J., "Prolonged Pharmacologic Activity of Neuroleptics," *Archives of General Psychiatry* 42:41, 1985.
11. Cotton, P., "Women's Health Initiative Leads Way as Research Begins To Fill Gender Gaps," *Journal of the American Medical Association* 267:469-470, 1992.
12. Council of Economic Advisors, *Economic Report of the President* (Washington, DC: U.S. Government Printing Office, 1992).
13. Goldman-Rakic, P.S., "Development of Cortical Circuitry and Cognitive Function," *Child Development* 58:601-622, 1987.
14. Goodman, D., "NIMH Grantee Finds Drug Responses Differ Among Ethnic Groups," *ADAMHA News* 18:15, Jan.-Feb. 1992.

15. Goodwin, F.K., and Jamison, K.R., *Manic-Depressive Illness* (New York, NY: Oxford University Press, 1990).

16. Henn, F.A., and McKinney, W.T., "Animal Models in Psychiatry," *Psychopharmacology: The Third Generation of Progress*, H.Y. Meltzer (ed.) (New York, NY: Raven Press, 1987).

17. Institute of Medicine, *Research on Mental Illness and Addictive Disorders: Progress and Prospects* (Washington, DC: National Academy Press, 1984).

18. Institute of Medicine, *Funding Health Sciences Research, A Strategy To Restore Balance* (Washington, DC: National Academy Press, 1990).

19. Janowsky, D.S., Glick, I.D., Lash, L., et al., "Psychobiology and Psychopharmacology: Issues in Clinical Research Training," *Journal of Clinical Psychopharmacology* 6:1-7, 1986.

20. Kane, J., Jeste, D., Barnes, T.R.E., et al., *Tardive Dyskinesia: A Task Force Report of the American Psychiatric Association* (Washington, DC: American Psychiatric Press, in press).

21. Kim, D., Pincus, H.A., and Fine, T., "Foundation Funding and Psychiatric Research," *American Journal of Psychiatry* 145:830-835, 1988.

22. Kimball, D.J., Brain Tissue Resource Center, McLean Hospital, Harvard Medical School, Belmont, MA, personal communication, Jan. 16, 1992.

23. King, F.A., Director, Yerkes Primate Research Center, Emory University, Atlanta, GA, personal communication, March 1992.

24. Kirch, D., National Institutes of Mental Health, Alcohol, Drug Abuse, and Mental Health Administration, U.S. Department of Health and Human Services, personal communication, October 1991.

25. Kirch, D., Wagman, A., and Goldman-Rakic, P., "Commentary: The Acquisition and Use of Human Brain Tissue in Neuropsychiatric Research," *Schizophrenia Bulletin* 17:593-596, 1991.

26. Kleinman, J., National Institute of Mental Health, Alcohol, Drug Abuse, and Mental Health Administration, U.S. Department of Health and Human Services, personal communication, October 1991.

27. Kraut, A., Executive Director, American Psychological Society, personal communication, December 1991.

28. Lash, L., Associate Director for Research Training and Research Resources, Division of Clinical Research, National Institute of Mental Health, Alcohol, Drug Abuse, and Mental Health Administration, U.S. Department of Health and Human Services, personal communication, December 1991.

29. Leshner, A., Acting Director, National Institute of Mental Health, Alcohol, Drug Abuse, and Mental Health Administration, U.S. Department of Health and Human Services, personal communication, 1991.

30. Lieber, C., President, Board of Directors, National Alliance for Research on Schizophrenia and Depression, personal communication, March 1992.

31. Lorei, T., Staff Assistant, Office of the Associate Chief Medical Director for Research and Development, Department of Veterans Affairs, Washington, DC, personal communication, February 1992.

32. Marvelle, K.J., and Scallet, L.J., *Report on Data on Research Activity and Post-Doctoral Research Training: Full-Time Department of Psychiatry Faculty* (Washington, DC: Policy Resources, Inc., 1990).

33. Mason, J.O., "From the Assistant Secretary for Health, U.S. Public Health Service: A National Agenda for Women's Health," *Journal of the American Medical Association* 267:482, 1992.

34. Morrison, A.R., Director, Office of Animal Research Issues, Alcohol, Drug Abuse, and Mental Health Administration, U.S. Department of Health and Human Services, personal communication, November 1991.

35. Nadelson, C.C., and Rabinowitz, C.B. (eds.), *Training Psychiatrists for the 90s: Issues and Recommendations* (Washington, DC: American Psychiatric Press, 1987).

36. Pardes, H., Sirovatka, P., and Pincus, H.A., "Federal and State Roles in Mental Health," *Psychiatry: Social, Epidemiologic, and Legal Psychiatry*, vol. 3 (Philadelphia, PA: Lippincott, 1984).

37. Pincus, H.A., American Psychiatric Association, personal communication, January-March 1992.

38. Pincus, H.A., and Pardes, H. (eds.), *The Integration of Neuroscience and Psychiatry* (Washington DC: American Psychiatric Press, 1985).

39. Pincus, H.A., West, J., and Goldman, H., "Diagnosis-Related Groups and Clinical Research in Psychiatry," *Archives of General Psychiatry* 42:627-630, 1985.

40. Pion, G.M., "A National Human Resources Agenda for Psychology: The Need for a Broader Perspective," *Professional Psychology, Research and Practice* 22:449-455, 1991.

41. Rice, D.P., Hodgson, T.A., and Capell, F., "The Economic Burden of Cancer, 1985: United States and California," *Cancer Care and Cost: DRGs and Beyond*, R.M. Scheffler and N.C. Andrews (eds.) (Ann Arbor, MI: Health Administration Press Perspectives, 1989).

42. Rice, D.P., Kelman, S., Miller, L.S., et al., *The Economic Costs of Alcohol and Drug Abuse and Mental Illness: 1985*, report submitted to the Office of Financing and Coverage Policy, Alcohol, Drug Abuse, and Mental Health Administration, U.S. Department of Health and Human Services (San Francisco, CA: Institute for Health and Aging, University of California, 1990).

43. Ridge, R., Pincus, H.A., Blalock, R., et al., "Factors That Influence State Funding for Mental Health Research," *Hospital and Community Psychiatry* 40:377-382, 1989.

44. Thom, T., Health Statistician, Division of Epidemiology and Clinical Application, National Heart, Lung, and Blood Institute, National Institutes of Health, personal communication, 1991.

45. Tourtellotte, W.W., and Rosario, I.P., National Neurological Research Specimen Bank, VA Wadsworth Medical Center, Los Angeles, CA, personal communication, January 1992.

46. U.S. Congress, Office of Technology Assessment, *Alternatives to Animal Use in Research, Testing, and Education*, OTA-BA-273 (Washington, DC: U.S. Government Printing Office, 1986).

47. U.S. Congress, Office of Technology Assessment, *Neural Grafting: Repairing the Brain and Spinal Cord*, OTA-BA-462 (Washington, DC: U.S. Government Printing Office, September 1990).

48. U.S. Congress, Office of Technology Assessment, *Federally Funded Research: Decisions for a Decade*, OTA-SET-490 (Washington, DC: U.S. Government Printing Office, May 1991).

49. U.S. Department of Health and Human Services, Alcohol, Drug Abuse, and Mental Health Administration, *ADAMHA, Research Training and Career Development Opportunities*, DHHS Pub. No. (ADM) 90-1641 (Washington, DC: U.S. Department of Health and Human Services, 1990).

50. U.S. Department of Health and Human Services, Alcohol, Drug Abuse, and Mental Health Administration, *Animals and Science*, DHHS Pub. No. (ADM) 91-1769 (Washington, DC: U.S. Department of Health and Human Services, 1991).

51. U.S. Department of Health and Human Services, Alcohol, Drug Abuse, and Mental Health Administration, National Institute of Mental Health, *Approaching the 21st Century: Opportunities for NIMH Neuroscience Research, The National Advisory Mental Health Council Report to Congress on the Decade of the Brain* (Washington, DC: U.S. Department of Health and Human Services, 1988).

52. U.S. Department of Health and Human Services, Alcohol, Drug Abuse, and Mental Health Administration, National Institute of Mental Health, *A National Plan for Schizophrenia Research: Report of the National Advisory Mental Health Council*, DHHS Pub. No. (ADM) 88-1571 (Washington, DC: U.S. Department of Health and Human Services, 1988).

53. U.S. Department of Health and Human Services, Alcohol, Drug Abuse, and Mental Health Administration, National Institute of Mental Health, *Research Infrastructure Task Force: Clinical Research Careers, Final Report*, internal document, November 1991.

54. U.S. Department of Health and Human Services, National Institutes of Health, "NIH/ADAMHA Policy Concerning Inclusion of Women in Study Populations," *National Institutes of Health Guide*, Aug. 24, 1990, p. 18.

55. U.S. Department of Health and Human Services, National Institutes of Health, "ADAMHA/NIH Policy Concerning Inclusion of Minorities in Study Populations," *National Institutes of Health Guide*, Sept. 28, 1990, p. 1.

56. U.S. Department of Health and Human Services, Public Health Service, *Action Plan for Women's Health*, DHHS Pub. No. PHS 91-50214 (Washington, DC: U.S. Department of Health and Human Services, September 1991).

57. Weiss, R.B., and Uhde, T.W., "Animal Models of Anxiety," *Frontiers of Clinical Neuroscience, Neurobiology of Panic Disorder*, vol. 8, J.C. Ballenger (ed.) (New York, NY: Alan R. Liss, 1990).

58. Zalcman, S.J., Chief, Neuroimaging and Applied Neuroscience Branch, National Institute of Mental Health, personal communication, December 1991.

Public Attitudes and Policy

CONTENTS OF CHAPTER 7

Boxes

Figure

Table

Public Attitudes and Policy

Researchers have partially uncovered the biological substrates of the mental disorders considered in this report and have propounded testable hypotheses as to causation. These scientific advances portend increased research opportunities as well as the development of improved treatments. But as is true for science in general, this research interacts with broad social and political factors (56,58). Support— or lack thereof—reflects social attitudes and the efforts of advocacy groups. The results of biomedical research also affect society. Improved understanding of the cause of a disorder can influence the public's response to individuals with a particular disorder as well as the direction of public policy.

This chapter attempts to tease out some of the social effectors of biological research into mental disorders and some of the implications of data arising from these studies. What factors have led to enthusiasm for biological research into mental disorders? What are the limitations of this approach? How might information about the biology of mental disorders influence public attitudes and policy? The

chapter begins with a general description of public attitudes toward mental disorders.

PUBLIC ATTITUDES TOWARD MENTAL DISORDERS

Mental disorders incur stigma, "a mark of disgrace or reproach" (72) (box 7-A). Surveys of 30 and more years ago showed that "the mentally ill are regarded with fear, distrust, and dislike by the general public" (41) and that persons labeled as mental patients tended to be stigmatized and shunned (51). And negative attitudes toward and ignorance of these disorders still abound (33). A sizable number of people continue to be frightened by the notion of mental illness and believe that others are frightened also, although it is becoming less socially acceptable to say so (50). A recent survey conducted for the National Organization on Disability (40) found that only a minority of persons polled (19 percent) felt very comfortable with a person with a mental disorder (figure 7-1).[1] Despite gains in knowledge about specific disorders and

---

Box 7-A—The Barriers Erected by Stigma: A Patient's Perspective

We had met under the most unusual circumstances, in a place we came to call "The Funny Farm. . . ." We were initiated into a stigmatizing sorority. . . .

[Having] experienced the problems and barriers that lie before us in "normal" society . . . the scene has been repeated in many different settings: a supervisor who viewed my work and abilities as outstanding and my rate of productivity as very high before my illness, but who recommended disability retirement when I was depressed and less productive; a university that graduated me with high honors, admitted me into its graduate program with outstanding recommendations, and then sent me a form letter in response to my request for readmission (following my illness) saying, "You do not meet our admission requirements;" and community mental health agencies that rejected my offers to be of assistance because I "scared" mental health professionals. . . .

The literature says little about us individually. Most researchers group us, thereby reinforcing the stigma. Some lay odds on our recovery and predict high rates of suicide. Some experiment with us, offering convincing evidence that we can be trained—rehabilitated. Others raise ethical concerns about studying us, but justify their actions by noting that useful data can be obtained by following us. Some have tried to document that public attitudes toward the mentally ill have changed.

If my own research and experiences are representative, public attitudes have not changed. From my perspective, researchers continue to define stigma with statistics. Physicians continue to locate emotional pain points with questions. Families continue to treat mental illness as a silent, shameful disease. Clergymen continue to preach that mental illness is the result of satanic influence. The barriers remain. They are real. . . .

SOURCE: Anonymous, *Schizophrenia Bulletin* 6:544-546, 1980.

---

[1] The survey included a random sample of 1,257 people interviewed by telephone between May 15 and June 18, 1991. The estimated margin of error was ± 3 percent.

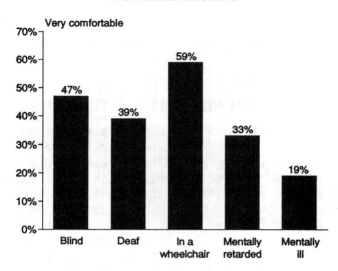

Figure 7-1—Level of Comfort With People With Mental Disorders

Very comfortable

Blind 47%
Deaf 39%
In a wheelchair 59%
Mentally retarded 33%
Mentally ill 19%

A survey conducted by Louis Harris & Associates, Inc., for the National Organization on Disability indicated that of all the disabilities asked about, people felt least comfortable with people with mental illness.

SOURCE: Adapted from National Organization on Disability, "Public Attitudes Toward People With Disabilities," survey conducted by Louis Harris and Associates, Inc., 1991.

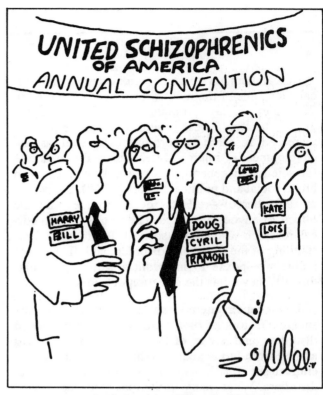

Credit: Copyright © Bill Lee. Reprinted with permission.

This cartoon, provided by O. Wahl, illustrates the commonly held misperception that schizophrenia is multiple personalities.

their treatment, considerable ignorance about mental disorders persists: For instance, 64 percent of college freshmen thought schizophrenia referred to multiple personalities (68). Data from research also have indicated that some providers of mental health care are themselves inadequately informed as to the diagnosis and treatment of mental disorders (for example, see 44,61,73).

While widespread and incontrovertible, the stigma attached to mental disorders is a difficult concept to define. Many stress the deliberate nature of stigma:

> Stigma refers to the process by which people who lack certain traits denigrate people who possess them, and it leads to individual differences in social interaction, prejudice, and discrimination (62).

Clearly, ignorance about mental disorders—their symptoms, treatability, or causes—can serve as a fertile breeding ground for negative attitudes. However, a lack of knowledge about mental disorders cannot explain all of the stigma that exists. For example, a 1990 national survey[2] of public attitudes toward people with chronic mental illness found

widespread evidence of the "not in my backyard" phenomenon, expressed as resistance to treatment and housing facilities in the community, with the incidence of opposition increasing with income and educational level (55). Even mental health care providers sometimes harbor negative attitudes toward individuals with mental disorders, especially those with severe and persistent conditions (8). In 1987, the American Psychiatric Association Task Force on the Chronic Mental Patient determined that

> among professionals such as ourselves, and among paraprofessionals, there are prevailing attitudes—that working with [chronic] patients is unrewarding and dull, and that ... prestige is not available for working in [chronic patient] programs (34).

While stigma is attached to many serious medical conditions, people with mental disorders are subject to much more rejection: Public attitudes toward mental disorders are more akin to those directed at drug addiction, prostitution, and ex-convict status

[2] Data from a telephone survey of approximately 1,300 Americans representative of the total population of adults 21 and older. In addition, four focus groups, two in Pennsylvania and two in Ohio, were conducted, as well as in-depth telephone interviews with 17 mental health opinion leaders.

than cancer, diabetes, and heart disease (2,33). The stigma reflects—in part—the fear or uneasiness evoked by individuals who display unusual or threatening behavior. Results from studies suggest that a sizable portion of the public harbors the belief that mental disorders are linked to violent behavior (35). As might be expected, the belief that people with mental disorders are more prone to violent acts leads to a strong rejection of people afflicted with these conditions (32).

The stigma attached to mental disorders, with all its variable expressions and sources, has important social implications. Afflicted individuals and their families suffer acutely from the stigma attached to mental disorders (28,71). Many family members feel uncomfortable talking about their problem and may feel responsible and isolated as a result (13, 29, 71). Ignorance and negative attitudes also interfere with successful treatment: Individuals with a mental disorder may avoid seeking treatment to avoid the associated stigma or simply because they are una- ware of its availability. And as mentioned above, providers themselves may be inadequately informed about the recognition or treatment of mental disor- ders, or may harbor negative attitudes toward people with these conditions (5, 9, 43, 73). Finally, data show that people with mental disorders react in a negative fashion, in the belief that other people view them negatively (10, 31)

The stigma attached to and ignorance of mental disorders is mirrored in the discrimination in the financing of treatment, housing, employment, and the funding of research, a topic considered in this report. Previous studies (21, 49) and mental health advocates (for example, see 17) have demonstrated the underfunding of research into mental disorders compared to their social cost, attributing the defi- ciency to the low priority assigned to these condi- tions by the public and policymakers. The Office of Technology Assessment's (OTA) analysis also shows that, relative to their social costs, cancer and heart disease research receive substantially more funding than mental disorders research (see ch. 6). Thus, while the 1980s did witness a significant increase in Federal funding for research into mental disorders and new private sources of funding, support for research into mental disorders still fell short of that for other conditions in relation to their cost to society.

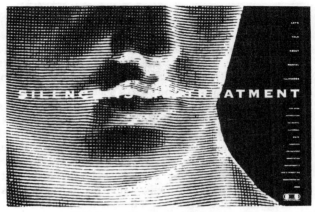

Credit: Courtesy of the American Psychiatric Association, 1992

A recent public education campaign, sponsored by the American Psychiatric Association, highlighted the negative impact of stigma on treatment-seeking.

Thus, the impact of stigma on public policy is compelling and undeniable. This finding echoes the results of a recent report by the Interagency Task Force on Homelessness and Severe Mental Illness (20):

> Stigmatization, fear, and mistrust regarding peo- ple with severe mental illnesses . . . are common- place in our Nation. Such reactions influence both the direct responses of community members to these individuals as well as the development of local, State, and Federal policies affecting them.

A conclusion that OTA draws from this analysis is that the dissemination of accurate knowledge about mental disorders—to the public at large, families, consumers, care providers, and policymakers—is essential to improving the lives of individuals with mental disorders and fair and informed policymaking (box 7-B).

The negative influence of stigma and ignorance on public policy cannot be offered as a simple or complete explanation for failures in public policy. Attitudes toward mental disorders reflect the influ- ence of a number of factors, ranging from beliefs about the origin of mental disorders, fear of individ- uals who are thought to be violent, and media portrayals. Furthermore, the way in which stigma contributes to policy formation is difficult, if not impossible, to distill precisely. The policy areas affected by negative public attitudes—research fund- ing, treatment, housing, mental health care finance, and employment—are not influenced by stigma alone, but by other factors, such as the structure of

Box 7-B—Educating the Public About Depression

Of the 15 million people who experience a major depressive disorder each year, four-fifths can be treated successfully; yet, only one-third of them seek treatment. Even when people seek treatment, symptoms of a depressive disorder are often unrecognized or inappropriately treated by health professionals. Given this level of ignorance, as well as the negative attitudes that surround mental disorders, the Federal Government sponsored its first major health education program about a specific mental disorder in 1986, with the initiation of the National Institute of Mental Health's (NIMH's) DEPRESSION Awareness, Recognition and Treatment (D/ART) program. The D/ART seeks to: 1) increase public knowledge of the symptoms of depressive disorders and the availability of effective treatment, 2) change public attitudes about depression so that there is greater acceptance of depression as a disorder rather than a weakness, 3) encourage changes in help-seeking behavior to reduce the number of untreated and inappropriately treated individuals, and 4) provide information to primary care physicians, mental health specialists, and medical students about advances in diagnosing and treating depressive disorders. The D/ART program will extend over a decade and consists of three components: a professional training program, a public education campaign, and a national worksite program.

For fiscal years 1986 to 1991, the D/ART program expended $4.5 million to train health professionals about recent advances in diagnosis and treatment of depressive disorders (table 7-1). Short-term training courses, developed for this purpose, have been used to train more than 11,000 primary care physicians, mental health professionals, and medical students about depressive disorders. In addition, the D/ART program sponsors continuing education programs in collaboration with professional associations.

In 1988, the D/ART program launched a two-part public education campaign consisting of a multimedia component to publicize messages about depressive disorders and a community partnership program to extend and reinforce the media messages at the local level. First, D/ART staff conducted 20 focus groups in nine geographically dispersed cities and contracted for a survey of 500 people in two cities (Indianapolis, IN and Sacramento, CA) to find out what people knew about depressive disorders. Furthermore, in the early stages of campaign development, the D/ART program organized a group of 45 campaign consultant organizations to advise about public education strategies. The group—comprised of representatives from the major mental health and medical professional associations as well as health and mental health organizations, businesses, labor, religious, and educational groups, mental health advocacy groups, foundations, and other Federal agencies—continues to provide advice on campaign policy matters and to disseminate information on depression.

The D/ART Public Education Campaign has expended $3.6 million in the past 5 years (table 7-1) to develop educational materials. For example, a total of 16 flyers, brochures, and booklets have been produced and distributed to more than 13 million people, with some of the publications geared toward the general audience and some to specific groups, such teenagers, college students, young African-Americans, and older people; some have been published in Spanish and five Asian languages. Also, close to 1,000 television and 9,000 radio stations have broadcast public service announcements (PSAs) about depression to as many as two-thirds of households nationwide. A number of the initial PSAs featured celebrity spokespersons to introduce the campaign.

A critical component of the D/ART program is its community partnership strategy. The Community Partnership Program consists of 32 mental health groups, mostly ''Mental Health Association'' and ''Alliance for the Mentally Ill'' organizations, located in 24 States and the District of Columbia. Community partners reproduce and distribute copies of print materials on depression; conduct public forums, worksite programs, and professional

Table 7-1—DEPRESSION Awareness, Recognition, and Treatment Program, Fiscal Years 1986-91

| Area | ($ thousands) | | | | | | Total |
	FY 86	FY 87	FY 88	FY 89	FY 90	FY 91	FY 86-91
Training	142	520	646	824	1,146	1,250	4,528 (53%)
Public education	292	924	447	745	616	631	3,655 (43%)
Worksite	N/A	N/A	50	50	100	100	300 (4%)
Total	434	1,444	1,143	1,619	1,862	1,981	8,483

SOURCE: I. Davidoff, Director, D/ART Campaign, National Institute of Mental Health, Rockville, MD, personal communication, Feb. 28, 1992.

seminars; develop videos; appear on television and radio talk shows; sponsor support groups and telephone hotlines, and carry out other varied educational activities, including brochure translations in five Asian languages. In 1990, the total dollar value of the programs that were offered and the partners' direct and in-kind contributions was estimated at nearly $1.3 million, about ten times the Federal investment in the Community Partnership Program. D/ART also recently initiated a Professional Partnership Program, through which depression-related community education activities similar to those offered by Community Partners will be developed by universities, foundations, and professional organizations.

In 1988, the D/ART program established a National Worksite Program as a collaborative effort between NIMH and the Washington Business Group on Health, a nonprofit health policy group composed of Fortune 500 employers. To date, $300,000 has been expended on this program component. The purpose of the worksite initiative is to assist employers in reducing the impact of depression on productivity, on health and disability costs, and on employees and their families. The program disseminates information about depressive disorders to employers and encourages corporate policies and programs that promote early recognition, quality cost-effective care, and on-the-job support for individuals experiencing depressive illnesses. The program has developed a "Management of Depression" model program and published a report based on the experience of seven large U.S. companies that contributed to development of the model. In 1992, the program will produce a training program for management personnel and occupational health professionals to improve early recognition and referral to appropriate care for depression.

Preliminary data suggest that the D/ART program has had some positive effects. For example, prior to the dissemination of any information, NIMH funded a 1987 telephone survey by the University of Michigan Institute of Social Research of 500 people (250 in Indianapolis, IN and 250 in Sacramento, CA) to determine the extent of their knowledge about depression. The survey found that most people believed that depressed persons could get better on their own rather than by seeking treatment. In 1990, the American Medical Association conducted a followup survey of the same group of 500 people. A total of 210 of the original group responded; 40 percent of the respondees in Indianapolis and 25 percent of the respondees in Sacramento said they knew more about depression because of the D/ART campaign. AMA also surveyed a new group of 500 people (250 people from each of the two cities). Of this group, 34 percent of those in Indianapolis and 30 percent of those in Sacramento said they were aware of the D/ART campaign and its messages. Another survey in North Dakota found that the number of adults treated for depressive disorders increased 1.5 times and the number of children treated increased 3 times in Human Service Centers (akin to Community Mental Health Centers) for fiscal years 1986 to 1991. The increase was attributed in part to the D/ART public and professional education programs and to a State program to develop treatment teams specifically for children within the Human Service Centers.

Has the D/ART program been a success? While the limited data on the effectiveness of the D/ART program preclude a quantitatively based answer to this question, several aspects of the program clearly deserve commendation. With limited resources and personnel (the entire D/ART program is managed by one- and one-half full-time Federal professional staff persons), the D/ART program established an educational campaign that is solidly rooted in research advances; the D/ART program carefully devises the messages to be relayed, uses diverse media to disseminate the messages, and coordinates its efforts with people in the community. D/ART has also trained substantial numbers of health and mental health care providers through its own efforts and through collaborations with public and private organizations. Advancement of this pioneering educational effort on a mental disorder by the Federal Government—via further study of its effect on the level of awareness, prevalence and treatment changes, expansion of the program into other communities, and adapting its techniques for educating the public about other conditions—will require some combination of increased funds and personnel, as well as highlighting this activity as a priority at the NIMH.

SOURCES: J.E. Barham, Mental Health Consultant, personal communication, May 4, 1992; R. Brown, Senior Scientist, Department of Mental Health, American Medical Association, personal communication, June 23, 1992; I. Davidoff, director, D/ART Campaign, National Institute of Mental Health, Rockville, MD, personal communication, June 1992; R. Kessler, Institute for Social Research, University of Michigan, personal communication, June 23, 1992; A. Koss, coordinator of State D/ART Program, Division of Mental Health, Department of Human Services, Bismarck, ND, personal communication, June 22, 1992; D.A. Regier, M.A. Hirschfeld, F.K. Goodwin, et al., "The NIMH Depression Awareness, Recognition, and Treatment Program: Structure, Aims, and Scientific Basis," *American Journal of Psychiatry* 145:1351-1357, 1988; D. Regier, Director, Division of Clinical Research, National Institute of Mental Health, personal communication, May 1992; U.S. Department of Health and Human Services, Public Health Service, Alcohol Drug Abuse and Mental Health Administration, National Institute of Mental Health, *Depression, Awareness, Recognition, and Treatment (D/ART) Fact Sheet*, DHHS Pub. No. (ADM) 90-1680 (Rockville, MD: U.S. DHHS, 1990).

service delivery, available treatments, economic constraints, and existing laws. Thus, influencing mental health policy requires not only dispelling the myths and negative attributes surrounding mental disorders but also paying attention to the other factors that affect these issues. For example, efforts to fight employment discrimination were focused on the inclusion of individuals with mental disorders in the recently passed Americans With Disabilities Act (ADA) (box 7-C). It is hoped that the ADA will have a profound effect on individuals with mental disorders by opening options in employment now unavailable to them.

THE IMPACT OF BIOLOGICAL RESEARCH

The ongoing revolution in neuroscience has invigorated research into mental disorders, leading to new discoveries about and increased emphasis on the biological underpinnings of these conditions. This is not the first time that the biological component of mental disorders has been emphasized— concepts of mental illness historically have been cyclic in nature (15,16,59). Nor have previous hopes concerning the curability or biological basis of mental disorders always correlated with improved public attitudes or care for those with these disorders. Current biological research into mental disorders is different from that done in previous eras, however. It is set on the stage of what has been called a new age of neuroscience (1).

> The research that is possible, or is already taking place, represents not just an extension of earlier efforts but a qualitative change. From a base of knowledge about the brain in general, neuroscience is now making the first exploratory inroads into the features that characterize us as humans: the ability to create and to calculate, to empathize, to recall and plan (Enoch Gordis quoted in 1).

General developments in brain research, complete with rapid technological advances and the contribution of a host of scientific areas, distinguish current biological research into mental disorders.

Most experts in the mental health field appreciate the fact that biological factors play an important role in the mental disorders considered in this report. Furthermore, advocates who focus on the biological

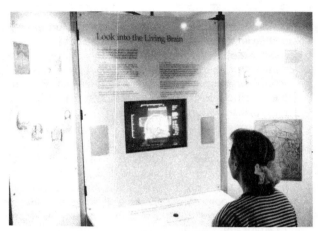

Photo credit: M. Catherine Sargent, 1992

Developments in neuroscience have received increasing attention, as illustrated in this exhibit of the American Psychological Association at the Smithsonian Institution.

aspects of mental disorders are an increasing force, joining and shaping the debate of policy issues. This section considers some of the social impacts of the biology of mental disorders—that is, how the gains from neuroscience research and the perception that mental disorders have a biological basis influence public attitudes toward mental disorders and mental health policy. The discussion is organized under two broad titles: Perceptions of Responsibility and The Link Between Mental Disorders and Medicine.

Perceptions of Responsibility

Despite the regular reemergence of biological explanations for mental disorders since the classical Greek period (48,57,59), these conditions have often been perceived as a sign of moral weakness or the manifestation of evil. The view that the antisocial, irrational, withdrawn, or unpredictable behavior sometimes produced by mental disorders stems from moral turpitude persists to this day, even among some medical researchers and caregivers (23). A key finding of a 1991 survey of public attitudes by the National Mental Health Association evidences these social beliefs or judgments: 43 percent of American adults see depression as a personal weakness (39).[3] Also, a 1988 survey by the Utah Division of Mental Health and the Alliance for the Mentally Ill found that 71 percent of respondents thought severe mental

---

[3] The National Mental Health Association poll is based on a nationwide telephone interview of 1,022 adults age 18 and older conducted between October 18 and 23, 1991.

Box 7-C—Americans With Disabilities Act: Employing People With Mental Disorders

The Americans With Disabilities Act of 1990 (ADA), which received the President's signature on July 26, 1990, is the most expansive civil rights legislation passed since the 1964 Civil Rights Act. Under the ADA, the estimated 43 million Americans with disabilities, including those with mental disorders, will be afforded protections from discrimination similar to those prohibiting discrimination based on race, sex, national origin, and religious affiliation. Equality of opportunity and protection from discrimination for individuals with disabilities is guaranteed in the areas of employment (Title I), public transportation and other State and local government services (Title II), public accommodations (Title III), and telecommunications (Title IV).

The ADA definition of a person with a disability applies to individuals meeting one of the following criteria: 1) having a physical or mental impairment that substantially limits one or more of the person's major life activities; 2) having a record of such an impairment; or 3) being regarded as having such an impairment. While the law refrains from delineating specific disabilities, it does define ''major life activities'': caring for oneself, performing manual tasks, walking, seeing, hearing, speaking, breathing, learning, and working. Thus, the act applies only to mental disorders that are severe enough to significantly affect a major life activity. Also, the law affords protection from discrimination based on health or treatment history to persons who have recovered from a physical or mental illness or have at some point been inappropriately diagnosed or misclassified as having a mental or physical disorder. Finally, the ADA directly addresses the negative impacts of the stigma associated with mental disorders, since it protects individuals from being denied employment on the basis of negative attitudes and misperceptions concerning mental disorders in the absence of a legitimate, job-related reason.

While the ADA covers almost every aspect of life in which people with disabilities might encounter discrimination, the employment provisions are likely to have the most profound impact on the lives of individuals with mental disorders. Title I of the ADA prohibits discrimination

> . . . against a qualified individual with a disability . . . in regard to job application procedures, the hiring, advancement, or discharge of employees, employee compensation, job training, and other terms, conditions, and privileges of employment.

Title I requires employers to provide reasonable accommodation to qualified employees, including physical modifications in order to make existing facilities used by employees readily accessible to and usable by individuals with disabilities. Alternatively, it may require nonphysical adjustments including job restructuring, part-time or modified work schedules, and other such modifications. Such nonphysical modifications may be especially important for people with mental disorders. Employers are required to make reasonable accommodations unless it can be demonstrated that the accommodation would impose an undue hardship on the operation of the business. This safeguards the viability of businesses and organizations by protecting employers from incurring unreasonable burden in the provision of needed accommodations. Such a burden may include the disruption of business as well as excessive financial expense.

Ironically, while the provisions of the ADA may serve to combat the stigma of mental disorders, they may also raise the specter of stigma—because coverage under ADA is dependent upon disclosure of disability. Persons with ''hidden disabilities''—those not apparent to an observer, such as mental disorders—are covered only if the disability is revealed. Individuals with a severe mental disorder or a history of mental disorder are often reluctant to disclose their disability, and the provisions of the ADA preclude preemployment inquiry into mental health history; however, employers are required to make reasonable accommodations only if the disability is known.

While this landmark act has the potential to benefit individuals with mental disorders greatly, hurdles remain in the ADA's implementation phase. Certain issues have yet to be resolved, including the determination of who exactly is covered, the precise definition of reasonable accommodation for individuals with mental disorders, the provision of an adequate definition of the role of medication in reasonable accommodation for individuals with mental disorders, and the promulgation of such information to both covered individuals and employers.

SOURCES: Americans With Disabilities Act of 1990, Public Law No. 101-336, 1990; House Report No. 101-485, Pt. 1 (Committee on Public Works and Transportation), Pt. 2 (Committee on Education and Labor), Pt. 3 (Committee on the Judiciary), and Pt. 4 (Committee on Energy and Commerce), all accompanying H.R. 2273; L.L. Mancuso, ''Reasonable Accommodation for Workers With Psychiatric Disabilities,'' *Psychosocial Rehabilitation Journal* 14(2):3-19, 1990; L.L. Mancuso, Director, Path Project, National Association of State Mental Health Directors, Alexandria, VA, personal communication, Feb. 21, 1992; National Mental Health Association, *A.D.A.: Americans With Disabilities Act of 1990 (Public Law 101-336)*, 1991; L.J. Scallet and C.F. Rohrer, *Analysis: Americans With Disabilities Act and Mental Health* (Washington, DC: Policy Resource Center, 1990).

illness was due to emotional weakness, 65 percent thought bad parenting was to blame, 35 percent cited sinful behavior, and 45 percent believed that the mentally ill bring on their illness and could will it away if they wished (67). These beliefs have contributed to the public condemnation of unusual or frightening behavior produced by mental disorders, as well as to the shame and guilt experienced by patients and their families.

A biological explanation of the unusual, erratic, or frightening behavior sometimes associated with mental disorders challenges the notion of moral turpitude directly. When atypical behavior is attributed to biological factors, an individual with a mental disorder is less likely to be perceived as the perpetrator of immoral actions than as the victim of forces beyond his or her control. Thus, a biological understanding of severe mental disorders may remove the blame for antisocial or atypical behavior from a person with the disorder.

While biological explanations may absolve individuals of some of the blame for their illness, such theories are not always associated with more benevolent treatment by society. Biological theories have led to abuses in the past, such as eugenic practices (see ch. 5). And other theories as to the origin of mental disorders—such as early childhood experiences—have been used to exculpate individuals from responsibility for their behavior. Furthermore, biological explanations may not be sufficient to overcome society's fear of violent or very bizarre individuals with mental disorders or the stereotype of the "berserk madman." The media spotlight on a hideous crime committed by an "ex-mental patient" reinforces the link in the public's mind between mental disorders and violence (box 7-D).[4]

Attributing behavior to biological, and especially genetic, factors may lead to the perception that human actions are predetermined. Biological explanations of behavior encroach uncomfortably on our sense of free will and moral agency (11).

[M]ost of us aren't comfortable with genetic explanations for our own or anyone else's behavior. We are proud of our freedom, individuality, and powers of self-determination (53).

American psychologist and philosopher William James struggled with this dilemma more than 100 years ago. James felt that our sense of self, needed to lend meaning to our existence, may be incompatible with the necessary assumption of psychology and neuroscience that the "prediction of all things without exception (including human behavior) must be . . . possible" (quoted in 11). Thus, neuroscience's exploration of the human brain challenges the way in which we think about the mind in general.

Individuals with mental disorders may be especially vulnerable when society is seduced by notions of biological reductionism and determinism. These notions can cause individuals with mental disorders to feel dehumanized, with less control over their minds. Insensitively labeling the way a person feels, thinks, or behaves as diseased can diminish his or her sense of "personhood" (36,60), as revealed in the following passage (37):

I have discussed the diagnostic label 'schizophrenia' with a number of patients. Interestingly, they often say that they do not mind the label itself, but it is the inaccurate attributions made to them because of it that they find objectionable. They know quite well when they are manifestly schizophrenic. They know it from their personal phenomenology at a point in time. They object to being *seen* as schizophrenic when they are not; they object to being treated as dependent children when it is not necessary; they object to having to lie to obtain work for which they are qualified; and they object to their not being listened to and taken seriously because they are, after all, 'schizophrenic.'

The extent to which persons are responsible for their actions—even if there is a biological underpinning—is far from resolved; it requires the consideration of social, philosophical, legal, and moral issues that are beyond the scope of this report. However, it is important to debunk the myth that modern neuroscience necessarily leads us to conclusions of biological reductionism and determinism. Recent advances in neuroscience do not suggest that our brains are biologically fixed or immutable; rather, results increasingly show the dynamic nature of nervous tissue and its responsiveness to environmental cues throughout life. And as Owen Flanagan

---

[4] While most individuals with a severe mental disorder are not violent, the question, "Are mental disorders linked to violence?" is a complex one. A psychotic episode can lead to a violent act. However, the relationship between mental disorders and violent acts is a complex one, being influenced by various factors, among other things the nature of the disorder, the availability of adequate treatment, and the law (35).

Box 7-D—Media Portrayals of Mental Disorders

Since the late 1950s and early 1960s, studies have consistently revealed a high incidence of media attention to mental disorders. While media attention contributed significantly to the end of mass warehousing of patients, often in cruel conditions, much of the information it provided about mental disorders was negative and inaccurate. Recent studies have shown that although there has been an increase in the frequency of portrayals of individuals with mental disorders, there has not necessarily been an increase in the accuracy of such portrayals. Surveys of images of mental disorders on prime-time television conducted in the 1980s found that between 17 and 29 percent of the shows had some portrayal of mental disorders. Unfortunately, much of that information concerning mental disorders is inaccurate and stigmatizing.

One of the most persistent and damaging inaccuracies conveyed by the media is the characterization of individuals with severe mental disorders as violent despite the fact that individuals with severe mental disorders are more likely to be withdrawn and frightened than violent and are more frequently victims than perpetrators of violent acts. Violence occurs on television at the rate of approximately six incidents per hour in prime time and 25 incidents per hour in children's daytime programming; a disproportionate number of these occurrences are either perpetuated by or against individuals identified as mentally disordered. In fact, characters labeled mentally disordered in television dramas are almost twice as likely as other characters to kill or be killed, to be violent or fall victim to violence. Efforts to combat this image are confounded by the fact that some individuals with mental disorders—particularly when untreated—are at risk of committing violent acts against themselves or others, or both. Perhaps more troubling is the fact that the stigmatizing equation of severe mental disorder with violence is not limited to fictional entertainment media. News stories and headlines identifying violent criminals on the basis of their mental health history, such as the recent Associated Press headline ''Woman Who Shot at Restaurant Previously Committed to Mental Hospital,'' saturate the news media, while stories of successful recovery are rare. Such news stories are damaging to individuals with mental disorders because they suggest both an inescapable connection between mental disorders and violence and the incurability of mental disorder (that is, even *former*, treated mental patients remain prone to violence).

Do these inaccurate and negative depictions of individuals with mental disorders adversely affect public attitudes? Research has shown that television is able to influence viewers' attitudes in subtle ways, through the repetition of images not necessarily labeled as factual. Knowledge specifically concerning the impact of media depictions of mental disorders on public opinions is limited. Some studies have revealed that programming intended to increase knowledge of and improve attitudes toward individuals with mental disorders has a positive impact. However, data indicate that the damaging effects of negative portrayals overwhelm the benefits of the media's positive efforts. Negative mass media portrayals of persons with mental disorders generate negative attitudes among viewers, and corrective information, or disclaimers, has been shown to be largely ineffectual.

Advocacy groups are working to reduce inaccurate and stigmatizing depictions of individuals with mental disorders in the mass media. For example, the Alliance for the Mentally Ill of New York State operates a Stigma Clearinghouse that records and responds to inaccurate or stigmatizing media depictions of individuals with mental disorders, and the National Alliance for the Mentally Ill may soon launch a similar program nationwide. In addition, the Carter Center in Atlanta, Georgia, has held two conferences addressing the problems of stigma and mental disorders and the role of the mass media and has subsequently launched a media initiative to address these issues.

SOURCES: *Stigma and the Mentally Ill: Proceedings of the First International Rosalynn Carter Symposium on Mental Health Policy*, Nov. 15, 1985 (Atlanta, GA: Carter Center, 1985); L.R. Marcos, ''Media Power and Public Mental Health Policy,'' *American Journal of Psychiatry* 146:1185-1189, 1989; A. Mayer and D. Barry, ''Working With the Media To Destigmatize Mental Illness,'' *Hospital and Community Psychiatry* 43:77-78, 1992; Robert Wood Johnson Foundation, Program on Chronic Mental Illness, ''Public Attitudes Toward People With Chronic Mental Illness,'' April 1990; O. Wahl, ''Mental Illness in the Media: An Unhealthy Condition,'' *The Community Imperative*, R.C. Baron, I.D. Rutman, and B. Klaczynska (eds.) (Philadelphia, PA: Horizon House Institute, 1980); O. Wahl, Professor, George Mason University, personal communication, February 1992; O. Wahl and J.Y. Lefkowitz, ''Impact of a Television Film on Attitudes Toward Mental Illness,'' *American Journal of Community Psychology* 17(4):521-528, 1989; O. Wahl and R. Roth, ''Television Images of Mental Illness: Results of a Metropolitan Washington Media Watch,'' *Journal of Broadcasting* 28:599-605, 1982.

Blaming the Brain

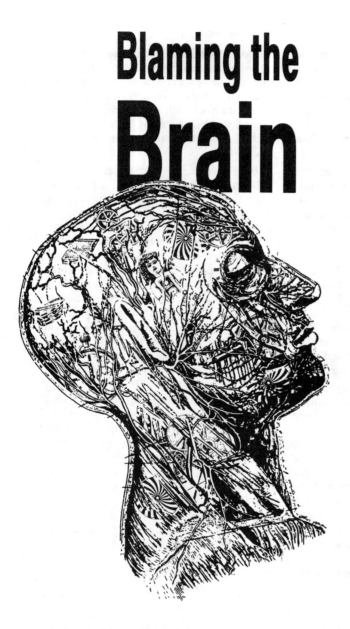

Credit: Illustration by Robin Applestein, reprinted by permission of R. Applestein and the Washington Times

Findings that biological factors underpin certain mental disorders help relieve individuals and their families from feelings of guilt.

(11) observes in his recent book, *The Science of the Mind*, science permits:

> . . . a model for conceiving of the mind that allows for the beliefs: that actions can be done on purpose; that action can be rational; that deliberation can result in free choice; that such choices can go against

very powerful desires and inclinations; that we can think of humans as responsible—all this without the paradoxical requirement that some actions, namely those of our free will, be totally uncaused.

The assertion that biological factors contribute to the development of mental disorders challenges the once reigning theory that they are caused by bad parenting. For example, psychoanalytic thought posited that psychic damage during early childhood produced schizophrenia and other mental disorders. This concept evolved into the focus on the "schizophrenogenic" mother—that is, a mother with overbearing tendencies, warped psychosexual development, and near-psychotic behavior who produces schizophrenia in her offspring (12). Since little or no scientific evidence supports these theories as sufficient or necessary causes of the severe mental disorders considered in this report, most experts reject them (14,25). However, the message that mental disorders are a response to cruel social and family conditions nonetheless continues to shape the attitudes of the public and even some experts (28). For example, data from a 1989 study showed that textbooks in abnormal psychology implicitly support the concept of the schizophrenogenic parent (69).

Given that family members are often viewed as the agents of mental illness, it is understandable that they embrace biological theories of mental disorders. When families belonging to the National Alliance for the Mentally Ill (NAMI) were asked what had helped them to cope with stigma, 73.2 percent indicated that "research findings which establish a biological basis for mental illness helped much or very much in dealing with stigma" (71). The concept that a biological defect causes a mental disorder largely exonerates family members and the individuals themselves from blame, placing it instead on a disease process (22). The solace found by families in biological explanations of mental disorders is revealed in this passage, written by the father of a son with obsessive-compulsive disorder (52):

> *It May Not Be Your Fault That You or Your Child Has Obsessive-Compulsive Disorder!* Early toilet training, a rigorously disciplined home environment, an unresolved oedipal complex, and endless demands that your child clean up her "disgusting" room may not be and is probably not the cause of this illness.

Obsessive-Compulsive Disorder, the flu, and diabetes may have at least one thing in common—

the cause. The disease is possibly biological; it may even be inherited from one generation to another, as suggested in my family's case. However, OCD manifests itself as strange behavior while the other two show up as physical illnesses. To my wife and me this understanding that there might be a physical cause was a great relief. . . .

At the same time, strict adherence to biological theories may impair psychosocial research into the development, relapse, and treatment of mental disorders. While beyond the scope of this report, it is important to note that some data suggest that psychosocial factors play a role in mental disorders. For example, research findings point out the role of what is called disruptive emotional expression, or EE, in schizophrenia. Studies suggest that people with schizophrenia who spend time in a stressful environment (that is, an environment with high EE) are more likely to suffer a relapse (24,27,64). The message from such studies is not a return to the cruel and stigmatizing concepts of family causation, but rather an acknowledgment that the emergence, symptoms, and course of mental disorders are multifactorial.

Genetic models of mental disorders may unintentionally recast the stigma and discrimination experienced by individuals with mental disorders and their families. With increased knowledge about the genetics of mental disorders, new questions emerge. Will individuals who pass on a gene or several genes predisposing their offspring to a mental disorder be viewed as blameworthy for having children? Will insurance coverage or employment be denied on the basis of a "positive" genetic test in the future?

Some groups and individuals interested in or afflicted by genetic diseases voice concerns about potential genetic discrimination—"the denial of rights, privileges, or opportunities on the basis of information gathered via genetic tests" (65). Eugenic policies in the past (see ch. 5) and popular support of prenatal testing for genetic diseases (and termination of the pregnancy in the event of a positive test) foster concern about possible genetic discrimination (47). It may be premature to raise concerns about genetic testing for mental disorders, given their complex and poorly understood genetic underpinnings (see ch. 5). However, that some mental disorders have a genetic component is strongly supported by research data. Therefore, tests for a genetic predisposition to some mental disorders may well be technically feasible in the future. Given

the stigma attached to individuals with mental disorders and their families, the chronic nature of disorders, and the current barriers to insurance and employment, genetic testing—or even the perception that genetics accounts for these conditions—could become a tool for discriminating against individuals with mental disorders and their families.

The Link Between Mental Disorders and Medicine

Intimately linked to the emphasis on biological aspects of severe mental disorders is the hope that biomedical research will lead to new treatments and, ultimately, cures for these disorders (19). As stated in NAMI's platform (38):

> For the purposes of research, the National Alliance has defined serious mental illnesses as those brain diseases that are at the present time neither preventable nor curable but are controllable with proper medication and support services. . . . Biomedical research will yield better treatment and a cure for these diseases.

Hope for a cure has accompanied many eras of mental health policy. In addition to the desire to eliminate the complicated problems associated with severe mental disorders, the current hopes for a cure spring from general optimism for biomedical research, the track record of biomedical research in finding treatment and cures for disease in general, the past and continuing development of drugs used to treat many individuals with mental disorders, and the neuroscience revolution. In light of the considerable advances of neuroscience research in general, it is hard not to be infected by this hope. A realistic viewpoint is necessary, however, to stay the course of what is likely to be a slow unraveling of the secrets of the brain. Furthermore, policymakers and advocates must also be wary of the danger, not always resisted in the past, of emphasizing research at the expense of providing adequate care for people with mental disorders.

Biological research on mental disorders has entered into the issue of mental health care finance. Currently, financial barriers limit access to treatment. Insurance coverage for mental health care is generally inferior to coverage for "physical" illnesses (3,42,54,66). Recently, advocates have lobbied for the designation of certain mental disorders as biological, or brain-based, in order to gain parity in insurance coverage (6,19,46). In the first case of its type, a father sued Arkansas Blue Cross and Blue Shield for increased coverage for the care of his daughter, who was hospitalized for bipolar disorder. His insurance policy provided for extensive coverage for physical conditions but limited coverage for "mental, psychiatric, or nervous" disorders. The plaintiff argued that bipolar disorder is a biological disorder and therefore should be considered "physical" under the terms of the policy. In this case, *Arkansas Blue Cross and Blue Shield* v. *Doe* (4), the courts ruled that bipolar disorder "is a physical condition within the meaning of the Blue Cross contract."

State legislatures also have begun to address the issue of providing equal treatment for biologically based mental disorders. For example, a bill that became law in Maine in 1992 requires group insurers that offer coverage for disorders of the brain to offer the same coverage for biologically based severe mental disorders. The law specifies all of the conditions included in this report: schizophrenia, bipolar disorder, major depression, panic disorder, and obsessive-compulsive disorder.

Advocates who would identify specific mental disorders as "brain-based" invoke the traditional medical model of illness as the most appropriate one for treatment in order to tap into society's perceived responsibility for providing health care. Will discovery that certain mental disorders are "brain-based"—or renaming them as such—achieve insurance parity? Clearly, pinpointing a diagnostic entity with a biological marker—coupled with treatment—can be useful for third-party payers, as expressed by William S. Custer, director of research at the Employee Benefit Research Institute (7):

One underlying problem with mental health benefits is the difficulty in defining an insurable event. An insurable event is whatever triggers benefit payment. Ideally that event should be out of the control of the insured individual or the individual's agent (in this case, the provider). The difficulty in insurance plan design for mental health benefits is that for at least some conditions, the need for mental health care is subjectively determined. More importantly, individuals seeking treatment must choose between several types of providers (psychologists, psychiatrist, social workers, etc.) and settings (hospitals, halfway houses, clinics, etc.), and more than 150

different modalities (45), with little information about the efficacy of treatment or quality of care. . . .

These problems could potentially be alleviated for those with mental disorders that have a biological cause and for which effective treatments can be found. For those illnesses, the detection of the biological cause would define an insurable event, for which an insurance plan could be designed which would more closely resemble those for other physical ailments.

In fact, since the mid-1970s, the treatment of severe mental disorders has increasingly reflected the medical model, with short-term hospitalization, the use of prescription drugs, and the development of a more reliable diagnostic classification system (63).

As indicated in this report, data point increasingly to the importance of biological factors in certain mental disorders. However, some mental health policy experts and advocates question whether labeling as such is necessary or appropriate, asserting that emphasizing the underlying causes of mental disorders is not necessary to gain care and will not guarantee adequate care; rather, what is needed is political will.

To accomplish some form of parity for insurance reimbursement of mental disorders requires no reliance on the brain disease theory or, indeed, on any theory of the cause or nature of mental disorders (60).

While the general view of what causes a disorder or problem can impact on policy approaches in dealing with it (58), simply renaming a condition may not be adequate for achieving such a goal. The court case previously described is illustrative: After the court ordered Arkansas Blue Cross and Blue Shield to pay for treatment of the daughter's bipolar disorder, the company rewrote its contract so that this disorder was specifically identified as a mental disorder, subject to the usual coverage limitations (42).

Another factor in this debate is the heightened concern about the cost of health care in general (30), which has led to an environment of restricting, not expanding, insurance benefits. For example, during the 1980s, the States began to mandate some type of mental health insurance coverage; the more recent trend in State legislatures is to waive mandates requiring such coverage (18). Concern also exists about what will happen to coverage of the other "nonphysical" disorders (26). Increased coverage of biological disorders could reduce even further coverage of psychological disorders that cannot demonstrate a clear biological foundation. Preventive efforts and stress-related disorders, for example, might be neglected (70). Another concern focuses on the definition of medical management, even for biologically based mental disorders.

> Skeptics view it as a prelude to eliminating insurance coverage for psychotherapy and fear that it will encourage unnecessary drug treatment and create an incentive to diminish the time spent talking to patients (63).

Although researchers are developing more effective biological approaches, psychosocial interventions are an important component of treatment and rehabilitation. Given the problems faced in obtaining adequate coverage for the care of severe mental disorders, as well as the complexities of the issues impacting on the health care and mental health care finance debate, a full consideration of these issues, which is beyond the scope of this report, is warranted.

SUMMARY AND CONCLUSIONS

While the last 30 years have seen an improvement in the public's knowledge of and attitudes toward mental disorders, stigma still abounds. People with mental disorders and their family members suffer acutely from that stigma. And negative public attitudes contribute to discrimination in research support, treatment availability, financing of care, housing, and employment.

The stigma attached to mental disorders, while compelling and undeniable, has manifold aspects. The notion of stigma embraces everything from willful denigration of those who are different to fear and ignorance. The social and public policy effects of stigma are also complex, being influenced by many different factors, including laws, the structure of service delivery, and economic constraints. Because of the complex nature of the stigma attached to mental disorders and the many relevant areas of public policy, OTA finds that a wide-ranging strategy will be necessary to bring about public policies that benefit persons with severe mental disorders. Educating the public about the nature of these conditions is one important tactic; vigilance in relevant policy areas, such as that evidenced in the passage of the Americans With Disabilities of Act, is another.

Concepts of what causes mental disorders influence public attitudes and policy. Modern neuroscience, which is undergoing revolutionary and rapid advances, is the primary influence on current understanding of the mental disorders considered in this report. Some skeptics point out that this trend is but another reincarnation of biological psychiatry, which historically has wielded influence from time to time—not always to the advantage of those with mental disorders. While many factors play a role, including professional self-interest, the perennial hope for a cure, and the optimism traditionally attached to biomedical research, the broad base of research into the function of the human brain distinguishes today's search for biological factors associated with mental disorders.

OTA identified several ways in which the data from biological research into mental disorders and perceptions of that data can affect public attitudes and policy. Biological explanations of mental disorders are used to counter the view that these conditions result from moral turpitude, thus exculpating individuals whose disorders may lead to unusual, erratic, or frightening behavior. Also, the assertion that biological factors contribute to the development of mental disorders debunks the stigmatizing notion that bad parenting is the essential cause. Biological data have been viewed as exonerating family members from blame and thus helping them to deal with stigma.

The increased emphasis on biological aspects of mental disorders, while helpful in dismantling some negative attitudes, is not without its limitations. As mentioned, perceptions of what causes mental disorders are not the sole reason for stigma. For example, fear of violent behavior, a simplistic image of mental disorders reinforced by the media, also shapes public attitudes. Furthermore, publicized data may be misinterpreted. The specious notion that a biological, especially a genetic, substrate for human behavior dissolves moral agency can be especially dehumanizing to persons with mental disorders. Also, while reproachful theories of causation, such as the schizophrenogenic mother, have been largely refuted, it is important to note that biological research has not ruled out the role of psychosocial factors in the development, course, and treatment of mental disorders. Finally, with rapid advances in molecular genetics, some sort of genetic test for mental disorders may become possible in the future; such a test—or simply the perception that these conditions are inherited—could prove to be a powerful tool for discrimination.

The emphasis on biological aspects of severe mental disorders is intimately linked to the hope that biomedical research will lead to new treatments and, ultimately, cures. While hopes for a cure have long accompanied new eras of mental health policy, this period bears the distinctive mark of the new age of brain research. A realistic viewpoint requires that we be patient and stay the course of what is likely to be a slow unraveling of the secrets of the brain. Similarly, policymakers must not be seduced into simplifying their consideration of mental disorders and focusing solely on research while ignoring the care needs of those currently afflicted with these disorders.

By highlighting the biological components of mental disorders, advocates seek more than treatment advances. As exemplified by recent court cases and State laws, attempts to obtain increased financial support for care also drive this trend. Identification of biological markers for certain mental disorders, along with effective treatments, can assist third-party payers for health care by enabling them to identify objectively an insurable event. However, other questions are raised by this trend, including concerns about the coverage of ''nonbiological'' disorders or interventions. A full consideration of mental health care and its finance is required to answer this issue.

CHAPTER 7 REFERENCES

1. Ackerman, S., *Discovering the Brain* (Washington, DC: National Academy Press, 1992).
2. Albrecht, G., Walker, V., and Levy, J., ''Social Distance from the Stigmatized: A Test of Two Theories,'' *Social Science and Medicine* 16: 1319-1327, 1982.
3. American Psychiatric Association, ''Coverage for Mental and Nervous Disorders: A Compendium of Public and Private Sector Health Insurance Plans,'' *The Coverage Catalog*, 2nd ed. (Washington, DC: American Psychiatric Press, 1989).
4. *Arkansas Blue Cross and Blue Shield* v. *Doe*, 1987. (22 Ar,.App.89 *Arkansas Blue Cross and Blue Shield, Inc., Appellant,* v. *John Doe as Parent and Next Friend of Jane Doe, Appellee*, No. CA 86-406, Court of Appeals of Arkansas, En Banc. July 29, 1987.
5. Atwood, N., ''Professional Prejudice and the Psychotic Client,'' *Social Work* 27:172-177, 1982.
6. Bergman, G.T., ''States Debate 'Parity' for Mental Illness Insurance Benefits,'' *State ADM Reports*, July-August 1991.
7. Custer, W.S., Director of Research, Employee Benefit Research Institute, Washington, DC, personal communication, 1992.
8. Dichter, H., ''The Stigmatization of Psychiatrists Who Work with Chronically Mentally Ill Persons,'' *Stigma and Mental Illness*, P.J. Fink and A. Tasman (eds.) (Washington, DC: American Psychiatric Press, 1992).
9. Eisenberg, L., ''Treating Depression and Anxiety in Primary Care: Closing the Gap between Knowledge and Practice,'' *New England Journal of Medicine* 326:1080-1084, 1992.
10. Farina, A., Fisher, J.D., and Fischer, E.H., ''Societal Factors in the Problems Faced by Deinstitutionalized Psychiatric Patients,'' *Stigma and Mental Illness*, P.J. Fink and A. Tasman (eds.) (Washington, DC: American Psychiatric Press, 1992).
11. Flanagan, O., *The Science of the Mind*, 2nd ed., rev. (Cambridge, MA: MIT Press, 1991).
12. Fromm-Reichmann, F., ''Notes on the Development of Treatment of Schizophrenics by Psychoanalytic Psychotherapy,'' *Psychiatry* 11:263-273, 1948.
13. Gantt, A.B., Goldstein, G., and Pinsky, S., ''Family Understanding of Psychiatric Illness,'' *Community Mental Health Journal* 25:101-108, 1989.
14. Gottesman, I.I., *Schizophrenia Genesis: The Origins of Madness* (New York: W.H. Freeman, 1991).
15. Grob, G., *Mental Illness and American Society, 1875-1940* (Princeton, NJ: Princeton University Press, 1983).
16. Grob, G., *From Asylum to Community: Mental Health Policy in Modern America* (Princeton, NJ: Princeton University Press, 1991).
17. Hatfield, A.B. (ed.), *Families of the Mentally Ill: Meeting the Challenges* (San Francisco, CA: Jossey-Bass, 1987).
18. *Health Benefits Letter*, ''Bare Bones Health Insurance: An Emerging Consensus in the States,'' May 23, 1991.
19. Howe, C.W., and Howe, J.W., ''The National Alliance for the Mentally Ill: History and Ideology,'' *Families of the Mentally Ill: Meeting the Challenge*, A.B. Hatfield (ed.) (San Francisco, CA: Jossey-Bass, 1987).
20. Interagency Council on the Homeless, *Outcast on Main Street: Report of the Federal Task Force on Homelessness and Severe Mental Illness* (ADM) 92-1904, 1992.
21. Institute of Medicine, *Research on Mental Illness and Addictive Disorders: Progress and Prospects* (Washington, DC: National Academy Press, 1984).
22. Johnson, D.L., ''Schizophrenia as a Brain Disease: Implications for Psychologists and Families,'' *Amer-*

ican Psychologist 44: 553-555, 1989.

23. Kanter, J.S., "Moral Issues and Mental Illness," *New Directions for Mental Health Services* 27:47-62, 1985.

24. Kavanagh, D.J., "Recent Developments in Expressed Emotion and Schizophrenia," *British Journal of Psychiatry* 160:601-620, 1992.

25. Keith, S.J., Matthews, S.M., and Schooler, N.R., "A Review of Psychoeducational Family Approaches," *Advances in Neuropsychiatry and Psychopharmacology: Schizophrenia Research*, vol. 1, C.A. Tamminga and S.C. Schulz (eds.) (New York, NY: Raven Press, 1991).

26. Koyanagi, C., National Mental Health Association, Alexandria, VA, personal communication, 1992.

27. Leff, J., and Vaughn, C., *Expressed Emotion in Families: Its Significance for Mental Illness* (New York, NY: Guilford Press, 1985).

28. Lefley, H.P., "The Stigmatized Family," *Stigma and Mental Illness*, P.J. Fink and A. Tasman (eds.) (Washington, DC: American Psychiatric Press, 1992).

29. Lefley, H.P., "Family Burden and Family Stigma in Major Mental Illness," *American Psychologist* 44:556-560, 1989.

30. Levit, K.R., Lazenby, H.C., Cowan, C.A., et al., "National Health Expenditures, 1990," *Health Care Financing Review* 13:29-54, 1991.

31. Link, B.G., "Understanding Labelling Effects in the Area of Mental Disorders: An Assessment of the Effects of Expectations of Rejection," *American Sociological Reviews* 52: 96-112, 1987.

32. Link, B.G., Cullen, F., Frank, J., et al., "The Social Rejection of Former Mental Patients: Understanding Why Labels Matter," *American Journal of Sociology* 92:1461-1500, 1987.

33. Link, B.G., Cullen, F.T., Mirotznik, J., et al., "The Consequences of Stigma for Persons with Mental Illness: Evidence from the Social Sciences," *Stigma and Mental Illness*, P.J. Fink and A. Tasman (eds.) (Washington, DC: American Psychiatric Press, 1992).

34. Minkoff, K., "Resistance of Mental Health Professionals to Working With the Chronic Mentally Ill," *Barriers to Treating the Chronic Mentally Ill*, A.T. Meyerson (ed.) (San Francisco, CA: Jossey-Bass, 1987).

35. Monahan, J., "Mental Disorder and Violent Behavior: Perceptions and Evidence," *American Psychologist* 47, 1992.

36. Mosher, L.R., Associate Director, Department of Addiction, Victim, and Mental Health Services, Montgomery County Government, Rockville, MD, personal communication, 1992.

37. Mosher, L.R., "Can Diagnosis Be Nonpejorative?" *The Nature of Schizophrenia*, L.C. Wynne (ed.) (New York, NY: John Wiley & Sons, 1978).

38. National Alliance for the Mentally Ill, Arlington, VA, 1991.

39. National Mental Health Association, "Depression: Misunderstanding Persists," *Focus: News From the National Mental Health Association*, winter 1992.

40. National Organization on Disability, "Public Attitudes Toward People With Disabilities," survey conducted by Louis Harris and Associates, Inc., 1991.

41. Nunnally, J.C., *Popular Conceptions of Mental Health* (New York, NY: Holt, Rinehart & Winston, 1961).

42. O'Keefe, A.M., *Handbook for Advocating Insurance Reform* (Arlington, VA: National Alliance for the Mentally Ill, June 1991).

43. Oppenheimer, K.C., and Miller, M.D., "Stereotypic Views of Medical Educators Toward Students With a History of Psychological Counseling," *Journal of Counseling Psychology* 35:311-314, 1988.

44. Ormel, J., van den Brink, W., Koeter, M.W.J., et al., "Recognition, Management, and Outcome of Psychological Disorders in Primary Care: A Naturalistic Follow-up Study," *Psychological Medicine* 20:909-923, 1990.

45. Orne, M.T., "Psychotherapy: Toward an Appropriate Basis for Reimbursement," *Cost Considerations in Mental Health Treatment: Settings, Modalities, and Providers*, Z. Taintor, P. Widem, and S.A. Barrett (eds.), (ADM) 84-1295 (Washington, DC: DHHS, 1984).

46. Peschel R., and Peschel, E., "A Medical Model for Specialists in Biologically Based Brain Disease," *Perceptual and Motor Skills* 72:96-98, 1991.

47. Pifer, L.K., "Genetic Markers for Schizophrenia: The Policy Context and Implications," *Biomedical Technology and Public Policy*, R.H. Blank and M.K. Mills (eds.) (New York, NY: Greenwood Press, 1989).

48. Porter, R., *A Social History of Madness: The World Through the Eyes of the Insane* (New York, NY: Weidenfeld & Nicolson, 1987).

49. *President's Commission on Mental Health*, vol. I, stock No. 040-000-00390-8 (Washington, DC: U.S. Government Printing Office, 1978).

50. Rabkin, J., "Determinants of Public Attitudes About Mental Illness: Summary of Research Literature," *Attitudes Toward the Mentally Ill: Research Perspectives* (ADM)-80-1031, J. Rabkin, L. Gelb, and J. Lazar (eds.) (Washington, DC: DHHS, 1980).

51. Rabkin, J., "Public Attitudes Toward Mental Illness: A Review of the Literature," *Schizophrenia Bulletin* 10(fall):9-33, 1974.

52. Rapoport, J.L., *The Boy Who Couldn't Stop Washing* (New York, NY: Penguin Books, 1989).

53. Restak, R., *The Brain Has A Mind of Its Own: Insights From a Practicing Neurologist* (New York,

NY: Harmony Books, 1991).

54. Ridgely, M.S., and Goldman, H.H., "Mental Health Insurance," *Handbook on Mental Health Policy in the United States*, D.A. Rochefort (ed.) (New York, NY: Greenwood Press, 1989).

55. Robert Wood Johnson Foundation, Program on Chronic Mental Illness, *Public Attitudes Toward People With Chronic Mental Illness*, 1990.

56. Robin, S.S., and Markle, G.E., "Let No One Split Asunder: Controversy in Human Genetic Engineering," *Politics and the Life Sciences* 6:3-12, 1987.

57. Roccatagliata, G., "The Idea of Melancholia in Classical Culture," *Psychiatry: The State of the Art*, vol. 8, P. Pichot, P. Berner, R. Wolf, et al. (eds.) (New York, NY: Plenum Press, 1985).

58. Rochefort, D.A., *American Social Welfare Policy: Dynamics of Formulation and Change* (Boulder, CO: Westview Press, 1986).

59. Rochefort, D.A., "Policymaking Cycles in Mental Health: Critical Examination of a Conceptual Model," *Journal of Health Politics, Policy and Law* 13:129-152, 1988.

60. Rubenstein, L., Executive Director, Mental Health Law Project, Washington, DC, personal communication, 1992.

61. Schulberg, H.C., and Burns, B.J., "Mental Disorders in Primary Care: Epidemiologic, Diagnostic, and Treatment Research Directions," *General Hospital Psychiatry* 10:79-87, 1988.

62. Sharfstein, S., President, Medical Director, and Chief Executive Officer, Sheppard and Enoch Pratt Hospital, Baltimore, MD, personal communication, 1992.

63. Sharfstein, S., and Goldman, H., "Financing the Medical Management of Mental Disorders," *American Journal of Psychiatry* 146:345-349, 19.

64. Strachan, A.M., "Family Intervention for the Rehabilitation of Schizophrenia: Toward Protecting and Coping," *Schizophrenia Bulletin* 12:678-698, 1986.

65. U.S. Congress, Office of Technology Assessment, *Cystic Fibrosis and DNA Tests: Implications of Carrier Screening*, OTA-BA-532 (Washington, DC: U.S. Government Printing Office, August 1992).

66. U.S. Department of Labor, *Employee Benefits in Medium and Large Firms*, Bull. 2363 (Washington, DC: Bureau of Labor Statistics, June 1990).

67. Utah Division of Mental Health, Task Force on Public Education, *Statewide Attitudes and Perceptions of Serious Mental Illness* (City: Pub., July 1988).

68. Wahl, O.F., "Public versus Professional Conceptions of Schizophrenia," *Journal of Community Psychology* 15:285-291, 1987.

69. Wahl, O.F, "Schizophrenogenic Parenting in Abnormal Psychology Textbooks," *Teaching of Psychology* 16:31-33, 1989.

70. Wahl, O.F, Associate Professor, George Mason University, Fairfax, VA, personal communication, 1992.

71. Wahl, O.F., and Harman, C.R., "Family Views of Stigma," *Schizophrenia Bulletin* 15:131-139, 1989.

72. Webster's New World Dictionary, 3rd College ed., V. Neufeldt and D.B. Guralnik (eds.) (New York, NY: Simon and Schuster, 1988).

73. Wells, K.B., Stewart, A., Hays, R.D., et al., "The Functioning and Well-Being of Depressed Patients: Results From the Medical Outcomes Study," *Journal of the Americal Medical Association* 262:914-919, 1989.

Decade of the Brain

Public Law 101-58
101st Congress Joint Resolution

Whereas it is estimated that 50 million Americans are affected each year by disorders and disabilities that involve the brain, including the major mental illnesses; inherited and degenerative diseases; stroke; epilepsy; addictive disorders; injury resulting from prenatal events, environmental neurotoxins and trauma; and speech, language, hearing and other cognitive disorders;

Whereas it is estimated that treatment, rehabilitation and related costs of disorders and disabilities that affect the brain represents a total economic burden of $305 billion annually;

Whereas the people of the Nation should be aware of the exciting research advances on the brain and of the availability of effective treatment of disorders and disabilities that affect the brain;

Whereas a technological revolution occurring in the brain sciences, resulting in such procedures as positron emission tomography and magnetic resonance imaging, permits clinical researches to observe the living brain noninvasively and in exquisite detail, to define brain systems that are implicated in specific disorders and disabilities, to study complex neuropeptides and behaviors as well as to begin to learn about the complex structures underlying memory;

Whereas scientific information on the brain is amassing at an enormous rate, and the field of computer and information sciences has reached a level of sophistication sufficient to handle neuroscience data in a manner that would be maximally useful to both basic researchers and clinicians dealing with brain function and dysfunction;

Whereas advances in mathematics, physics, computational science, and brain imaging technologies have made possible the initiation of significant work in imaging brain function and pathology, modeling neural networks, and simulating their dynamic interactions;

Whereas comprehending the reality of the nervous system is still on the frontier of technological innovation requiring a comprehensive effort to decipher how individual neurons, by their collective action, give rise to human intelligence;

Whereas fundamental discoveries at the molecular and cellular levels of the organization of the brain are clarifying the role of the brain in translating neurophysiologic events into behavior, thought, and emotion;

Whereas molecular biology and molecular genetics have yielded strategies effective in preventing several forms of severe mental retardation and are contributing to promising breakthroughs in the study of inheritable neurological disorders, such as Huntington's disease, and mental disorders, such as affective illnesses;

Whereas the capacity to map the biochemical circuitry of neurotransmitters and neuromodulators will permit the rational design of potent medications possessing minimal adverse effects that will act on the discrete neurochemical deficits associated with such disorders as Parkinson's disease, schizophrenia, and Alzheimer's disease;

Whereas the incidence of neurologic, psychiatric, psychological, and cognitive disorders and disabilities experienced by older persons will increase in the future as the number of older persons increases;

Whereas studies of the brain and central nervous system will contribute not only to the relief of neurologic, psychiatric, psychological, and cognitive disorders, but also to the management of fertility and infertility, cardiovascular disease, infectious and parasitic diseases, developmental disabilities and immunologic disorders, as well as to an understanding of behavioral factors that underlie the leading preventable causes of death in this Nation;

Whereas the central nervous and immune systems are both signaling systems which serve the entire organism, are direct connections between the nervous and immune system, and whereas studies of the modulatory effects of each system on the other will enhance our understanding of diseases as diverse as the major psychiatric disorders, acquired immune deficiency syndrome, and autoimmune disorders;

Whereas recent discoveries have led to fundamental insights as to why people abuse drugs, how abused drugs affect brain function leading to addiction, and how some of these drugs cause permanent brain damage;

Whereas studies of the brain will contribute to the development of new treatments that will curtail the craving for drugs, break the addictive effects of drugs, prevent the brain-mediated "high" caused by certain abused drugs, and lessen the damage done to the developing minds of babies, who are the innocent victims of drug abuse;

Whereas treatment for persons with head injury, developmental disabilities, speech, hearing, and other cognitive functions is increasing in availability and effectiveness;

Whereas the study of the brain involves the multidisciplinary efforts of scientists from such diverse areas as physiology, biochemistry, psychology, psychiatry, molecular biology, anatomy, medicine, genetics, and many others working together toward the common goals of better understanding the structure of the brain and how it affects our development, health, and behavior;

Whereas the Nobel Prize for Medicine of Physiology has been awarded to 15 neuroscientists within the past 25 years, an achievement that underscores the excitement and productivity of the study of the brain and central nervous system and its potential for contributing to the health of humanity;

Whereas the people of the Nation should be concerned with research into disorders and disabilities that affect the brain, and should recognize prevention and treatment of such disorders and disabilities as a health priority;

Whereas the declaration of the Decade of the Brain will focus needed government attention on research, treatment, and rehabilitation in this area: Now, therefore, be it *Resolved by the Senate and House of Representatives of the United States of America in Congress Assembled*, that the decade beginning January 1, 1990, hereby is designated the "Decade of the Brain," and the President of the United States is authorized and requested to issue a proclamation calling upon all public officials and the people of the United States to observe such decade with appropriate programs and activities.

Approved July 25, 1989.

Legislative History—H.J. Res. 174 (S.J. Res. 173):
Congressional Record, vol. 135 (1989):

June 29, 1989, considered and passed House
July 13, 1989, considered and passed Senate

Acronyms and Glossary of Terms

Acronyms

ADA	—Americans with Disabilities Act
ADAMHA	—Alcohol, Drug Abuse, and Mental Health Administration
APA	—American Psychiatric Association
APA	—American Psychological Association
APS	—American Psychological Society
CAT	—computerized axial tomography
CDC	—Centers for Disease Control
CSF	—cerebrospinal fluid
D/ART	—DEPRESSION Awareness, Recognition and Treatment
DBBBS	—Division of Basic Brain and Behavioral Sciences
DCR	—Division of Clinical Research
DHHS	—U.S. Department of Health and Human Services
DOD	—Department of Defense
DOE	—Department of Energy
DSM-III	—Diagnostic and Statistical Manual of Mental Disorders, 3rd edition
DSM-III-R	—Diagnostic and Statistical Manual of Mental Disorders, 3rd edition, revised
DST	—dexamethasone-suppression test
ECA	—Epidemiologic Catchment Area
ECT	—electroconvulsive therapy
EEG	—electroencephalograph
ELSI	—Ethical, Legal, and Social Implications
FCCSET	—Federal Coordinating Council for Science, Engineering, and Technology
FDA	—U.S. Food and Drug Administration
GABA	—gamma aminobutyric acid
IRB	—institutional review board
LSD	—lysergic acid diethylamide
MAOI	—monoamine oxidase inhibitors
MRI	—magnetic resonance imaging
NAMI	—National Alliance for the Mentally Ill
NARSAD	—National Alliance for Research on Schizophrenia and Depression
NASA	—National Aeronautics and Space Administration
NCI	—National Cancer Institute
NE	—norepinephrine
NEI	—National Eye Institute
NIA	—National Institute on Aging
NIAAA	—National Institute on Alcohol Abuse and Alcoholism
NICHD	—National Institute on Child Health and Human Development
NIDA	—National Institute on Drug Abuse
NIDOCD	—National Institute on Deafness and Other Communication Disorders
NIDR	—National Institute of Dental Research
NIEHS	—National Institute on Environmental Health Sciences
NIMH	—National Institute of Mental Health
NINDS	—National Institute of Neurological Disorders and Stroke
NMHA	—National Mental Health Association
NSF	—National Science Foundation
OCD	—obsessive-compulsive disorder
PCP	—phencyclidine
PET	—positron emission tomography
PHS	—U.S. Public Health Service
PKU	—phenylketonuria
RDC	—Research Diagnostic Criteria
REM	—rapid eye movement
SAD	—seasonal affective disorder
SAMHSA	—Substance Abuse and Mental Health Services Administration
SPECT	—single photon emission computed tomography
SPEM	—smooth-pursuit eye movements
UAGA	—Uniform Anatomical Gift Act
USDA	—U.S. Department of Agriculture
VA	—Department of Veterans Affairs

Glossary

Acetylcholine: A chemical messenger in the nervous system. See *neurotransmitter.*

Adoption study: The attempt to separate the influence of genes from that of the environment by comparing the presence of a trait in biological versus adoptive family members. Compare *family study, twin study.*

Affective disorder: See *mood disorder.*

Agoraphobia: Fear of being in public places from which escape might be difficult. This condition frequently accompanies panic disorder. See *panic disorder.*

Allele: A version of a gene at a particular locus on the chromosome; one allele is inherited from each parent. If the two alleles at a locus are identical, the organism is homozygous for that gene; if they are different, heterozygous. See *genotype, phenotype.*

Animal model: An animal that shares, or in which can be replicated or approximated, features of human disorders and that is used in studies of these disorders. Although animal models cannot duplicate human mental disorders completely, they can be used to study basic brain structure and functions, mechanisms that may contribute to particular symptoms, hypothesized causes of a disorder, and drugs for treatment of the disorder.

Animal rights: The concept that animals have intrinsic rights that are equal to humans' rights. Compare *animal welfare.*

Animal welfare: In the context of scientific research, provision of proper food, shelter, care, and treatment of animals used in experiments. Compare *animal rights.*

Antianxiety drug: Medication, such as benzodiazepines, used to treat symptoms of anxiety disorders.

Antidepressant: Medication used to treat depressive symptoms. See *tricyclic antidepressant, monoamine oxidase inhibitor (MAOI), fluoxetine.*

Antipsychotic, antipsychotic drug: Medication used to treat psychosis, for example in schizophrenia. See *chlorpromazine, clozapine.*

Anxiety: Commonly experienced apprehension, tension, or uneasiness from anticipation of danger, the source of which is largely unknown or unrecognized. See *anxiety disorder.*

Anxiety disorder: Any of several mental disorders characterized by anxiety, including agoraphobia, obsessive-compulsive disorder, and panic disorder. See *agoraphobia, anxiety, obsessive-compulsive disorder, panic disorder.*

Autoreceptor: A protein (receptor) in the wall of a nerve cell that binds a neurotransmitter released by that cell. Autoreceptors act as a feedback mechanism to regulate a neuron's activity. See *neurotransmitter;* compare *receptor.*

Axon: The long extension of a nerve cell along which electrical impulses travel. See *neuron.*

Basal ganglia: A group of nuclei in the upper part of the brain that, among other functions, help mediate movement. See *nuclei.*

Base pairs: Two complementary nucleotides held together by weak bonds. Two strands of DNA are held together in the shape of a double helix by the bonds between base pairs. The base adenine pairs with thymine, and guanine pairs with cytosine. See *DNA.*

Behavioral sensitization: The increasing response of a laboratory animal to repeated administration of the same dose of a stimulant drug. Compare *kindling.*

Behavioral therapy: A form of psychotherapy that focuses on modifying faulty behavior rather than basic changes in the personality. Instead of probing the unconscious or exploring the patient's thoughts and feelings, behavior therapists seek to eliminate symptoms and to modify ineffective or maladaptive patterns by applying basic learning techniques and other methods. (Examples: relaxation therapy, self-control therapy, social skills training.) This mode of treatment is used for depression and obsessive-compulsive disorder.

Benzodiazepines: A class of drugs used to treat some anxiety disorders by increasing the action of the inhibitory neurotransmitter GABA. See *anxiety disorder, GABA, neurotransmitter.*

Biological rhythm: Change in a physiological or behavioral function that repeats at regular intervals and provides a framework of temporal organization for an organism. Alterations in biological rhythms have been associated with mood disorders. See *circadian rhythm, mood disorder.*

Bipolar disorder: A severe mood disorder characterized by manic and major depressive episodes, with periods of recovery generally separating the mood swings. Psychosis may be present during manic episodes. Bipolar disorder usually begins in the mid 20s and is chronic. See *depression, mania, mood disorder;* compare *major depression.*

Candidate gene: A gene suspected of causing or being otherwise closely linked to a disorder; the location of the gene is then sought by linkage analysis. See *linkage analysis.*

Catecholamine: A class of neurotransmitter including norepinephrine, epinephrine, and dopamine. See *dopamine, neurotransmitter, norepinephrine.*

Causative factor: The biological substance or activity that causes a disorder. Compare *correlated factor.*

Cerebral cortex: The upper portion of the brain, consisting of layers of neurons and the pathways connecting them. The cerebral cortex is divided into four lobes on each side and is the part of the brain responsible for higher-order thinking and decisionmaking.

Cerebrospinal fluid (CSF): Fluid manufactured in the brain and contained within the brain and spinal cord; it circulates in the central nervous system.

Chlorpromazine, *Thorazine*: A traditional antipsychotic drug, first introduced in the 1950s, used to treat psychotic symptoms. Chlorpromazine can produce side effects typical of traditional antipsychotic drugs. See *antipsychotic, traditional antipsychotic drugs.*

Chromosome: The rod-shaped body that contains genes and intervening regions of DNA that do not code for proteins. Each human cell except gametes (eggs and sperm) contains 23 pairs of chromosomes: 22 pairs of autosomes and one set of sex chromosomes. See *DNA, gene.*

Circadian rhythm: A biological rhythm, such as body temperature, that repeats approximately every 24 hours. See *biological rhythm.*

Clomipramine, *Anafranil*: A medication commonly used to treat obsessive-compulsive disorder; it inhibits the reuptake of the neurotransmitter serotonin. See *serotonin.*

Clozapine, *Clozaril*: A newer antipsychotic agent used to treat symptoms of schizophrenia in persons who do not respond to traditional antipsychotic drugs. Clozapine ameliorates both positive and negative symptoms of schizophrenia; it does not seem to produce tardive dyskinesia. Clozapine can result in agranulocytosis, a potentially fatal decrease in the number of white blood cells, which fight infection. See *antipsychotic, tardive dyskinesia, traditional antipsychotic drugs.*

Cognition: The processing of information by the brain; specifically, perception, reasoning, and memory.

Cognitive therapy: A psychotherapeutic approach based on the concept that emotional problems are the result of faulty ways of thinking and distorted attitudes toward oneself and others. The therapist takes the role of an active guide who helps the patient correct and revise his or her perceptions and attitudes by citing evidence to the contrary or eliciting it from the patient. The therapist uses cognitive and behavioral techniques to correct distortions of thinking associated with depression, that is, pessimism about oneself, the world, and the future. Brief treatment.

Comorbidity: The occurrence of two or more mental disorders at the same time. The disorders may occur independently of each other, or one may occur as a consequence of the other.

Compulsion: An insistent, intrusive, and unwanted action that is repeated over and over. See *obsessive-compulsive disorder.*

Computerized axial tomography (CAT): A type of imaging used to scan the living brain that uses computers to combine series of x-rays; CAT scans provide clearer pictures of the brain than x-rays alone.

Correlated factor: A biological substance or activity that is linked to a disorder and may result in some of its symptoms. Compare *causative factor.*

Corticotropin-releasing factor: A hormone produced by the brain that controls cortisol levels; elevated levels appear to be associated with depression.

Delusion: A belief that is clearly implausible but compelling and central to an individual's life.

Dendrite: One of several branched fibers extending out of a nerve cell that receives impulses from another neuron. See *neuron.*

Depression: When used to describe a mood, depression is characterized by feelings of sadness or dejection. Depression may be a symptom seen in a variety of disorders, including bipolar disorder and major depression, and be characterized by extreme feelings of sadness or irritability, inactivity, withdrawal from society, and difficulty concentrating. See *bipolar disorder, major depression.*

Dexamethasone-suppression test (DST): Developed as a test of hormone functioning, it has been studied as a possible diagnostic tool in depression. In healthy individuals, administration of the drug dexamethasone suppresses the concentration of cortisol in the blood. Approximately 40 to 50 percent of persons diagnosed with major depression have an abnormal DST in that they do not suppress cortisol in response to dexamethasone. See *depression.*

DNA (deoxyribonucleic acid): The molecule that encodes genetic information. DNA is a double-stranded helix held together by weak bonds between base pairs of nucleotides. See *base pairs, chromosome, gene.*

Dopamine: A chemical messenger in the brain. This neurotransmitter appears to play some role in schizophrenia and perhaps other mental disorders. See *neurotransmitter, schizophrenia.*

Electroconvulsive therapy (ECT): Electric shock treatments used to treat persons with severe depression.

Electroencephalograph (EEG): An instrument for measuring electrical waves generated by neurons in the brain.

Eugenics: Attempts to improve inherited qualities through selective breeding. Positive eugenics is the systematic attempt to increase the transmission of desired traits by promoting the reproduction of individuals carrying the genes for such traits; negative eugenics is the systematic attempt to minimize the transmission of undesirable traits by preventing or reducing the reproduction of individuals carrying the genes for such traits.

Family study: The attempt to determine whether a trait runs in a family, and thus may be heritable, by studying as many members of the family as possible in several generations. Compare *adoption study, twin study.*

Fluoxetine, *Prozac:* The most widely prescribed antidepressant in the United States, it acts on the neurotransmitter serotonin. Prozac produces fewer serious side effects than MAOIs or tricyclic antidepressants. Side effects associated with Prozac include nausea, tremor, insomnia, nervousness, and occasionally agitation or anxiety. See *antidepressant, serotonin.*

GABA (gamma aminobutyric acid): A major neurotransmitter implicated in anxiety disorders. See *anxiety disorder, neurotransmitter.*

Gene: The fundamental physical and functional unit of heredity. Each gene is made up of an ordered sequence of base pairs, is located on a particular position on a particular chromosome, and codes for (determines the structure of) a particular protein. See *base pairs, DNA, chromosome, protein.*

Genetic counseling: A clinical service that provides an individual, and sometimes his or her family, with information about heritable conditions. At present, genetic counseling can provide only a general estimate of risk for a mental disorder, not an accurate assessment of individual risk.

Genetic heterogeneity: The phenomenon whereby a disorder is caused by one gene in some individuals but a different gene in other individuals.

Genotype: The genetic constitution of an organism. Compare *phenotype.*

Glutamate: A neurotransmitter that stimulates nerve cells and may play a role in certain mental disorders. See *neurotransmitter*.

Hallucination: A perception without an objective basis, often an imaginary voice, vision, taste, or smell.

Hippocampus: A nucleus in the brain crucial to learning and memory; part of the limbic system. See *limbic system, nuclei*.

Hypothalamus: A group of nuclei in the brain that regulate hormones and such behaviors as eating, drinking, and sex. See *nuclei*.

Incomplete penetrance: Failure of a trait to be expressed, even though the gene coding for it is present.

Informed consent: The agreement of a person to participate as a subject in an experimental procedure after rationally weighing the possible benefits and risks of the procedure. The nature of some mental disorders may render individuals incompetent to give informed consent and, therefore, unable to participate in research projects.

Interpersonal psychotherapy: A form of psychotherapy in which the therapist seeks to help the patient to identify and better understand his or her interpersonal problems and conflicts and to develop more adaptive ways of relating to others. The therapist focuses on client's current interpersonal relationships. Helps clients learn more effective ways of relating to others and coping with conflicts in relationships. Brief, focused treatment.

Kindling: The creation of seizures in an area of the brain by subjecting it to repeated, low-level electrical stimulation; eventually, the area becomes so sensitive that seizures will occur spontaneously, with no electrical stimulus. Compare *behavioral sensitization*.

Limbic system: A network of structures in the brain (including the hippocampus and part of the temporal lobes) associated with control of emotion and behavior, specifically, perception, motivation, gratification, memory, and thought. See *hippocampus*.

Linkage analysis: A technique for determining whether a major gene produces a trait and, if so, where on the chromosomes that gene is located (but not which gene it is or what its function is). Linkage analysis uses markers (such as genetic traits or DNA sequences) whose loci are known and calculates the probability that the loci for the marker and the gene being sought are linked.

Lithium carbonate: The most common medication used to treat bipolar disorder, lithium is used to diminish manic symptoms and to prevent future episodes. Side effects include increased thirst and urination, memory problems, tremor, and weight gain. Long-term treatment, which is commonly required, can have toxic effects on the thyroid gland, the kidneys, and the nervous system; lithium can also cause fetal abnormalities.

Locus ceruleus: A nucleus in the brain that is involved in, among other things, the body's response to stressful situations, such as the fight-or-flight response. See *nuclei*.

Magnetic resonance imaging (MRI): A technique that constructs images of the living human brain by detecting molecular changes in neurons exposed to a strong magnetic field.

Major depression: A mood disorder characterized by profound depression, that is, complete loss of interest or pleasure in activities. Other common symptoms include weight gain or loss, insomnia or excessive sleepiness, slowed or agitated movement, intense feelings of guilt or worthlessness, diminished ability to concentrate, and recurrent thoughts of death or suicide. Bouts of depression commonly recur. Psychosis may also accompany major depression. The typical age of onset is the late 20s. See *mood disorder*; compare *bipolar disorder*.

Mania: A mood disorder characterized by expansiveness, elation, talkativeness, hyperactivity, and excitability. See *bipolar disorder*.

Manic depression, manic-depressive disorder: See *bipolar disorder*.

Melancholia: A severe form of depression in which there is a nearly complete loss of interest or pleasure in activities, accompanied by somatic symptoms such as weight loss and early morning wakening.

Metabolite: A compound that results from the chemical breakdown of a neurotransmitter in the space between nerve cells. See *neurotransmitter*.

Monoamine: A group of neurotransmitters; namely, norepinephrine, epinephrine, serotonin, and dopamine. See *dopamine, neurotransmitter, norepinephrine, serotonin*.

Monoamine oxidase inhibitor (MAOI): A class of antidepressants that acts by prolonging monoamine activity; generally used to treat persons who do not respond to tricyclic antidepressants. MAOIs can interact with certain foods and other medications to produce potentially fatal hypertension. See *monoamine*.

Mood disorder: A mental disorder characterized by extreme or prolonged disturbances of mood, such as sadness, apathy, or elation. Mood disorders are divided into two major groups: bipolar, or manic-depressive, disorders, characterized by depression and mania; and unipolar, or depressive, disorders, characterized by depression only. See *major depression, bipolar disorder*.

Negative eugenics: See *eugenics*.

Neuroendocrine system: Hormones that influence the activity of neurons and glands. Many symptoms associated with depression may be related to changes in the hormones secreted by these glands, particularly the pituitary, adrenal, and pineal glands.

Neuron, nerve cell: The basic functional unit of the nervous system, neurons carry on information processing in the brain. The neuron consists of a relatively compact cell body containing the nucleus, several branched extensions (dendrites), and a single long fiber (the axon) with twig-like branches along its length and at its end. Information in the form of electrical impulses generally travels from the dendrites, through the cell body, and along the axon to other cells via neurotransmitters. See *axon, dendrite, neurotransmitter.*

Neuroscience: The study of the nervous system and how it is affected by disease. Neuroscience draws from numerous fields, including anatomy, physiology, physics, electronics, genetics, biochemistry, optics, pharmacology, psychology, neurology, psychiatry, neurosurgery, and computer science, and is based on the concept that behavior, thought, and emotion are the result of nerve cell interaction.

Neurotransmitter: Specialized chemical messenger synthesized and secreted by neurons to communicate with other neurons. A neurotransmitter is released into th' space between neurons (synapse), moves across that space, and attaches (binds) to a specific protein (receptor) in the outer wall of a neighboring neuron. Some neurotransmitters stimulate the release of neurotransmitters from other neurons (excitatory neurotransmitters), while others inhibit the release of neurotransmitters from other neurons (inhibitory neurotransmitters). See *neuron, receptor.*

Non-REM sleep: The four stages of sleep during which the sleeper does not experience rapid eye movement. Compare *REM sleep.*

Norepinephrine: A chemical messenger in the brain. Alterations in this neurotransmitter have been implicated in several mental disorders. See *neurotransmitter.*

Nuclei, nucleus: Groups of neurons in the brain that are located in the same region and that share, to varying degrees, the same function. Axons extending from nuclei convey information between and among nuclei throughout the brain. See *neuron.*

Obsession: Irrational thought, image, or idea that is irresistible and recurrent, if unwanted. See *obsessive-compulsive disorder.*

Obsessive-compulsive disorder (OCD): A mental disorder characterized by recurrent and persistent thoughts, images, or ideas perceived by the sufferer as intrusive and senseless (obsessions) and by stereotypic, repetitive, purposeful actions perceived as unnecessary (compulsions). The average age of onset is 20. OCD is generally chronic, with symptoms waxing and waning. The disorder frequently occurs with depression and Tourette's syndrome, a neurological disorder. See *anxiety disorder, depression.*

Panic disorder: A mental disorder characterized by sudden, inexplicable bouts, or attacks, of intense fear and strong bodily symptoms, namely, increased heart rate, profuse sweating, and difficulty breathing. Panic attacks occur twice a week, on average. The disorder is usually chronic, with symptoms waxing and waning, and the average age of onset is 24. Antidepressants and antianxiety drugs, as well as psychotherapy, are often used to treat panic disorder. See *anxiety disorder.*

Peptides, neuropeptides: Chemicals, including some hormones, that act as messengers in the brain. Neuropeptides modulate the activity of many other neurotransmitters. See *neurotransmitter.*

Phenocopy: Nongenetic production of the symptoms of a disorder that mirror those of the genetically derived disorder.

Phenotype: The manifestation of a genetic trait. See *allele, genotype.*

Positive eugenics: See *eugenics.*

Positron emission tomography (PET): Imaging technique that creates computerized images of the distribution of radioactively labeled materials in the brain in order to show brain activity. PET scans of labeled drugs that attach to specific receptors show the distribution and number of those receptors.

Protein: A large molecule composed of chains of smaller molecules (amino acids) in a specific sequence, proteins are required for the structure, function, and regulation of the body's cells, tissues, and organs. Each protein has a unique function. Examples are hormones, enzymes, and antibodies.

Psychodynamic psychotherapy: Any form or technique of psychotherapy that focuses on the underlying, often unconscious factors (drives and experiences) that determine behavior and adjustment.

Psychopharmacology: The study of the action of drugs on the mind.

Psychosis: A mental state characterized by extreme impairment of the sufferer's perception of reality, including hallucinations, delusions, incoherence, and bizarre behavior. Psychosis is a prominent symptom of schizophrenia. See *delusion, hallucination, schizophrenia.*

Raphe nuclei: The major serotonin-containing nuclei in the brain, they regulate sleep and are involved with behavior and mood. See *nuclei.*

Receptor, receptor molecule: Protein embedded in the wall of nerve cells that binds neurotransmitters. Each receptor binds a specific neurotransmitter, thereby turning a particular biochemical or cellular mechanism on or off. Receptors are generally found in the dendrites and cell body of neurons. See *dendrite, neuron, neurotransmitter;* compare *autoreceptor.*

Recombination: The exchange of segments of chromosomes during the production of egg and sperm; the exchange site is called crossover.

REM (rapid eye movement) sleep: Stage of sleep during which the eyes move rapidly, brain activity resembles that observed during wakefulness, heart rate and respiration increase and become erratic, and vivid dreams are frequent. Compare *non-REM sleep.*

Reuptake: Removal of a neurotransmitter from the synapse by the neuron that released it. Compare *metabolite*; see *neurotransmitter, synapse.*

Schizoaffective disorder: A mental disorder involving symptoms of both schizophrenia and mood disorders. See *mood disorder, schizophrenia.*

Schizophrenia: A mental disorder characterized by disturbance of cognition, delusions and hallucinations, and impaired emotional responsiveness. The disorder consists of positive symptoms (delusions, hallucinations, illogical thought, and bizarre behavior) and negative symptoms (blunting of emotion, apathy, and social withdrawal). The positive symptoms of schizophrenia are also typical of psychosis. Schizophrenia usually begins in the late teen years or the early 20s. The disorder cannot now be cured or prevented, but its symptoms can be treated. See *psychosis.*

Seasonal affective disorder (SAD): A depressive disorder in which the onset of depression occurs during the winter months, with remission or mania during the spring. Symptoms of SAD are generally treated with phototherapy, that is, bright artificial light in the early morning, in the evening, or at both times.

Sensitization: See *behavioral sensitization, kindling.*

Serotonin: A chemical messenger in the brain. This neurotransmitter has been implicated in several mental disorders, including mood disorders. See *mood disorder, neurotransmitter.*

Single photon emission computed tomography (SPECT): An imaging technique that shows brain activity by tracking the distribution of radioactively labeled substances in the brain.

Somatic: Physical, as opposed to mental; for example, somatic symptoms of a mental disorder.

Substance abuse: A maladaptive pattern of psychoactive substance use indicated by either: 1) continued use despite knowing that it causes or exacerbates a persistent or recurrent social, occupational, psychological, or physical problem, or 2) recurrent use in situations in which it creates a physical hazard (such as driving when intoxicated). Abuse refers to relatively mild, transient symptoms. Compare *substance dependence.*

Substance dependence: Impaired control over use of a psychoactive substance and continued use of the substance despite adverse consequences. Dependence can include physiological tolerance to a substance and is more serious and persistent than substance abuse. Compare *substance abuse.*

Supportive psychotherapy: A treatment technique that helps a patient reduce stress and cope with his or her disorder without probing disturbing thoughts or emotions. Compare *behavioral therapy, cognitive therapy, interpersonal psychotherapy, psychodynamic psychotherapy.*

Synapse: The site at which an impulse is transmitted from the axon of one nerve cell to the dendrite of another nerve cell, typically by a neurotransmitter. See *neurotransmitter.*

Tardive dyskinesia: A side-effect of traditional antipsychotic drugs. This side-effect, which involves abnormal involuntary movements of the face, tongue, mouth, fingers, upper and lower limbs, and occasionally the entire body, usually appears after taking the drug for some time and occurs in at least a mild form in 25 to 40 percent of patients on antipsychotic agents. Tardive dyskinesia may be severe or irreversible in 5 or 10 percent of cases. See *traditional antipsychotic drugs.*

Traditional antipsychotic drugs, Typical antipsychotic drugs: Medication used to treat psychosis, for example in schizophrenia. These medications can have various side effects including dry mouth, constipation, blurring of vision, weight gain, restlessness, and tremor. The most serious side effect is tardive dyskinesia. Traditional antipsychotic drugs were introduced for the treatment of psychosis in the 1950s and act by binding to a dopamine receptor (D2). See *chlorpromazine, tardive dyskinesia.*

Trait: A genetically determined characteristic. See *allele, genotype, phenotype.*

Tricyclic antidepressant: Traditional medication for depression that acts by blocking reuptake of monoamines. Side effects include dry mouth, constipation, sedation, nervousness, weight gain, and diminished sex drive. See *monoamine.*

Twin study: The attempt to determine whether a trait is genetic by comparing how often identical twins (sharing the same genes) who are raised in the same environment share that trait with how often fraternal twins (having different genes) raised in the same environment share the trait. A high rate of trait-sharing among identical, but not among fraternal, twins usually demonstrates that the trait is genetic. Compare *adoption study, family study.*

Index

Index

Interagency Task Force on Homelessness and Severe Mental Illness, 26, 153
Interpersonal psychotherapy, definition of, 59

James, William, 158

Kennedy, Edward M., 39
Kindling and sensitization hypothesis of bipolar disorder, 10, 87
Kraepelin, Emil, 45, 50

Legal issues surrounding neuroscience advances, 23-24, 26, 39
Linkage analysis, 105-6, 109-12
Lithium, 9, 10, 56, 58, 84-85, 93
LOD score, 106
LSD (lysergic acid diethylamide), 78

Magnetic resonance imaging (MRI), 76, 77, 79, 86
Major depression. *See* Depression, major
Mania. *See also* Bipolar disorder
    animal models of, 135
    characterization of, 9, 54
    course of, 56
    diagnosis of, 55
    medication for, 9, 58
Manic-depressive illness. *See* Bipolar disorder
MAOIs. *See* Monoamine oxidase inhibitors
Marital status
    mood disorders and, 56
    schizophrenia and, 50
Media portrayals of mental disorders, 20, 153, 159
Melancholia, 55
Mendel, Gregor, 101
Mental disorders. *See also* Anxiety disorders; Bipolar disorder; Depression, major; Mood disorders; Obsessive-compulsive disorder; Panic disorder; Schizophrenia
    animal models of, 134-36
    brain structure and function and, 74-77
    challenges for genetic mapping of, 14, 109-12
    classification of, 39, 46-47
    comorbid substance abuse and, 57
    cost of, 3-5, 16, 35-36
    creativity and, 56, 115
    definition of, 45-46
    eugenics and, 25, 104
    evidence of biological factors involved in, 13, 93-94, 101
    genetic counseling for, 113-15
    homelessness and, 35
    impact of biological research, 18-19, 21, 156-63
    media portrayals of, 20, 153, 159
    medical model of, 162
    methods of study of, 71-77
    prevalence of, 3, 35
    psychosocial factors and, 13, 71, 112, 161
    risk of, 113

    stigma attached to, 3, 5, 26, 151-53, 163
    study of genetics of, 103-5, 113-16, 161
    suicide and, 6-7, 52
    treatment of, 92-93
    violence and, 20, 158, 159
Mental health care, insurance coverage for, 18-19, 161-63
Mental health professionals, 45
    cost of care provided by, 4, 36
    D/ART program training for, 28, 154
    negative attitudes toward persons with mental disorders, 26, 152
    shortage and training of clinician-researchers, 18, 23, 141-44
Mental health services
    cost of, 4, 36
    government funding for, 5, 37
Microscopy, 38
Molecular biology, 38, 71, 74
Monoamine oxidase inhibitors
    action of, 82
    generic and brand names, 58
Monoamines. *See also* Norepinephrine; Serotonin
    mood disorders and, 10, 82-84
Mood disorders. *See also* Bipolar disorder; Depression, major
    biochemistry of, 10, 82-85
    brain structure and function and, 85-86
    characterization of, 8, 53
    circadian rhythms and, 10, 87
    classification of, 54-55
    comorbidity and, 56, 57
    genetics of, 10, 107-8
    hormonal abnormalities and, 10, 85
    immune and viral factors, 88
    prevalence of, 8-9, 56
    sleep disturbances and, 10, 86-87
    social correlates of, 56
    suicide and, 7, 52
    symptoms of, 10, 53-55
    treatment of, 8-9, 56, 58-59

National Advisory Mental Health Council, 39, 130
National Alliance for Research on Schizophrenia and Depression (NARSAD), 15, 132
National Alliance for the Mentally Ill (NAMI), 15, 37, 132, 154, 156, 160, 161
National Depressive and Manic Depressive Association, 132
National Institute of Mental Health (NIMH)
    D/ART program, 27-29, 154-55
    genetic counseling and, 114
    genetic research investment, 101
    mental disorder research funding, 14-17, 21-22, 123-29
    neuroscience research and, 6, 21-22, 38, 123-30
    research budget, 14-15, 17, 39, 124-25
National Institute on Aging, 124
National Institutes of Health (NIH), 130-31, 138

REA's **Problem Solvers**

The "PROBLEM SOLVERS" are comprehensive supplemental text-books designed to save time in finding solutions to problems. Each "PROBLEM SOLVER" is the first of its kind ever produced in its field. It is the product of a massive effort to illustrate almost any imaginable problem in exceptional depth, detail, and clarity. Each problem is worked out in detail with a step-by-step solution, and the problems are arranged in order of complexity from elementary to advanced. Each book is fully indexed for locating problems rapidly.

ADVANCED CALCULUS	HEAT TRANSFER
ALGEBRA & TRIGONOMETRY	LINEAR ALGEBRA
AUTOMATIC CONTROL	MACHINE DESIGN
SYSTEMS/ROBOTICS	MATHEMATICS for ENGINEERS
BIOLOGY	MECHANICS
BUSINESS, ACCOUNTING, & FINANCE	NUMERICAL ANALYSIS
CALCULUS	OPERATIONS RESEARCH
CHEMISTRY	OPTICS
COMPLEX VARIABLES	ORGANIC CHEMISTRY
COMPUTER SCIENCE	PHYSICAL CHEMISTRY
DIFFERENTIAL EQUATIONS	PHYSICS
ECONOMICS	PRE-CALCULUS
ELECTRICAL MACHINES	PSYCHOLOGY
ELECTRIC CIRCUITS	STATISTICS
ELECTROMAGNETICS	STRENGTH OF MATERIALS &
ELECTRONIC COMMUNICATIONS	MECHANICS OF SOLIDS
ELECTRONICS	TECHNICAL DESIGN GRAPHICS
FINITE & DISCRETE MATH	THERMODYNAMICS
FLUID MECHANICS/DYNAMICS	TOPOLOGY
GENETICS	TRANSPORT PHENOMENA
GEOMETRY	VECTOR ANALYSIS

If you would like more information about any of these books,
complete the coupon below and return it to us or visit your local bookstore.

RESEARCH & EDUCATION ASSOCIATION
61 Ethel Road W. • Piscataway, New Jersey 08854
Phone: (908) 819-8880

Please send me more information about your Problem Solver Books

Name _____

Address _____

City _____ State _____ Zip _____

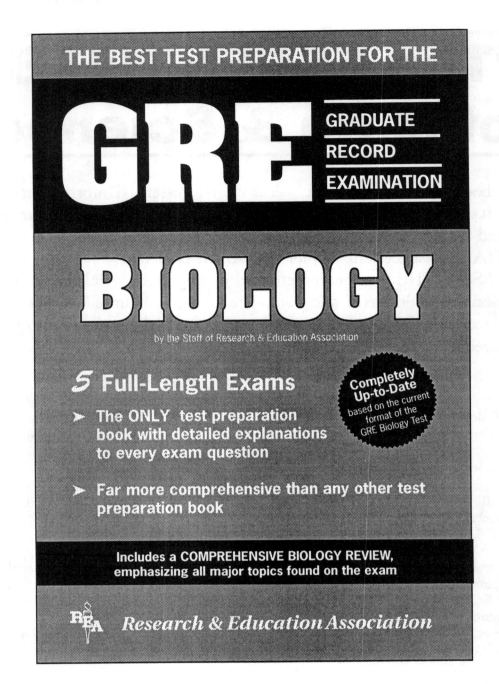

THE BEST TEST PREPARATION FOR THE

GRE
GRADUATE
RECORD
EXAMINATION

BIOLOGY
by the Staff of Research & Education Association

5 Full-Length Exams

Completely Up-to-Date
based on the current format of the GRE Biology Test

➤ The ONLY test preparation book with detailed explanations to every exam question

➤ Far more comprehensive than any other test preparation book

Includes a COMPREHENSIVE BIOLOGY REVIEW, emphasizing all major topics found on the exam

Research & Education Association

Available at your local bookstore or order directly from us by sending in coupon below.

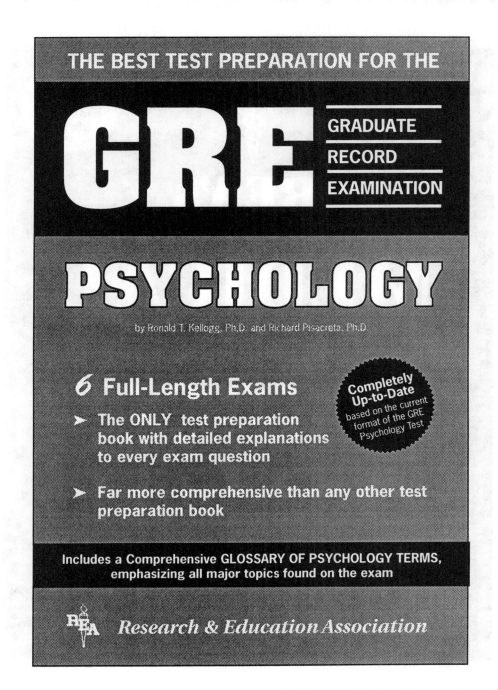

THE BEST TEST PREPARATION FOR THE

GRE

GRADUATE
RECORD
EXAMINATION

PSYCHOLOGY

by Ronald T. Kellogg, Ph.D. and Richard Pisacreta, Ph.D.

6 Full-Length Exams

Completely Up-to-Date based on the current format of the GRE Psychology Test

➤ The ONLY test preparation book with detailed explanations to every exam question

➤ Far more comprehensive than any other test preparation book

Includes a Comprehensive GLOSSARY OF PSYCHOLOGY TERMS, emphasizing all major topics found on the exam

Research & Education Association

Available at your local bookstore or order directly from us by sending in coupon below.

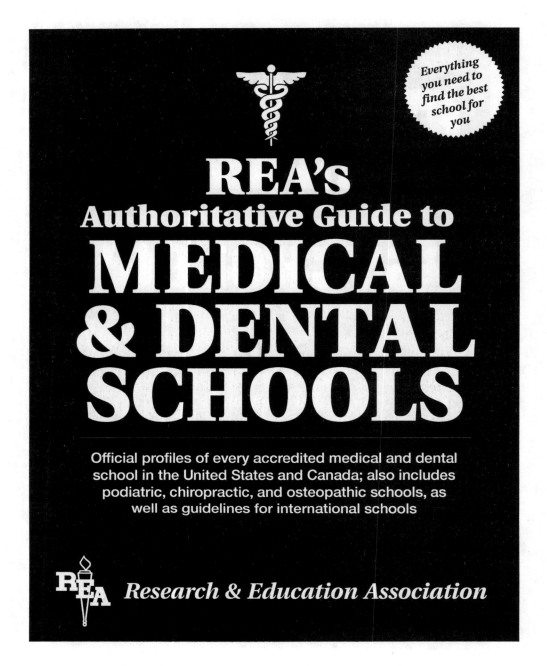

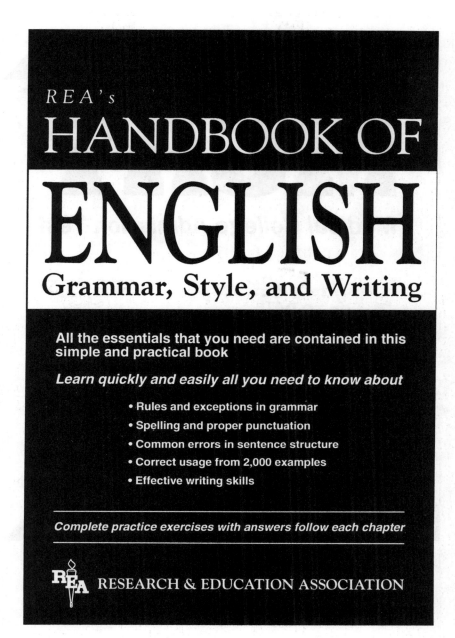

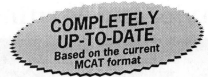
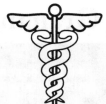